Spa Business Strategies

A Plan for Success

Janet M. D'Angelo

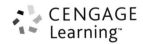

Australia • Brazil • Japan • Korea • Mexico • Singapore • Spain • United Kingdom • United States

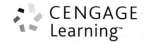
CENGAGE
Learning™

Spa Business Strategies, Second Edition

Janet M. D'Angelo

President: Milady Dawn Gerrain

Publisher: Erin O'Connor

Acquisitions Editor: Martine Edwards

Senior Product Manager: Philip Mandl

Editorial Assistant: Elizabeth Edwards

Director of Beauty Industry Relations:
Sandra Bruce

Senior Marketing Manager: Gerard McAvey

Production Director: Wendy Troeger

Senior Content Project Manager:
Nina Tucciarelli

SeniorArt Director: Joy Kocsis

For product information and technology assistance, contact us at
Cengage Learning Customer & Sales Support, 1-800-354-9706

For permission to use material from this text or product,
submit all requests online at **www.cengage.com/permissions**
Further permissions questions can be emailed to
permissionrequest@cengage.com

Library of Congress Control Number: 2009926527

ISBN-13: 978-1-4354-8209-8

ISBN-10: 1-4354-8209-3

Milady
Executive Woods
5 Maxwell Drive
Clifton Park, NY 12065
USA

Cengage Learning is a leading provider of customized learning solutions with office locations around the globe, including Singapore, the United Kingdom, Australia, Mexico, Brazil, and Japan. Locate your local office at **www.cengage.com/global**

Cengage Learning products are represented in Canada by Nelson Education, Ltd.

To learn more about Milady, visit **milady.cengage.com**

Purchase any of our products at your local college store or at our preferred online store **www.cengagebrain.com**

Printed in the United States of America
2 3 4 5 6 7 16 15 14 13 12

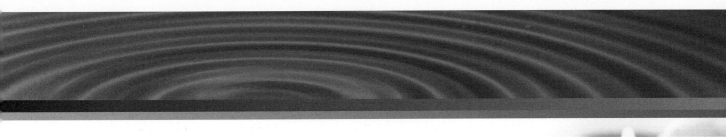

CONTENTS

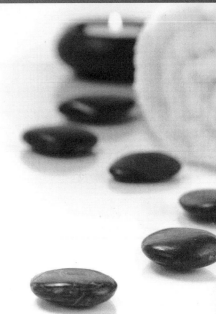

CHAPTER 5: ARCHITECTURE AND DESIGN
OF YOUR SPA 91

CHAPTER 6: PURCHASING PROFESSIONAL
PRODUCTS AND EQUIPMENT 125

CHAPTER 7:   TECHNO-SAVVY: USING
                 COMMUNICATION SYSTEMS IN THE SPA 175

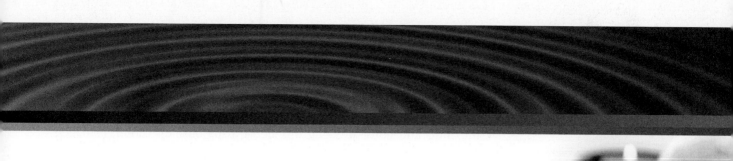

FOREWORD

Janet D'Angelo has developed a comprehensive, thoughtful, and timely volume in the second edition of *Spa Business Strategies: A Plan for Success.* Her passion for education and communication is unparalleled in our skin care industry today. Page by page you will hear Janet's voice speaking to you as an intelligent, critical-thinking, spa business owner or spa professional as she shares information based on research and experience, much of which can be immediately applied to your business.

This volume arrives at a point in our evolution as spa professionals where we are in need of sophisticated vehicles for applying technology; possessing business acuity and financial acumen, and ramping up professionalism. She also implies the value in using tried-and-true qualities and virtues such as patience and persistence and utilizing one's intuition.

Janet D'Angelo describes in eloquent, yet straightforward terms what it takes to be victorious in today's tumultuous spa milieu. She stresses the importance of having a clear vision and mission for your spa; acquiring continuing and advanced education; and in possessing advanced certification and licensure. She advocates goal-setting and developing assessments for both client retention and staff growth. Additionally, Janet describes the significance of understanding one's personal work style to facilitate relationship-building, employing exemplary customer service, and in finding support for skills or talents that team members may bring to round out the business.

Spa Business Strategies: A Plan for Success offers the tools you will need to be a prosperous spa owner in an interactive format which includes worksheets, tables, and marketing materials designed to inspire your creativity.

You will find clear directives that move beyond a theoretical or didactic approach, and discover a path for administering practical applications to the "nuts and bolts" of living the life of a spa business owner, manager, and/or practitioner.

The future of the spa business will require having a sound business plan, keeping abreast of trends and technological advancements, as well as having the flexibly to change direction, expand one's comfort zone, and to grow with the vengeance of an enthusiastic student. Many savvy spa enthusiasts will have as much information as the spa professional, and the bottom line remains in having the readiness to meet their needs and demands. *Spa Business Strategies: A Plan for Success* is the platform for making it happen!

Many blessings to Janet D'Angelo and to all of you!

Sallie Deitz

student, clinical aesthetician, author, and educator

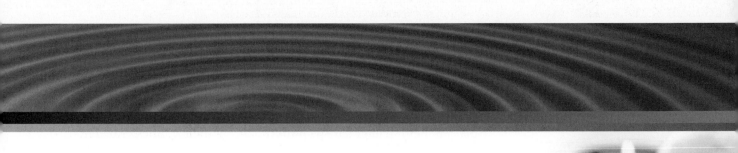

PREFACE

About 13 years ago, I had an interesting conversation with two graduate students from Harvard Business School who were conducting research on the spa industry. Eager to learn more about leveraging buildups, they raised questions about the economic feasibility of the spa business. Shortly after that, I received a call from a colleague who was studying the career path of estheticians and looking for similar information, including job placement, salary ranges, and business training programs available to those looking for a career in spa therapies. Back then, I was marketing esthetic education programs and eager to provide those entering the field with as much information as possible on these important spa business topics. Unfortunately, there was little organized research available to give prospective spa owners, managers, and business developers an overall view of the spa business.

Despite a lack of data to substantiate the growth of the spa business, it was nevertheless clear that a lot of people were becoming interested in the health and beauty field. Much of the increased attention given to the spa sector was the result of a growing interest in collaborative efforts between medical and beauty professionals. As skin care salons turned into day spas and a new generation of service providers began to infiltrate medical practices, there was a real sense that the spa industry and particularly day spas were emerging as a major force in the health, beauty, and wellness movement.

In the relatively short time span since then, a number of spa professionals, market research analysts, journalists, and trade organizations have worked hard to shed light on the status of the spa industry, giving us a much better understanding of the demographics of the spa-goer and the number of spas that currently exist. Today industry leaders are also eager to provide statistics on other relevant business topics, such as compensation practices that will help smaller day spa owners manage their businesses better.

Still, one of the most prevalent complaints I receive from spa owners, managers, students, product and equipment vendors, spa designers, and other professionals working in the field is the lack of information available on how to manage a successful spa business. In an industry that has encouraged service providers to open their own small businesses, I too have been frustrated by the lack of data, education, and tools available to those looking to become day spa owners. As competition for spa dollars increases and the smaller day spa owner is forced to compete with larger corporate entities, my concerns have increased. In writing the first edition of *Spa Business Strategies,* I hoped to answer many of the questions I have received from entrepreneurs and business people looking to develop and market a profitable day spa. Today I am grateful for the opportunity to continue along this path with a second edition of *Spa Business Strategies* that provides new information on financial management; cost projections, taxes, market value and feasibility; and updates statistics, marketing techniques and the technological tools needed to help business owners and managers meet the ever-increasing demands of this dynamic field.

Because day spa business owners and managers are often looking for clear directives, this book takes a thoughtful and interactive approach to working through many of the issues the spa owner or director will encounter, offering suggestions, checklists, practical examples, and targeted worksheets to help simplify what is sometimes rather dry and complex subject matter. I hope that you will find this technique easy to follow; it is intended to help you move beyond business theory to address the practical business matters that are vital to the day-to-day operation of a successful spa business. If you already own a spa, the material in this book is certainly worth reviewing and may also help you to improve or consider new options for maintaining your current business.

Beginning with the exercises in Chapter 1, which are designed to help the entrepreneur define that all-important vision and focus his or her intention, you will be encouraged to think thoughtfully about your career path, the opportunities, challenges, rewards and practical business management skills needed to become a successful day spa owner or manager. Subsequent chapters follow a natural sequence to guide the prospective spa owner through all of the stages of developing a spa business plan, including finding the right location, financing, architecture and design, purchasing professional products and equipment, marketing, and operations. Working through the material in these chapters, you will notice the emphasis on planning, the primary ingredient necessary for maintaining a healthy business.

All of these exercises are designed to help you along your entrepreneurial journey; however, it is my hope that you will view this book as more than a set of business guidelines. With the spa business often touted as one of the fastest growing fields, it is important that you carefully evaluate the current and future state of the industry. In these competitive times, I would encourage you to take a global perspective and become thoroughly informed about all aspects of the business, including what you can expect in terms of profit and the personal demands involved in business ownership *before* going into business. Those who are able to focus their intention and develop critical thinking skills are in a prime position to achieve success. Best wishes and many blessings to you as you embark on your spa journey!

NEW TO THIS EDITION

Companion Workbook

Many of you reported that it would be helpful to have a separate business journal to work through the topics presented in the text, so I am pleased to say that a companion *Spa Business Strategies Workbook* is now available for this purpose.

Instructor Course Management Guide CD-ROM

We also heard from a number of educators who were eager to integrate the material in this text in the classroom, prompting the creation of an additional *Course Management Guide CD-ROM* that contains all the materials spa educators need to teach spa business management in an easy-to-use format. This innovative instructional guide written solely with educators in mind includes comprehensive lesson plans and a computerized test bank specifically designed to transform classroom management and increase student interest and understanding.

Instructor Support Slides on CD-ROM

Additional PowerPoint slides are available to aid the instructor in presenting the material in the classroom.

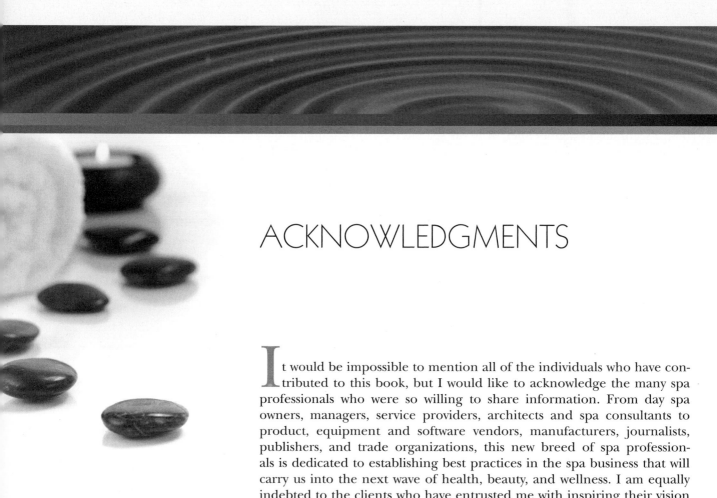

ACKNOWLEDGMENTS

I t would be impossible to mention all of the individuals who have contributed to this book, but I would like to acknowledge the many spa professionals who were so willing to share information. From day spa owners, managers, service providers, architects and spa consultants to product, equipment and software vendors, manufacturers, journalists, publishers, and trade organizations, this new breed of spa professionals is dedicated to establishing best practices in the spa business that will carry us into the next wave of health, beauty, and wellness. I am equally indebted to the clients who have entrusted me with inspiring their vision and to the many prospective spa owners, educators and colleagues who have provided me with input on how they are using this book to support their individual goals.

A special thanks goes to my father who instilled in me the importance of education and a strong work ethic and to Nadia Tagliavento, Jenny Dugan, my friends, family and associates who graciously contributed in one way or another to the completion of the first edition of *Spa Business Strategies*.. To the following people and organizations who took time out of their busy schedules to share their expertise, offer insight and/or information that helped me to refine the second edition of this text—thank you. I am very grateful for your willingness to support me in this effort – Shungo!

Adeena Babbitt, the American
    Society for Aesthetic Plastic
    Surgery
Belvedere USA Corporation

Beth McCoy
Bruce Schoenberg
Carolyn Lee
Cary Collier

David Suzuki
David Smotrich
Elaine H. Johnson
Esther Feit
Gary Henken
Gary Rayberg
Jane Segerberg
Jim Larkey
Joel Friedman
Joyce Hampers
Judy Singer
Lesley Shammus
Mark Roselle
Marti Morenings
Nancy White, Natural Marketing Institute

Pam Williams
Peter Anderson
Peter Lebovitz
Polly Johnson
Randy Schreck
Rhonda Cummings
Roberta Burd
Ruby Gu
Sallie Dietz
Shelby Jones, International Spa Association
Ted Ning, LOHAS
Wendy Shaya
William Caligari

To the many high-tech gurus, professional service providers, government agency and business associates who have helped me to understand printing and production, electrical wiring, telephone systems, building codes, architecture and design, contracts, and legal matters and so forth over the years, I thank you for your patience and support.

I would also like to express my gratitude to Marcia Yudkin, who encouraged me to broaden the scope of my writing, and Cody Bideaux who spurred me on, always managing to show up with an encouraging word at exactly the right moment.

Finally, my sincere and heartfelt thanks goes to the entire staff at Milady who work so hard, especially Martine Edwards, who has continually supported my efforts to refine and broaden the scope of this text with additional resources and educational tools; Philip Mandl, who attended to all of the many details that went into writing the second edition of this book; and Nina Tucciarelli, who supervised the production and artwork. To Pam Lappies, Judy Roberts, and Jessica Burns, who were there at the beginning and without whose support the first edition would not have come to fruition. Thanks also to Kimberley Comiskey, owner of Kimberley's Day Spa who graciously shared her spa vision, and to photographers Paul Castle and Christopher Morris, who worked so very hard to capture its essence. Last but certainly not least, a huge thanks to Lois Woods who helped to bring my vision for "Successful Day Spa" to life.

The publisher and author wish to thank all of the reviewers who contributed their insights, comments, and suggestions in the development of this book.

Linda G. Cowin, Touch of Excellence Body, Hair and Skin Care, WA
Shannon Smith, Steiner Education Group, FL
Sheryl Baba, Solstice Day Spa, MA
Lenore Brooks, Brooks & Butterfield Ltd., MA
Sadie Cousins, Marinello Schools of Beauty, CA
Linda Craig, Looking Good Hair & Nail Salon, CA
Nancy Phillips, Stylist, IL
Jeffrey Pippitt, Western Nebraska Community College, NE
Cheryl Sacks, RS&C Enterprises, PA

PHOTOGRAPHY AND LOCATION

Spa location:
Kimberley's A Day Spa Ltd.
982 New Loudon Road
Latham, NY 12110

Location Photography by:
Paul Castle, Castle Photography, Inc.
Troy, NY
www.castlephotographyinc.com

Figures 2-1, 4-1, 6-1: Photos courtesy of Getty Images.

Figures 2-2, 6-8, 8-1, 9-6: Photos courtesy of PhotoDisc.

Figure 2-3: Image copyright Leah-Anne Thompson, 2009. Used under license from Shutterstock.com.

Figure 2-5: Mii amo is a 24,000 square foot destination spa opened in 2001 by Sedona Resorts in Sedona, Arizona.

Figure 2-6: Photo courtesy of The Raj Ayurveda Health Spa, Vedic City, IA (*www.theraj.com*).

Figure 2-7: Photo courtesy of Kohler Waters Spa, Kohler, WI.

Figure 2-8: Photo courtesy of Canyon Ranch Health Resorts, SpaClubs, and Canyon Ranch Living.

Figure 4-1: Image copyright Stephen Coburn, 2009. Used under license from Shutterstock.com

Figure 4-2a: Photo courtesy of Oasis Day Spa, at JFK Airport, New York (*www.oasisdayspanyc.com*)

Figure 4-2b: Photo courtesy of Emerge Day Spa and Salon, Newbury Street, Boston, Massachusetts.

Figure 4-2c: Photo courtesy of Absolute Nirvana Spa, Santa Fe, New Mexico.

Figure 4-2d: Photo courtesy of Tranquility Day Spa and Salon, Manassas, VA.

Figure 4-2e: Photo courtesy of Sen Spa, San Francisco, CA

Figure 5-1: Photo courtesy of Image Source Limited.

Figures 5-2, 5-3, and 5-4: Spa Blueprints courtesy of the Belvedere USA Corporation.

Figures 5-6 and 6-10: Photo courtesy of Essential Therapies Day Spa, Bolton, MA.

Figure 5-7: Photo courtesy of Edit EuroSpa, Denver, Colorado.

Figure 6-2: Photo courtesy of Lady Burd® Exclusive Private Label Cosmetics

Figure 6-3: Photo courtesy of EditEuro Spa, Denver, CO.

Figure 6-4: Photo courtesy of Canfield Imaging.

Figure 6-5: Photo courtesy of Aesthetic Technologies.

Figure 6-6: Photos Courtesy of Bio-Therapeutic, Inc.

Figure 6-7: Photo courtesy of SpaEquip, Inc.

Figure 6-8: Photo courtesy of Cosmopro.

Figure 6-9: Photo courtesy of Oasis Day Spa.

Figure 6-12: Photo courtesy of Essential Therapies Day Spa, Bolton, MA.

Figure 6-14: Photo courtesy of Golden Ratio Woodworks, Inc.

Figure 6-15: Photo courtesy of Stock Studio Photography, Saratoga Springs, NY.

Figure 11-3: Image copyright Liv Friis-Larsen, 2009. Used under license from Shutterstock.com

For participation as models in the photo shoot:

Sarah Boone	Lisa Rosenthal
Crystal M. Bruno	Anne Ruege
Kimberley Ann Comiskey	Kyle C. Schlesinger
Janet M. D'Angelo	Robert Serenka
Jennifer S. French	Holly Siola
Niamh Matthews	Melissa Strife
Colleen McCue	Courtney Troeger
Christopher Morris	Nina Tucciarelli
Fehma Naz	David W. White
Sarah Pollack	Stacey Wiktorek

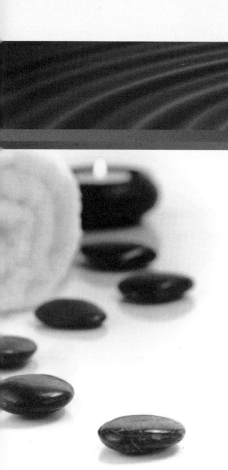

ABOUT THE AUTHOR

Janet M. D'Angelo, M.Ed, is founder and president of J. Angel Communications, LLC, a marketing and public relations firm specializing in the health, beauty and wellness industry. In this practical guide to building a spa business, she imparts more than 25 years of hands-on experience developing business administration, management, sales, marketing, and public relations strategies for various spa and related industry businesses including day spas, medical spas, salons, educational institutions, nonprofit organizations, technology, product and equipment manufacturers and vendors.

An educator at heart, Janet has enthusiastically lent her support to the development of business resources and has worked tirelessly to raise industry awareness and promote professional standards in the spa and skin care industries throughout her career, serving on trade association advisory boards and research committees, addressing legislative boards, conducting business seminars at trade shows and conferences and writing articles for numerous magazine and trade publications. In addition to *Spa Business Strategies*, she is also a contributing author of *Milady's Standard Esthetics Fundamentals* (Cengage Learning ©2009); *Milady's Standard Esthetics Advanced* (Cengage Learning ©2010) and *Milady's Standard Comprehensive Training for Estheticians* (Thomson Delmar Learning, ©2003). She can be reached at janet@jangelcommunications.com

PLEASE NOTE: The author has taken care in the preparation of this book, but makes no express or implied warranty of any kind to the reader and assumes no responsibility to the reader for errors or omissions. The author

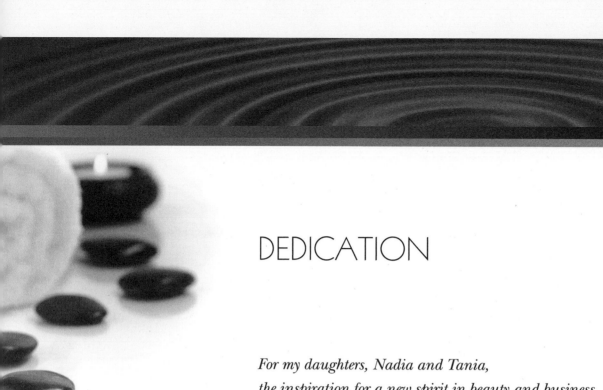

DEDICATION

For my daughters, Nadia and Tania,
the inspiration for a new spirit in beauty and business.

WHAT IS YOUR VISION?

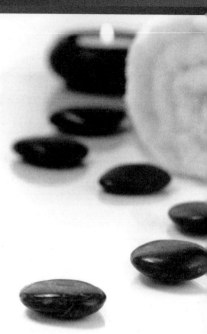

As a marketing consultant, it is my job to inspire the vision of my client. Before I can do that, I need to be clear about what that vision is. Whether the client is involved in a start-up operation or has an established spa, the first order of business is to understand what the client hopes to achieve.

To form a better understanding of the client's goal, I ask them to fill out a detailed questionnaire, encouraging them to define both the practical and theoretical aspects of their work. The questionnaire covers three key areas. First, I want to know something about the client's background and what led them to opening a spa. Did they start out as a service provider, or were they involved in some other business prior to contemplating spa ownership? Second, I want to know what role they intend to play in their spa business. Are they focused on *healing others,* do they intend to *manage operations* or will they act as CEO with little hands-on involvement? Third, I want a clear picture of the products and services they currently offer or intend to offer and what they might be looking to incorporate down the road. All of this information is vital to marketing their spa and developing long-term business goals.

DEFINING A STRATEGY

As I begin to understand each client's vision, I also look to establish the best way for us to work together. Did they enjoy writing their thoughts down and elaborate at length, or were their responses short and to the point? Did they call to ask for clarification as they completed the questionnaire? Seek additional time to explain their responses? Did they nix the idea of responding to the questionnaire on their own altogether and ask to review it jointly?

Sometimes clients will question the importance of putting their answers down on paper; however, once they have had time to process the exercise, their reaction is generally the same. Typical comments are: "I never really gave it much thought until now," "This really helped me to collect my thoughts," and "Once I started putting my philosophy down on paper, my mission became clear." They are equally surprised when their personal goals and ideas are woven into the fabric of marketing materials and advertising campaigns. Sometimes the simplest remark can become the basis of their mission statement, an exciting tag line, or an eye-catching ad. Before we go any further, let's work through several simple but important preliminary exercises.

The Entrepreneurial Journey

Our world is so full of distractions that it is often hard to hear our own thoughts. It can be even more difficult to find the time to tune into them. If you are not already a spa owner, you will soon learn that running your own business will afford you even less time to yourself. Because I want clients to think thoughtfully about the evolution of their spa, I encourage them to complete the business development questionnaire at a time when they are feeling relaxed and in a space where they are comfortable and will not be distracted. Although the preliminary exercises in this chapter are more introspective in nature, they are based on the same concept and are designed to set the tone for what will hopefully become a regular time and space that you can call your own. Learning to listen to that all-important inner voice is one of the most valuable exercises you will perform as a business owner.

Focusing Your Intention

> As you set the stage for this exciting journey, I would also encourage you to be mindful of what could ultimately be the single most significant factor in your success—your attitude.

Much has been written about the power of our thoughts, or the law of attraction, a centuries-old and universally acclaimed principle which states that *like attracts like,* and expresses how our thoughts, feelings, words, and actions affect our intentions.

As you consider the ramifications of this profound philosophy, I strongly urge you to take a thoughtful look at your own intentions. Are you truly focused on building a lucrative business? Do you have a can-do attitude? Do you have faith in your own abilities? Do you look to see what you can learn in any given situation? If it is truly your intention to create a successful business, it is important to become conscious of how your own thinking, both personally and professionally, impacts all of your actions.

Even if you don't have all of the skills and resources required to open or manage a successful spa immediately available to you, remember that you can take control of your attitude. Believe in yourself. Have faith that the right opportunities, the right resources, consultants, teachers, employees, clients, financing, etc. will show up and that you will understand the best way to utilize them. This is the law of attraction. As you learn to see every lesson as an opportunity for growth, and to focus your intention on developing positive outcomes, your vision will expand into what I hope will be one of the best experiences of your life.

> ## Affirmation for Spa Success
>
> It is my deepest desire to bring forth good health, beauty, and wellness to all those who enter my spa.

EVALUATING YOUR PERSONAL QUALIFICATIONS

To begin your entrepreneurial journey, you will need a quiet space, a notebook, and a pen or pencil. Be sure to remove yourself from all of the stresses of everyday life. Turn off the radio, television, and computer, and tune out your children, your spouse, and anything else that might distract you. Find an uncluttered space where you will feel relaxed and settle into a comfortable position. Some like to incorporate certain rituals, such as lighting a candle or playing soothing music, to promote relaxation and create a positive energy flow.

PLAN FOR SUCCESS

Setting the right intention is an important part of any plan for success. Before beginning your entrepreneurial journey take a few minutes to create your own intentions:

It is my strong desire to _____

I attract the financial resources needed to _____

I attract consultants/advisors/teachers who _____

I attract employees who _____

I attract clients who _____

Character Traits

The first part of this exercise involves an assessment of your personal character traits. Start by taking a few moments to breathe deeply and clear your mind of all other concerns. Once you have achieved a relaxed state, think about those characteristics that most closely identify who you are. Perhaps you consider yourself an optimist, a cheerful person, and a hard worker. You might also think of yourself as a procrastinator or someone who has a hard time budgeting. We all possess strengths and weaknesses. Do not filter or analyze anything. Simply state what is unique to your personality as you fill in the following Personal Inventory Checklist. Identifying the strengths and weaknesses in your character will help you to become a better spa owner or manager.

Accomplishments

The next part of this exercise involves drafting a list of your accomplishments. Looking back at some of the major milestones in your life will help you to get started. Are you a high school or college graduate? A licensed esthetician, massage therapist, or cosmetologist? Do you have a job? Work for someone else or yourself? How many jobs have you held over the years? Were all of them in the same field, a related field, or a different field altogether? What do you feel were your most valuable contributions in each of these roles? Have you received any special honors or awards? Many times we do not stop to reflect on the personal impact our lives have on others. Perhaps you are also a parent or work as a volunteer in your community. There is no doubt you have accumulated a number of personal and professional triumphs. Use the following worksheet to list the most significant achievements in your life. Then take some time to reflect upon which you have found most rewarding and why.

PERSONAL INVENTORY CHECKLIST

My Top Five Strengths	My Top Five Weaknesses
1. _____	1. _____
2. _____	2. _____
3. _____	3. _____
4. _____	4. _____
5. _____	5. _____

INVENTORY OF ACCOMPLISHMENTS

Personal Accomplishments

1. *Example: Volunteer for American Cancer Society*

2. _____

3. _____

4. _____

5. _____

Professional Accomplishments

1. *Example: Spa Director at Urban Day Spa for over five years*

2. _____

3. _____

4. _____

5. _____

FUTURE GOALS

Reflecting upon past achievements is often a good way to uncover what you would like to do next. Are you considering opening your own spa? Expanding your current operation? Will you operate your spa as a sole proprietor or have a partner? Maybe you are interested in obtaining a management position and working for someone else for awhile. Will this be a new role for you? What attracted you to the spa business in the first place? What do you like most about it? Are there specific tasks within your current job description that you enjoy more than others? Which is your least favorite? These are just some of the questions to consider as you lay the groundwork for the next phase of your career.

FUTURE GOALS

Over the next five years, I would like to accomplish the following.

For example:

1. *Open my own spa.*
2. *Broaden the range of services I currently provide.*
3. *Obtain a massage therapy license.*
4. *Become computer literate.*
5. *Improve my business and management skills.*

1. _____
2. _____
3. _____
4. _____
5. _____

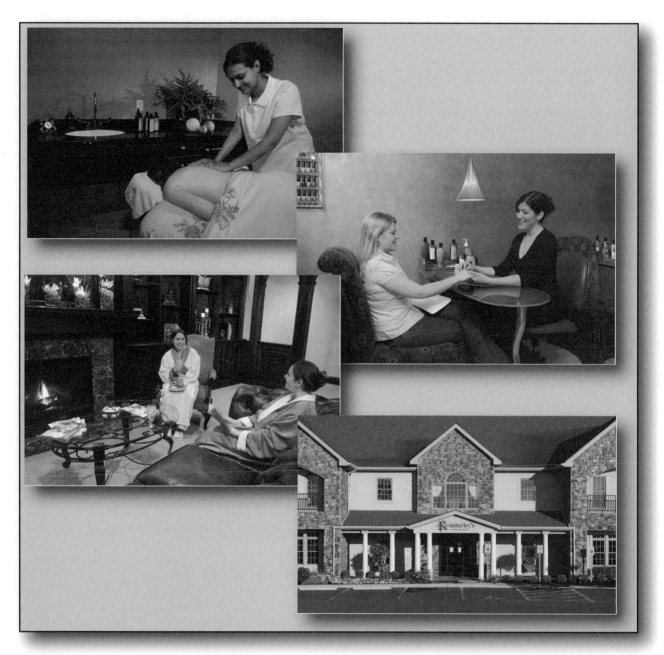

FIGURE 1-1   A clear vision of the type of spa you want to own is the first step in developing a plan for success.

ESTABLISHING BUSINESS GOALS

The next exercise involves focusing more intently on your business goals. If you could imagine the perfect spa setting, what does that look like? Be specific. In what type of spa work environment would you be comfortable? Is it a small, medium, or large spa facility? Would you like to own or manage a day spa, health and wellness center, or a medical aesthetics practice? Perhaps you would like to work in a destination spa or develop an amenity spa within a hotel or resort (Figure 1-1). Think about the number of treatment rooms your spa will incorporate. Who will work in those rooms? What kind of treatments will they perform? Will your spa be geared toward health or beauty practices? Will you incorporate hydrotherapy? Will that take the shape of a Swiss shower, Vichy shower or hydrotherapy tub? What equipment and technology will you use—microcurrent, light therapy, or microdermabrasion? What kind of atmosphere would you like to create— sleek, charming, or restful? What colors appeal to you? Will your employees wear uniforms? Are there flowers, plants, waterfalls, music, and/or chimes? What professional products, complementary books, CDs, and videos will you sell? Who will receive your services? How will you treat them? Are there certain policies you feel are fundamental to running a good business? Are there any that would be difficult for you to enforce? How will you handle employee issues? There are many things to think about.

Sound overwhelming? It doesn't have to be. Giving these questions some serious thought is the first step in your plan to succeed. Putting your ideas down on paper is the next step to bringing them closer to reality. Use the following space to describe your ideal spa. If sentences or phrases do not come easily, just write the first words that come to mind. Be sure to welcome the questions that have no answers, leaving space to add information as it comes to you. Many find it helpful to designate a special notebook or spa journal specifically for this use. This is an excellent way to commit those "lightbulb moments" to memory. Referring to your spa journal from time to time is also a good way to measure your progress and keep your spa vision on track.

Describe your ideal spa in 100 words or less.

_____

_____

_____

_____

_____

_____

_____

_____

_____

_____

Are You an Entrepreneur?

Now that you have a general idea of the type of spa business you would like to build, let's shift to what it will take to turn your dream into a reality. Although some believe that entrepreneurs are born, not made, this is not necessarily true. The motivation for starting your own business can be the direct result of any number of situations. For example, losing your job, feeling unfulfilled or undervalued, or simply not making enough money are all common reasons for taking the entrepreneurial route. In some cases, _luck_ or _fate_ plays a role. How many times have you heard a successful business owner say "I was just in the right place at the right time"?

If you are an independent type with good instincts and the skills necessary to operate your own business, you too have a good chance of running a successful spa business.

WHAT'S _YOUR_ MOTIVATION?

The desire to make more money and the need to be recognized for the contributions that one makes to the success of an operation are two of the more popular incentives for going into business for oneself. Working hard for someone else without any of the benefits or prestige has driven more than one employee to establish their own business. Others simply may have difficulty taking orders from higher-ups or feel that they could do a better job managing the business where they now work. Perhaps none of these fit your particular situation, and being your own boss has always been your dream. Whatever your reasons are, clarifying them is a critical part of realizing your plan for success.

As you contemplate the following checklist, consider your personal reasons for becoming a spa owner. If your motivation includes factors that are not listed here, be sure to add them. Keep this list in a safe place as a positive reminder of your goals and intentions. This will help you to maintain your focus, especially on those days when things do not go according to plan.

MOTIVATION FOR BECOMING SELF-EMPLOYED

Check all that apply; then rate each of your reasons from 1 to 5, with 1 being the most important and 5 being the least important.

☐ Desire to make more money   1 2 3 4 5

☐ Need to feel more fulfilled   1 2 3 4 5

☐ Want more control over my career   1 2 3 4 5

☐ Dislike taking direction from someone else   1 2 3 4 5

☐ Desire to create my own schedule   1 2 3 4 5

☐ Realization that clients come to the spa
  to see *me*   1 2 3 4 5

☐ Frustration over the way the spa I presently
  work in is being managed   1 2 3 4 5

☐ Crave the prestige that comes from owning
  my own business   1 2 3 4 5

☐ Other _____   1 2 3 4 5

What have you discovered about yourself? Write one sentence that best describes your reason for opening your own spa business.

_____

_____

_____

ASSESSING YOUR BUSINESS SKILLS

Once you understand the primary reasons you chose to open your own spa, you are ready to tackle one of the most difficult tasks that you will face in starting your own business—taking stock of your individual strengths and weaknesses. Although many are intimidated by self-evaluation, knowing how your entrepreneurial qualifications stack up can be a *freeing* experience. As Michael Gerber, author of *The E Myth Revisited: Why Most Businesses Don't Work and What to Do About It,* points out, one of the biggest problems entrepreneurs face is that they fail to realize the difference between working in a business and making that same type of business work. Applying this philosophy to the spa business, we can see that being a good service provider does not necessarily equate to managing a spa business well. To start the self-evaluation process, let's begin with three important questions.

1. *What skills are necessary for starting a spa business?*

2. *Do I have these skills?*

3. *If not, how will I acquire them?*

Although it is not mandatory that a spa be owned by a licensed service provider, such as a licensed esthetician or massage therapist, chances are you may have those credentials. It is probably also safe to assume that if you are a service provider, you are probably a good one. In fact, that may be the reason you chose to open your own spa in the first place. Having knowledge of the ingredients that make for a good facial or body treatment are important to understanding the business, but the ability to perform a facial or body treatment well is not the only thing needed to operate a successful spa. As the owner, president, or CEO of your spa business, you will be required to perform and/or supervise a variety of tasks. Some of these tasks will be practical or technical in nature, and others will be administrative. Before you enter the marketplace, it is imperative that you are keenly aware of all the duties and responsibilities of spa ownership and understand exactly where your specific strengths and weaknesses lie. Those entering the spa industry from the business side, as investors, owners, and managers, should be equally diligent, gathering as much information about the culture, spa treatments, and the specific business skills required as possible.

INGREDIENTS FOR SUCCESS

We have already determined that entrepreneurs are not necessarily born; they can also be shaped or molded. In some cases, new business owners have the opportunity to learn from previous management. Others may seek higher levels of education to assist them in assuming the responsibilities of operating a business. However, most successful entrepreneurs possess certain general character traits. Use the following worksheet to assess your personal qualifications. Then rate your capabilities on a scale of 1 to 5, with 1 being excellent and 5 indicating that you have work to do in that area.

CHARACTER TRAITS OF THE SUCCESSFUL ENTREPRENEUR

Rating Scale

1 Excellent; 2 Very Good; 3 Average; 4 Less than Adequate; 5 Need to Develop

Trait	1	2	3	4	5
☐ Disciplined	1	2	3	4	5
☐ Confident	1	2	3	4	5
☐ Self-motivated	1	2	3	4	5
☐ Passionately committed to achieving goals	1	2	3	4	5
☐ Possess tremendous energy	1	2	3	4	5
☐ Comfortable with change	1	2	3	4	5
☐ Recover from setbacks easily	1	2	3	4	5
☐ Enjoy working with people	1	2	3	4	5
☐ Have a strong work ethic	1	2	3	4	5
☐ Possess excellent organizational skills	1	2	3	4	5
☐ Possess excellent communication skills	1	2	3	4	5
☐ Have a clear vision of business goals	1	2	3	4	5
☐ Have a clear vision of personal goals	1	2	3	4	5
☐ Ability to stay focused on short- and long-term projects	1	2	3	4	5
☐ Ability to motivate others	1	2	3	4	5
☐ Ability to work cooperatively with others	1	2	3	4	5
☐ Ability to manage and direct others with integrity	1	2	3	4	5
☐ Balance work and personal life	1	2	3	4	5
☐ Manage stress well	1	2	3	4	5
☐ Practice effective time management	1	2	3	4	5
☐ Possess strong leadership skills	1	2	3	4	5

TABLE 1-1	BUSINESS SKILL ANALYSIS		
Business Task	**Experienced**	**Feel Confident Could Learn**	**Need Professional Help**
1. Understanding of the industry			
2. Accounting/bookkeeping			
3. Managing information technology systems (computers, telephone, fax, credit card machines, etc.)			
4. Handling telephone communications			
5. Conducting sales transactions			
6. Scheduling appointments			
7. Managing payroll			
8. Scheduling employees			
9. Maintaining client records			
10. Developing customer policies			
11. Developing employee policies			
12. Handling human resources (interviewing, hiring, firing, developing compensation and benefits packages)			
13. Developing procedural guidelines			
14. Evaluating employee performance			

Business Qualifications

When it comes to business skills, many novices fall short of the experience required to own or manage a spa. This is perfectly natural. It would be hard for any one person, particularly those who have never owned their own business or held a management position, to possess *all* the skills required to operate a successful spa business. Table 1-1 will help you to evaluate the skills needed to run your spa business, determine those which you are most adept at, and work on those that you need to hone or outsource.

TABLE 1-1	BUSINESS SKILL ANALYSIS CONTINUED		
Business Task	Experienced	Feel Confident Could Learn	Need Professional Help
15. Problem solving			
16. Resolving conflicts			
17. Purchasing property/negotiating a lease			
18. Managing finances			
19. Maintaining inventory control			
20. Complying with local and state business laws			
21. Understanding of the technical skills of *all* service providers			
22. Marketing			
23. Promoting sales			
24. Handling public relations			
25. Advertising			
26. Working with product vendors			
27. Merchandising			
28. Managing retail sales			
29. Educating clients			
30. Recommending products			

As you review the list of items, remember that *smart* entrepreneurs realize they cannot wear all hats well. *Wise* businesspeople develop a general understanding of all the tasks that go into running a business and then decide which they will focus on and which they will delegate to others. For example, you may decide that you like the idea of marketing and promotion but do not have all the skills necessary to perfect the pieces that will give your business a polished professional image. In this case, you may decide to consult with someone who can turn your ideas into a successful marketing campaign while you maintain the internal operations necessary to implement and measure the success of such efforts. You might also like the idea of managing day-to-day operations, crunching numbers to assess the spa's success, or measuring employee progress. If so, installing systems that can help you keep track of sales, employee commissions, and general business reports is a good place to start. Still, you are likely to hire a professional accountant who is more knowledgeable to assist you with balancing your budget or a break-even analysis and to ensure that your business complies with state and federal tax laws.

DELEGATING RESPONSIBILITY

Many spa owners function strictly in a management capacity. However, it is not uncommon for a spa owner who is also a licensed service provider to devote a certain amount of time to performing services and a certain percentage of time to managing day-to-day business operations. Other spa owners are perfectly comfortable spending most of their time in the treatment room while supervising a front desk manager and outsourcing a large percentage of the tasks listed in Table 1-1. Whichever path you choose, you will need to make an honest assessment of where your talents lie and how you wish to channel your energy. There are no absolute *do's* and *don'ts* here, with the exception that every spa business owner should be aware of all the facets that go into running a business and be prepared to make the critical decisions necessary to execute these tasks for the best possible outcome.

THINK IT OVER

If at this point you are asking yourself what these exercises have to do with operating your own business, go back and reevaluate each one. Having a complete vision of your personal and professional goals and understanding your individual strengths and weaknesses is the first step in your journey to becoming the best spa owner or manager you can be.

THE SPA BUSINESS

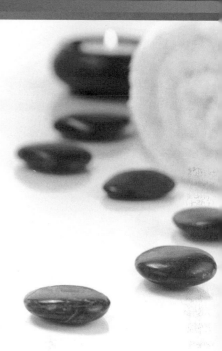

I f your vision included being part of a life-changing experience, you are about to meet your destiny. In the last two decades, the popularity of esthetic beauty and spa services has soared, transforming the spa industry into a multibillion-dollar business that has changed the way people think about health, beauty, and wellness.

Receiving prime coverage from all facets of media, including major television networks and print publications such as the *Wall Street Journal* and *Newsweek,* spa treatments and age management products are frequently in the news. Whether the topic is nutritional skin care, spa body treatments, the increasing number of men receiving spa services, or the integration of medical and holistic health practices, the world seems to be fascinated with spa therapies.

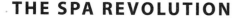

THE SPA REVOLUTION

Although it is difficult to extract precise data and growth rates, you will be hard pressed to find a report that does not point to the increasing number of spas and people using them. Given highly publicized data from government agencies, trade publications, industry organizations, marketing gurus, and research analysts, the spa business continues to be a *hot* commodity. Still, those interested in opening a spa are cautioned to look closely at all available data, weighing the overall rate of growth and the revenue stream attributed to each of the main spa categories against previously published data and current economic indicators.

As you gather your own information, consider the following:

- According to a 2008 study conducted by the International Spa Association (ISPA), the U.S. spa industry generated an estimated $10.9 billion dolars in gross revenue in 2007. [ISPA 2008 Spa Industry Update]

- In June 2008, the total number of spas in the United States was estimated at 18,100 with 80 percent of those spas reportedly day spas. [ISPA 2008 Spa Industry Update]

- The U.S. Census Bureau Economic Census reports that the number of hair, skin, and nail establishments totaled 92,440 in 2006.

- While the majority of spa-goers are still female, ISPA's 2006 Spa-Goer Study indicates that the number of men using spa services is increasing, with the male population now accounting for approximately 31 percent of all spa-goers.

- A Natural Marketing Institute (NMI) study on the Lifestyles of Health and Sustainability [LOHAS], indicates that LOHAS consumers currently account for 19 percent of the total U.S. consumer market (U.S. adults). Further investigation of this market segment indicates that spa-goers are 60 percent more likely to be LOHAS consumers than the general population, and 92 percent of this population believe there is a definite connection between mind, body, and spirit. [Natural Marketing Institute 2007 LOHAS Consumer Trends Database™]

- According to the National Center for Complementary and Alternative Medicine (NCCAM), 36 percent of adults in the United States, ages 18 years or older use some form of complementary or alternative medical and health care therapies.

- The American Society for Aesthetic Plastic Surgery reports that 11.7 million cosmetic surgical and nonsurgical procedures were performed in the U.S. in 2007, with the number of nonsurgical procedures such as Botox injections, hyaluronic acid, laser hair removal, microdermabrasion, and IPL laser treatments procedures having risen by 754 percent since 1997. [American Society for Aesthetic Plastic Surgery 2007]

- The market for personal care and cosmetics continues to grow with the expansion of new retail concept stores devoted exclusively to the sale of cosmetic products and an increase in electronic shopping marts (e-commerce). [U.S. Economic Census data for 2006 indicates a total of 13,591 cosmetic, beauty supply and perfume stores in 2006.]

Spa Origins

Why the seemingly sudden and overwhelming interest in spa therapies? Actually, the origins of most spa therapies can be traced to ancient times, when the curative aspects of natural elements, particularly plants, herbs, hot water, and mineral springs, were highly regarded (Figure 2-1).

The health and beauty practices of such early civilizations as the Egyptians, Romans, Greeks, Chinese, and Indians demonstrate a strong connection to the earth and an extreme reverence for spiritual principles and practices. These ancient civilizations took a holistic approach to the human condition, embracing what is now commonly referred to as the *mind-body-spirit connection.*

Equally invested in both the physical and emotional well-being of the individual, these ancient cultures were not only interested in curing illnesses, they were intent on preventing them. More importantly, they expected the individual to assume responsibility for their own health and well-being and advocated the use of several modalities.

History offers many examples of what we now consider spa therapies, alternative health and skin care practices that were not considered alternative at all; instead, they were viewed as a vital part of a comprehensive health program that, rather than competing with, complemented the

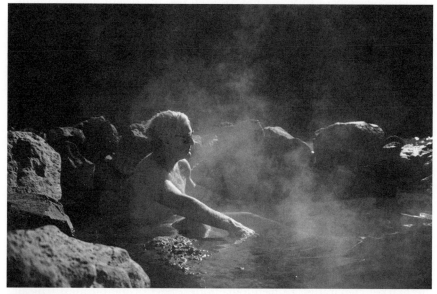

FIGURE 2-1 Natural spa therapies such as warm mineral springs have been popular for centuries.

wisdom of conventional medicine. This fascinating topic has been addressed in numerous articles and textbooks and is worthy of further exploration in understanding the spa revolution that is taking place around the globe today.

What is important to remember for those opening spas in the 21st century is that spa-goers are once again seeking a more inclusive approach to health, beauty, and wellness. Amid breakthroughs in science and technology, people in modern-day cultures are looking to achieve balance and harmony in their lives to counteract what has become for many a hectic and stressful lifestyle. It is not surprising then that we are experiencing a renaissance in the interconnectedness of mind, body, and spirit.

PHILOSOPHICAL SHIFT

Here in the United States, the spa industry has come full circle. Although U.S. spa therapies were originally founded on basic principles of health, relaxation, and nature cures, they eventually became more focused on beauty pampering, weight loss, and fitness. Today, many U.S. spas are returning to their roots as they move beyond the traditional beauty pampering experience to adopt more health- and wellness-oriented practices. Many are also placing a greater emphasis on natural healing methods and spiritual principles.

This new way of thinking has fostered two important new paradigms. First, it has generated a variety of creative alliances among esthetic and medical professionals. Blending Eastern and Western philosophies, we are seeing an increasing number of day spas, medical spas, and wellness centers that are successfully integrating traditional and alternative practices. Along with the conventional beauty fare and medical aesthetic procedures, it is common to see elements of ayurveda, yoga, shiatsu, naturopathy, and aromatherapy included in spa treatments. Second, this new outlook has changed the public's perception of spas. No longer seen as an indulgence of the rich and famous, the new-age spa has gained credibility as an essential part of an inclusive health and wellness program.

INCREASED DEMAND FOR SPA SERVICES

Demand for spa services is on the rise for several reasons. Perhaps the most significant is directly correlated to the growth of the skin care segment of the market. Separating from the glamour aspect of the business typically associated with traditional hair and nail salons, *estheticians* began opening their own skin care clinics and salons in the 1970s. Like many of their most influential predecessors, including cosmetic mavens Helena Rubenstein and Elizabeth Arden, who at the turn of the 20th century were thoroughly entrenched in a holistic approach, these forward-thinking entrepreneurs once again legitimized the connection between health and beauty.

As skin care became a predominant theme in the world of beauty, the role of the esthetician expanded, opening the door to a new and more inclusive way of thinking about spa therapies. Adopting many of the practices reserved for a trip to the destination or resort spa, the *day spa* breathed new life into a genre eager to restore itself. This provided the spa industry with even greater credibility and became the impetus for an increasing number of viable new business options, including the medical spa and wellness center.

SCIENTIFIC BREAKTHROUGHS

The public's increasing interest in spa therapies has been coaxed along by several important scientific, cultural, and economic developments. For example, breakthroughs in science and technology have played a major role in eliminating disease and increasing human longevity; and as people begin to live longer, many are searching for ways to improve the quality of that life. The quest for a healthier, more invigorating, and ageless lifestyle has generated more than a passing interest in preventive medicine; it has literally changed the way people think about the aging process, subsequently introducing many new esthetic products, equipment, and techniques to spas around the globe.

Working from a long list of high-powered *pharmaceutical, cosmeceutical,* and *botanical* ingredients, manufacturers are now turning out a number of more efficient, results-oriented products that are capable of correcting more challenging conditions. In addition, technology has produced a wide array of powerful delivery systems and advanced aesthetic procedures such as phonophoresis, microdermabrasion, microcurrent, and photomodulation that are helping many to improve their self-image.

Advances in medical aesthetic specialties such as cosmetic surgery and dermatology have influenced spa services as well. Once a topic discussed behind closed doors, cosmetic surgery and age management techniques are now the subject of daily news and casual conversation. This increased acceptance of more aggressive age management procedures has supported a cooperative relationship between medical professionals and spa therapists that shows no sign of slowing down.

THE BABY BOOMERS

Baby boomers have played a significant role in promoting spa services (Figure 2-2). This well-educated, take-charge generation, born between 1946 and 1964, has almost single-handedly changed the way we view age in this country. Possessed by an age-defiant attitude and armed with the greatest disposable income of our time, baby boomers are destined to become one of the oldest populations in our living history and will no doubt continue to set lifestyle trends that will influence generations to come. While this group has demanded to look as good as they feel, they have also taken a far more open-minded approach. Their willingness to experiment with new techniques and embrace the healthy aging practices of other cultures has played an important role in promoting alternative therapies and integrating Eastern and Western philosophies in the spa.

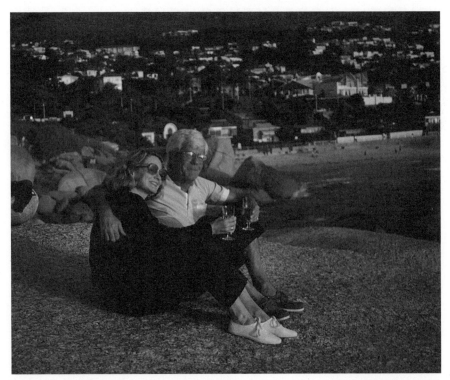

FIGURE 2-2 The baby boomer generation has played a significant role in promoting spa services.

HEALTH CARE CONCERNS

The rising cost of health care and increasing environmental concerns have also played a role in the spa's evolution, encouraging the movement toward holistic and alternative approaches, such as homeopathic or naturopathic remedies. Consider the direct correlation between the depletion of the ozone layer and the increased rate of skin cancer. Not only have such findings brought about an increased awareness of the need for sun protection, but they have also encouraged many to reevaluate their lifestyle and seek preventative or alternative methods to maintain skin health. For example, environmental hazards have prompted the rising use of vitamin or antioxidant therapy to replenish the skin and combat the visible signs of sun damage. The threat of skin cancer has also popularized new products and techniques such as self-tanners and spray tanning machines.

Other psychosocial influences related to automation and lifestyle changes, the increased threat of violence, and uncertainty brought about by war and terrorist attacks have also contributed to the allure of spas. Aside from stress relief associated with the demands of a fast-paced work style and leisure life, we are also discovering that people are simply looking to spas as a safe haven from the *real* world—a telling sign of the volatile times in which we live.

Market Analysis

"Unquantified," "completely fragmented," "lacking comprehensive statistical analysis," "reliable data needed to leverage market position and sustain growth"

All of these words and phrases have been used to describe the spa business, but that is changing. The spa business is no longer plagued by a lack of data. As spa therapies blend into the mainstream fabric of our society, market analysis has become big business with many looking to quantify and subsequently qualify the spa industry. This trend is welcome news, particularly to those interested in entering or expanding the market; however, a good deal of groundwork must continue to be laid before information is truly indicative of reality. One of the challenges in the United States is the lack of a national standard and an integrative method of accounting. With so many variations on the spa theme, it is nearly impossible to report emphatically on the state of the industry. This has increased the demand for valid statistics.

MAKING SENSE OF STATISTICS

Just what are statistics, and why should we study them? Open the pages of any magazine, nonfiction book, or newspaper publication, and you are bound to find a reference to statistics. *Statistics* are a vital part of research that helps us to calculate and make inferences about any number of things, including groups of people or even behavior patterns. For example, statistics on the spending habits of teenagers are likely to have tremendous value for many organizations and businesses, including spas and, of course, parents.

Numerous statistics are relevant to the spa industry, such as the number of spas located in a particular section of the country or the number of times the average person is likely to visit a spa in a year. The average gross revenue of day spas is another statistic that is likely to resonate with potential spa owners. What would you like to know more about before opening a spa? Make a list of general questions you feel are important to your understanding of the spa industry. Now think of the ways in which you might use such information. Finally, think about how you would go about obtaining this information. Use the examples in Table 2-1 to help you get started.

Validity

As you set out to find answers to your questions, it is important to remember that valid statistics follow standardized procedures to gather and measure information before any inferences or generalizations can be made. In calculating data, statisticians use a certain scientific protocol for collecting, organizing, and summarizing their findings. Some measurements, such as descriptive statistics, are fairly straightforward, while others, such as inferential statistics, are more complex. For example, *descriptive statistics* may simply state the number of spas in the country. They may also supply an annual income for those spas. On the other hand, *inferential statistics* make inferences about a particular group based on information supplied by a smaller subset of that group. For example, the number of times a representative segment of the population went to a spa in one year may be used to project future attendance or make a statement about the increasing popularity of spa services. To comprehend the meaning of descriptive or inferential statistics, it is also important to know how the study was conducted, who conducted it, exactly who or what was measured, and how those interpreting the data arrived at their hypotheses or inferences. The source of funding is another important piece of information that should not be overlooked.

TABLE 2-1 SPATISTICS		
As a potential spa owner, what do I need or want to know about the spa business?	**How will this information help me to further my business?**	**Where will I find this information?**
Example:	*Example:*	*Example:*
1. How *many* spas are there in the geographic area in which I am looking to open a spa?	1. Determining the number of spas in a specific area will help me to evaluate the competition.	1. State or local business directory and/or licensing boards; research studies.
2. What *types* of spas are established in the geographic area I am considering?	2. Understanding the type of spa businesses that already exist will help me to develop a unique selling position.	2. The Internet or spa brochures; research studies.
3.	3.	3.
4.	4.	4.
5.	5.	5.

Buyer Beware

We have touched on the bare basics here, but it is important to keep in mind that statistics is a complex subject. In reviewing data, it is always wise to be cautious. Formulating the right questions is just as important as how the data is collected and the results are interpreted.

Those new to research and statistics should also be aware of the credibility factor when reviewing or purchasing any information. Studies can be expensive, and all research is not equal. Keep in mind that some researchers may simply recognize an economic opportunity, while others may have a vested interest in portraying their findings in a certain light. Some reports offer little more than an exercise in data analysis with information provided representing only a small or skewed segment of the population. We must be particularly cautious as we become more comfortable with online research, which raises yet another area of concern. While the Internet may provide a population of eager and willing participants and almost instantaneous results, particularly when there is a reward for participation, qualifying respondents and the validity of data are far from finessed.

It is nevertheless an exciting time for the spa industry. Market studies are long overdue and point to a new direction, with many working hard to supply long-awaited answers that will ultimately broaden the scope of the industry and raise professional standards. When research is conducted in an objective and systematic way using sound scientific methods, statistics can give us a solid basis for interpreting information and drawing reasonable conclusions. In your search to find valid answers to your spa business questions, it is important to look for carefully designed research studies from reputable resources that contain a thoughtful analysis of the data.

DEMOGRAPHICS

Today more than ever, marketing analysts are relying on demographics to develop a better understanding of consumers and predict future trends. *Demographics* is the study and analysis of the characteristics of a particular group of people or population, including age, sex, education level, and economic status. This information has become a major part of market research. It has also prompted us to look beyond the basics at a more detailed analysis of who is buying what, how, and why. Demographics can be instrumental in supplying marketing professionals with valuable information to uncover trends and formulate predictions about future spending habits.

In the spa industry, many are using demographics to determine such facts as how many men go to spas, how much disposable income teenagers have, and what effect these segments of the population have on retail sales. Let's take a look at several prominent trends and how savvy marketing gurus use this information to leverage marketing power.

MARKET TRENDS

It seems that not too long ago the entire world wanted to blur sexual identity, with virtually every business, including spas and salons, taking on a *unisex* attitude that pronounced equality and loosened sexual boundaries. Today, we are witnessing an explosive counterculture that seems far happier espousing gender differences, particularly between men and women. What happened?

The Female Consumer

One answer is the feminist revolution. As women developed a powerful voice in their own right, they no longer needed to make a statement about similarities. Today, rather than make a case for equality, women appear to be more comfortable highlighting the virtues that helped them to arrive safely at the helm of many business and economic opportunities. What role do demographics play in all this? Using demographic information available from a variety of resources, we can begin to make a case for understanding, targeting, and winning the female segment of today's market. For example, when it comes to understanding women in the United States, did you know that:

- Women comprised 51 percent of our nation's population in 2008.
- Women have constituted the majority of college students since 1979.
- Women earned 57 percent of all bachelor's degrees awarded in 2006–2007.
- The rate of women earning master's degrees rose from 40 percent in 1970–1971 to 61 percent in 2006–2007.
- In 1948, women represented only 31.3 percent of the workforce; that figure rose to 56.2 percent in 2008.
- Women workers held 51 percent of all management and professional occupations in 2007.
- Fifty-nine percent of women in the labor force in 2007 had children under the age of three.

- Women owned 6.5 million businesses in the United States in 2002.
- Women account for approximately 80 percent of all consumer purchases.

Now you may be thinking, what difference does all of this data make in the esthetics and spa industry, which has a long history of being dominated by the female population. The truth is that marketing to today's female consumer is quite different from marketing to previous generations of salon and spa-goers (Figure 2-3).

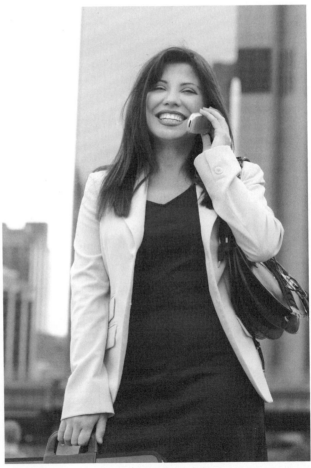

FIGURE 2-3   The modern female consumer has different needs than previous generations of spa-goers.

In analyzing these statistics, we can make several important inferences about female consumers. First, the current population of women is better educated and accounts for a far greater number in the workforce than any previously recorded generation of women in the history of our country. They also have greater spending power and are juggling far more responsibilities than most of their mothers did, including child-rearing. How does this information influence the way you market to women? With stress levels increasing along with the size of their paychecks, many women are looking to spas to help them relax.

However, relaxation is not the only motivation for a woman's visit to the spa. Women go to spas for any number of reasons that are driven by a variety of needs and wants. They may be looking to jump-start a weight loss program or remedy a skin condition. In meeting those needs, spa therapists must take into account the female value system. For example, women believe in education and like to be part of the decision-making process; so don't shy away from telling them all about the latest treatments and techniques or enlisting them in choices.

Women today are also challenging traditional concepts of beauty. Certainly, many are still interested in appearances, but "being beautiful" no longer holds the same power over women that it did in the past. To be sure, women still have facials, face lifts, Botox injections, body wraps, liposuction, and manicures and pedicures in record numbers, but nowadays women are more inclined to think of beauty in terms of their overall health and well-being or presenting a polished professional image. Most would like to eliminate stereotypes and see a broader, more inclusive definition of beauty that respects all cultures and life cycles. Looking and feeling their best is part of an overall attitude that helps women to achieve what has been coined as their "personal best." Appearances are definitely still important, but they are no longer a woman's ticket to the world.

Gender Differences

The topic of marketing to women seems to be at the forefront these days, but we are also charting new territory when it comes to the male market. This is particularly true in the spa industry as we look for ways to encourage men to appreciate the many benefits that women have derived from spas for years. Fortunately, along with understanding what women want, researchers are eager to explore the male psyche and particularly to cite differences in male and female communication, purchasing, and relaxation patterns, which are important subjects for the spa owner.

Open any spa trade publication and you are bound to find a good deal of material on these topics, with any number of industry-specific articles expounding advice on how to understand and reach your share of the male market. For spa owners currently faced with the predicament of figuring out ways to attract male consumers without alienating women, studying psychosocial differences can prove extremely useful in creating a more thoughtful sales and marketing approach.

Beyond gender differences, demographics also help us to track other equally important social and economic phenomena. For example, demographics can help us to translate data and track trends related to minority populations, aging, health care issues, salary levels, geographic mobility, and technology, just to name a few. The impact of retiring baby boomers is yet another social phenomenon that will have a significant impact on spa revenues as we transition to the very different set of values and spending habits of *generations x and y*. All of these things ultimately impact the way we conduct business and allow us to anticipate customer needs and position or reposition the way we market our products and services.

MAKING IT REAL

Being conscious of the broader social and economic climate is an important piece of developing an inclusive business plan, but to fully appreciate the role of demographics, you needn't look further than your own database.

Before you can develop an effective marketing plan, it is important to take a look at the needs and wants of your customers. This means taking the time to investigate the cultural and economic situation in your community. Many times, spa owners are puzzled by the lack of enthusiasm their clients have for certain products or services that they assumed would be a big hit. Frequently, this is due to a lack of understanding of what their customers really want. You cannot sell something to someone who doesn't want it or need it. This does not mean you cannot introduce something new successfully; it just means that you have to understand the most effective way to position your product to reach your target market.

For those thinking about opening a spa for the first time, investigating the demographics of the community beforehand can prove to be one of the greatest marketing tactics you employ. Finding out who lives in the community, how much money they make, and what is most important to them will help you to position, price, and promote your services in a way that is geared to their income level and value system. It can also save you a great deal of time, effort, energy, and money, if it turns out that the community is not a good fit for your spa design or philosophy; for example, even with the best intentions, trying to force a rural community with modest income levels, embedded in natural health and well-being, to embrace trendy, high-ticket items that are glamour-focused probably will not work.

For those already doing business, a study of the demographic and lifestyle habits of the community may serve as a reality check that helps to fine-tune current marketing and promotional efforts. For example, you may want to consider volunteering to apply makeup for the local theater group, if it seems that activity is held in high regard in your community. Or perhaps you will get involved in environmental concerns or support skin cancer awareness. You might also consider offering budget-conscious services or sales promotions if most of the population earns a rather modest income. Maybe your spa is located in an affluent suburban community. In which case, you may want to promote services that are more status-oriented or sophisticated, highlighting the fact that you offer all the ambience of a trendy urban spa without the hassle of traveling into the city, or that you carry products that are seen in magazines like *Vogue* or *In Style,* if that's what your clients read.

Finding the Information You Need

How will you find such detailed information about people? It is not as hard as you might think. There are many ways to learn about a community and its inhabitants, but it is often helpful to begin with the big picture. Those interested in relocating or finding out more about a particular region might begin by studying *demographic clusters*. Cluster analysis is available through public and private agencies that extract and publish specific demographic data on geographic locations around the country.

Local resources such as town hall and state government agencies like the Department of Labor are easily accessible and can be helpful in supplying you with important data, such as the number of people living in the community, average income, and family and work status. Are inhabitants mainly families or single dwellers? Blue-collar or professional workers? Two-career families? While tax rates and the selling price of homes are public information, real estate agents can be a good source of information on other important aspects of the community, such as lifestyle habits, number of churches, civic and social groups, shopping centers, and recreational opportunities. You can also learn a great deal by simply observing and conversing with people. Have breakfast at the local coffee shop, browse through retail shops, talk to other merchants, and attend public functions and town meetings.

If you are already in business, take a closer look at who your clients are. Collecting your own statistical data will help you to analyze important information such as the primary age range of your clients, professional status, and the male-to-female ratio. A detailed analysis of which services are most popular and how much clients spend on retail per visit will also help you to better understand and fulfill client needs.

UNDERSTANDING YOUR CLIENTELE

- ☐ Total number of clients _____
- ☐ Average age _____
- ☐ Average income _____
- ☐ Number of women _____
- ☐ Number of men _____
- ☐ Number of teenagers _____
- ☐ Employment status _____
- ☐ Most sought-after service _____
- ☐ Average monthly/yearly service expenditure per client _____
- ☐ Average monthly/yearly retail expenditure per client _____

RETAIL TRENDS

In addition to understanding your target market, it is important to keep an eye on related market trends, particularly those affecting the sale of spa goods and services. For example, new retail concepts, such as beauty super-stores like Sephora® and Bath and Body Works® and the influx of medical aesthetic boutiques in shopping malls, all have some bearing on the spa market. Other products aimed at bringing the spa experience home, such as whirlpool tubs, spa bath products and accessories, aromatherapy candles, scrubs, and massage oils, are also likely to have an impact on the amount of revenue spa-goers bring in to the spa.

BUSINESS CONSIDERATIONS

To maintain a competitive edge in this continually evolving market, it is also important to be aware of the latest economic trends and how they directly affect your spa. This is especially true for the small business owner, who must stay ahead of the curve to survive. No matter what type of spa you operate, it is imperative that you are educated on new products and methods of delivery. You should also be aware of the increasing number of new business protocols that are affecting the way spas operate. Creating alliances and cross-merchandising are a big part of building a solid marketing strategy. Keeping abreast of global and geographic economic conditions as well as general market trends and cultural shifts is another important consideration in maintaining a broader market perspective. Ups and downs in the Dow Jones, Nikkei, and European stock exchanges are bound to influence investors. As you apply this knowledge to your spa business, it will enable you to develop a more meaningful approach to daily operations.

Best Practices in Spa Development

Industry leaders have made great strides in developing an inclusive spa classification system. However, a tremendous amount of work needs to be done before we can make unilateral statements about the spa business. In the United States, the development of national standards at the economic census level including a separate category for spas in the North American Industry Classification System (NAICS) is an important goal that should be at the forefront of this effort. Such standards will allow for more credible research. Otherwise, words like *fragmented* will continue to plague the spa business, preventing both esthetic and medical-aesthetic components from moving forward in the best possible way.

Another important concern, particularly for the day spa owner, is the need for information to assist in developing better business practices and professional standards. As data collection becomes a priority, industry leaders should not lose sight of their constituents. Many spas, particularly day spas, have evolved as independently owned small businesses. As more powerful enterprises compete for a share of the market, useful, affordable information will become critical to their survival.

DEFINING THE SPA

Along with tracking demographic trends and client needs, one of the biggest questions currently being raised in the spa industry is "What defines a spa?" With everything from destination and day spas to wellness centers, medi-spas, and even "quickie" convenience and kiosk spas, it seems that no two spas are alike these days. No wonder entrepreneurs and research analysts are scratching their heads. Significant variations notwithstanding, defining the type of spa business you envision is the first step in developing a successful business or marketing plan.

Search any spa directory or trade publication and you are likely to find a diverse collection of spa businesses. These incorporate a seemingly endless array of services and treatments and may use an even wider range of equipment and service providers. Some spas offer hair and beauty services, while others focus strictly on skin care. Some spas are medically based, while others take an alternative health or fitness approach.

You are also likely to find several broad categories of spas, including day spas, destination or resort spas, wellness centers, and medical spas (Figures 2-4 to 2-7). These can be categorized further as small independent practices, franchises, or larger corporate facilities. Spas can also vary in terms of the size of the facility and the number of treatment rooms and personnel. So how on earth can we develop a classification that includes all of them?

The word *spa* is used so loosely today that many are frustrated by the lack of clear identifying criteria. Although the U.S. Census Bureau lists a distinct NAICS (formerly SIC) category for hair, nail, and skin care services, there is still no standard industry code that separates spas or day

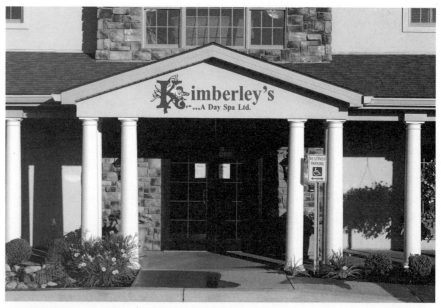

FIGURE 2-4   Many options are available to those looking for a career in the spa industry. Pictured here is Kimberley's Day Spa, Latham, New York.

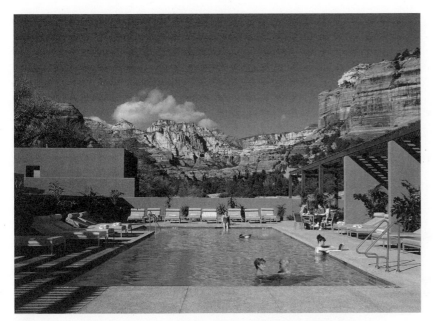

FIGURE 2-5   Mii Amo, Destination Spa. Mii amo, Sedona, Arizona.

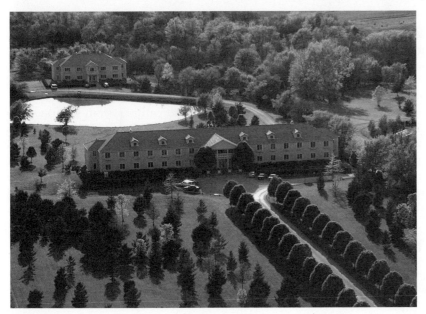

FIGURE 2-6   The Raj Ayurveda Health Spa, Medical Spa, Fairfield, Iowa.

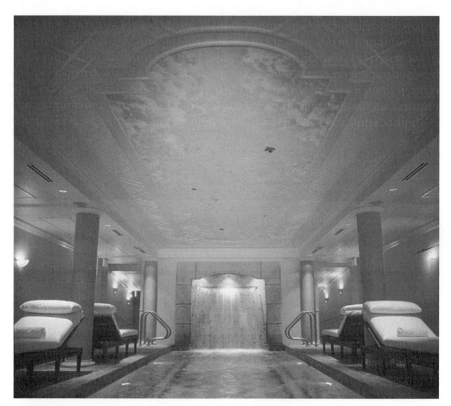

FIGURE 2-7   Kohler Waters, Resort Spa, Kohler, Wisconsin.

spas from resort spas or other related facilities, such as fitness and wellness centers. Similarly, no specific trade classification system separates the skin care clinic from a beauty salon that offers skin care services and calls itself a day spa. Due to the lack of definition, many of the industry's leading trade associations, publications, and educators have attempted to set guidelines and categorize spas in a way that supports further analysis of the industry. The following categories are generally accepted as representing the broader spectrum of spas.

The Day Spa

Day spas are currently the most popular type of spa. Although many beauty salons and skin care clinics have adopted the term *day spa* to note the addition of facials and/or body treatments, a true day spa by most expert standards means that the spa offers patrons shower facilities and some other

energy or body work therapies, and herbal remedies to prevent and/or treat illness, they may also integrate more traditional methods, including physical therapy, exercise programs, and nutrition counseling. Yoga, meditation, lifestyle, and longevity programs are some of the modalities you may encounter within such an establishment. Wellness centers tend to be subjective in their approach to preventative care and healing, but when integrated with spa therapies, such as massage and skin care, this format lends credibility to the concept of whole health and once again brings us back to the true origins of spa therapy focused on treating the whole person.

Future Spa Trends

Inspired by a powerful vision, those dedicated to the advancement of spa therapies have taken several giant steps in recent years; however, the most significant progress has come from a public relations standpoint. With spa therapies now linked to health, nutrition, and environmental factors, the spa, predominantly the day spa, has literally changed the face of the health and beauty industry and has fostered a number of formidable new partnerships. Today, we are at yet another crossroad that will require an energetic new wave of visionaries to address changing protocols, strengthen business alliances, and build solid client relationships. What can we expect?

Charting new territory is invigorating and exciting. It can also be challenging. Successful ventures require insight, vision, and strong leadership skills. They also demand patience and a willingness to persevere to accomplish one's goals. Faced with new challenges, the spa industry will need creative thinkers and dynamic leaders to shape public opinion.

The opportunities for spas appear to be limitless. However, new tools, new players, and new prototypes will continue to challenge traditional roles and urge us to sharpen our vision. The following trends bear particularly close watching over the next few years.

NEW ALLIANCES, NEW MODELS, AND NEW STANDARDS

The administration of new prototypes is a crucial consideration. New alliances and models will no doubt continue to include a varied group of esthetic, health, and wellness professionals: estheticians, medical doctors, nurses, nutritionists, naturopathic physicians, chiropractors, acupuncturists, massage therapists, and fitness instructors. We can also expect to see a number of new disciplines integrated into spas, including physical therapists, psychotherapists, lifestyle counselors, and personal image consultants and coaches.

Medical spas will continue to grow and are likely to be directed by an even broader range of physicians, such as general internists, gynecologists, obstetricians, cardiologists, allergists, and orthopedic specialists looking to enhance their profitability under the constraints of managed care. We can also expect more nurses and allied health professionals, such as nutritionists, to become strong contenders in the area of beauty and wellness, with more of them taking on entrepreneurial roles in the development of medically oriented lifestyle spas.

Not only will these new alliances and protocols increase the demand for new business structures, but they will also force the issue of standards. At this point, many are challenging a number of antiquated laws that govern the industry. This is placing additional strain on already over-programmed state boards, perplexed by the new treatments and procedures that are fast becoming part of the current health and beauty culture. As estheticians, nurses, physicians, and alternative health care providers all seek to garner a share of the market, we will be forced to come to terms with some of the more hotly debated issues around licensing and regulations; for example, who should be allowed to perform chemical peels, microdermabrasion, and laser hair removal, laser- and light-based rejuvenation procedures, or administer Botox and collagen injections? Should such treatments occur only under the direct supervision of a physician? Should that doctor be on the premises at the time of service or a phone call away? With many pushing the limits of their licensure, these questions and the issue of regulation are likely to command more creative models of supervision that will ultimately require an alliance of esthetic and medical professionals.

With so much at stake, expect to see an ongoing number of power struggles and the rise of many grassroots organizations looking to sway legislative opinion; however, the role of the consumer should not be overlooked. Public demand will play an important role in dictating new standards as better-educated consumers, in some cases more knowledgeable than practitioners, begin to take a stand on the administration of healthy aging treatments.

Hopefully, territorial issues will give way to new integrative and creative alliances that recognize the contribution of a varied group of professionals. However, this is likely to require the mediation efforts of a number of professionals, including public health administrators and strategic business planners.

INCREASED TRAINING AND EDUCATION STANDARDS FOR SPA PROFESSIONALS

The revision of new laws and licensing regulations is challenging many in the industry to rethink current teaching practices, with "more education" becoming the mantra for spa professionals as a new age in beauty, health, and wellness emerges.

We have reached a point where advances in science and technology have exceeded the curriculum development of many vocational or career training facilities preparing spa professionals for licensing, such as estheticians and massage therapists. This is occurring at a time when other well-educated professionals, such as registered nurses, are looking to stake a claim in the marketplace. As these budding entrepreneurs seek additional licenses to practice skin care and open medical spas, we are witnessing an increasingly competitive situation.

This highlights a major problem that continues to plague the industry—the lack of a unified and more inclusive program for "spa therapists," a virtual misnomer as there is no such licensed professional. Typically, nonmedical personnel performing face and body treatments in spas are either massage therapists, estheticians, cosmetologists, or nail technicians. Each of these spa service providers requires a separate license. With the increasing demand for practitioners to perform a wider range of more involved and crossover treatments, as well as the influx of students already possessing business and nursing degrees, the industry is witnessing a growing number of advanced training programs designed to fill in the gaps. While postgraduate education has its place, particularly when it comes to enforcing continuing education credits, the time is right to rethink current education protocols.

The Evolution of Spa Education

Before the advent of sophisticated technology and medical spas, most education for spa personnel in the United States took place in proprietary career or vocational training schools with the focus on preparing students for licensing, a process typically regulated by state boards, such as the Board of Cosmetology. These generally included licensing programs for estheticians, cosmetologists, and massage therapists, each of which required a set number of clock hours to measure competency.

Because standards set for spa professionals in the United States have historically been lower than those of their European counterparts from which they originated (for example, the average number of hours for esthetics training is 600 hours across the U.S.), many frustrated spa professionals and school owners began seeking additional credentials from outside agencies to enhance their standing. The Comité International d'Esthétique et de Cosmétologie (CIDESCO) has been the choice of many estheticians interested in acquiring internationally acclaimed credentials. Those graduating from this program, typically referred to as CIDESCO diplomats, are required to adhere to very strict standards that generally exceed most state requirements for estheticians in the United States.

Today other agencies like the International Therapy Examination Council (ITEC), one of the largest international boards of its kind, which offers a wide range of qualifications in the fields of esthetics, sports and fitness, and holistic and massage therapies, are also becoming popular in the United States.

Organizations like the National Certification Board for Therapeutic Massage & Body Work, the National Coalition of Estheticians, Manufacturers & Distributors, & Associations (NCEA), the National Interstate Council of State Boards of Cosmetology, and the Federation of State Massage Therapy Boards are working hard to enforce national standards that would allow graduates increased recognition and mobility across state borders.

As state boards give the go-ahead to replace clock hour curricula with credit hour programs, many others are beginning to embrace a new level of education, this time at the college level. Degreed programs in hotel and hospitality management have long been a natural choice for those interested in managing destination, resort, and amenity spas. These courses have a strong business component that is now filtering into the spa industry as universities and colleges join ranks with vocational training programs, to offer special business courses to unenrolled spa and salon managers and service providers interested in increasing their business skills. This is welcome news to the spa industry, but it has not been the most practical way to address the growing need for a well-rounded spa curriculum that addresses the needs of those who enter the business as "licensees."

This has given rise to yet another phenomenon and the birth of several new and innovative degreed programs that are actually combining all of the necessary skills needed to succeed in the spa business, including academic and business courses, and licensing programs for estheticians and massage therapists. But more are needed. Establishing degreed programs that combine technical skills with increased academic requirements and business skills will not only increase credibility at the consumer level, it will also help to build collegial confidence among spa and medical professionals. It is also likely to force the issue of more inclusive programming, opening the doors to college-level administrators with a desire to develop new programs in medical aesthetic and holistic health care.

Similar to other strong technical programs, such as those for medical laboratory technicians, I believe that the next wave of spa professionals will have at least associate degree status. Eventually, we may also see four-year degreed programs in spa therapy, each with its own specialty, such as a concentration in naturopathic or traditional medical aesthetics practices.

CONTINUED USE OF TECHNOLOGY AND DEMOGRAPHIC ANALYSIS

The trend toward a more thoughtful analysis of industry trends and statistics will continue with industry trade associations, vendors, and publishers taking a more active role in developing studies that address the needs of their constituents. Although they will continue to rely on the expertise of marketing and research analysts to assist them in conducting research, leaders within the industry will develop a much stronger voice as they seek to control their own interests and monitor the high price of being informed.

Demographic analysis will continue to affect the way we do business, taking on a significant role in how we market new treatments and products. Along with the greater use of technology, this will lead to the development of better business practices; however, it will also force many smaller spas, unwilling or unable to expand their efforts and adapt to new technology, out of business. Those unable to use customized software programs to assist with accounting, marketing, and client and personnel management will quickly become extinct.

As spas become more sophisticated and better equipped, we can definitely expect them to become more business savvy. Many spa owners who are also service providers will trade scrubs and rubs for desktops, as they opt to devote less time to performing treatments and more time to developing business and tending to sales, marketing, and client and personnel management. Those established spa owners who prefer to remain in the treatment room must be willing to expend more capital to hire better-qualified front desk managers who will add customer service and marketing tasks to their job descriptions.

RECOGNITION OF CONSUMER NEEDS AND WANTS

Expect consumers to have a lot more input in coming years as they insist on better treatments and service. Frustrated by rising costs and a diminished health care system, consumers will look to spas to fulfill their desire for health and wellness. Although they may be willing to pay for personalized services that recognize and support individual agendas, they will also demand to have a greater say in the quality of care they receive.

But before spa owners can supply consumers with the standard of care they desire, they must understand what consumers want—before they even know they want it. In an effort to understand the needs and wants of spa-goers, owners and managers will expect therapists to build solid relationships with clients. Built-in callback and call-in times will become standard practice as the influx of medical professionals prompts spas to adopt more of the protocols used in that field to build patient confidence.

Spa managers will also go direct, providing incentives for clients to fill out practitioner "report cards" after receiving services. Even those spas attracting a transient clientele will seek more creative methods for learning what clients really want. Expect interactive surveys, focus groups, and the Internet to play an important role in accessing such information. These will be used in conjunction with ongoing demographic analysis to evaluate all facets of the industry, from customer service, pricing, and the type of products used to how well the spa has addressed cultural concerns.

Although consumers will expect practitioners and spas to know what they want and need before they do, they will also take responsibility for lobbying for those things that are near and dear to them. Results-oriented, healthy aging products and services are bound to be at the top of this list. An ecologically concerned society will also insist that manufacturers and spas be held accountable for providing natural, environmentally safe products. As age boundaries continue to blur, special advocacy groups will also push spas to take a stand on ethical and moral issues, such as age management and self-image, particularly those that affect the self-esteem of an increasingly younger population of spa-goers.

THE GREENING OF SPAS

With concerns about global warming and economic and environmental sustainability at an all-time high, spas have already begun taking on yet another important role: protecting the earth and its inhabitants from toxic chemicals and excessive waste. This phenomenon has led to the greening of spas on just about every level, including architecture and design, water and energy conservation, noise and pollution control, organic product ingredients and related growing and manufacturing practices, product packaging, recycling, housekeeping, etc. It has also raised the bar for those looking to attract an increasing number of LOHAS consumers.

Supporting eco-friendly business practices certainly makes sense in an industry focused on health and wellness, and as LOHAS consumers continue to gain a significant voice in the spa community we can expect this practice to take on even greater economic importance. We can also expect to see a real interest on the part of the entire spa industry to partner with environmental protection agencies and special interest groups, particularly when it comes to sustaining natural resources for organic skin care products, a growing segment of the personal care industry that is increasingly in demand by today's ecologically conscious spa consumer.

LIFESTYLE CENTERS

Combating the effects of a stress-weary world, lifestyle centers will become the popular new genre for health and wellness. These facilities will offer the convenience of spa therapies, such as skin care, massage, exercise, and nutritional counseling, and then some, to create a mega-spa atmosphere. Blending traditional and alternative therapies, you will be able to find just about anything you're looking for in terms of health and wellness, including but not limited to medical aesthetics, herbal remedies, vitamins, chiropractic care, acupuncture, yoga classes, lifestyle counseling, and psychotherapy. With something for everyone, clients will be able to achieve their personal best in the modality with which they are most comfortable.

Expect these *superspas* and *lifestyle centers* to pop up in urban and suburban malls, with extra amenities such as child care and pediatric clinics to accommodate the demands of working mothers. With so many of these lifestyle facilities staffed and endorsed by medical professionals, expect retail centers not only to provide over-the-counter cosmetics and beauty prescriptions, but also to conduct mini medical aesthetic procedures, such as Botox and collagen injections.

The Spa Life

What was only a dream a few short years ago has suddenly blossomed into a full-blown reality with spa living accommodations cropping up in urban and suburban landscapes across the country. Baby boomers will continue to steer this market as they look to spas to set new standards for addressing their needs as senior citizens. In this vein, expect to see spa philosophies and amenities incorporated into a growing number of planned retirement communities to help keep boomers fit and mobile as they enter their twilight years—although we can certainly expect those years to contain more vitality than ever before (Figure 2-8).

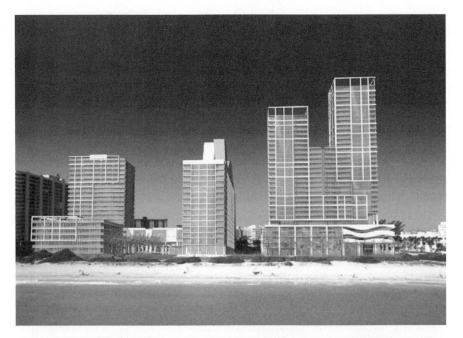

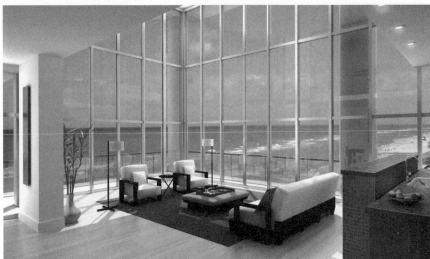

FIGURE 2-8 A AND B   Lifestyle condominium complexes such as this one developed by Canyon Ranch in Miami, Florida, will become a way of life for those invested in healthy living.

The male market will continue to flourish as men buy into the philosophy of looking and feeling good. This will manifest in an increasing number of spas devoted strictly to providing men with services in a way that protects both their privacy and their masculinity.

THINK IT OVER

As you contemplate many of the thought-provoking issues raised in this chapter, consider also the short time in which the spa industry has grown and developed into a powerful economic force. With so many new options and challenges ahead of us, the next wave promises to be even more exciting. As you consider your role in the scheme of spas to come, remember that true visionaries are always one step ahead—ahead of the competition and ahead of the trends.

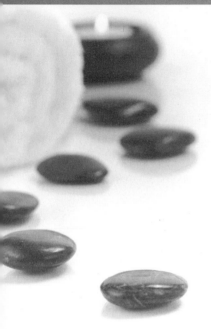

GETTING DOWN TO BUSINESS

Small Business Administration statistics indicate that about two-thirds of all new small businesses survive the first two years; less than half survive four.[1] While about one-third of new small businesses are reportedly successful at the time of closure, these figures are nevertheless a warning to those looking for more than a 50/50 shot at long-term success.

There are many reasons why some businesses manage to survive those critical first few years and some don't, but in actuality the success or failure of most small businesses is likely to reflect either a superior or extremely inadequate ability to deal with the realities of running a business.

WHY BUSINESSES FAIL OR SUCCEED

Even with all systems in place, the road to success is typically a bumpy one. No matter how well qualified you are, at first you can expect to put in long hours for little pay. Not everyone is willing to endure this challenge. If you are a person who requires instant gratification, think twice before starting your own business. Although the satisfaction derived from promoting health and wellness may be rewarding, it may not afford you

---

[1] The U.S. Small Business Administration Office of Advocacy defines a *small business* as one with fewer than 500 employees.

the luxurious lifestyle you imagined, especially in the early stages of your spa's development. To avoid the common pitfalls that most new business owners make, consider the following reasons why many businesses fail. If you can manage all of these things well, you have a great chance at achieving success.

Top 20 Reasons for Business Failure

1. No real vision
2. Poor planning
3. Poor financial and business management strategies
4. Limited managerial experience
5. Lack of information management systems
6. Insufficient knowledge of the market
7. Economic conditions
8. Inability to establish an inclusive sales and marketing program
9. Sales "anxiety" or uneasiness with selling your products and services
10. Human resource problems
11. Inexperienced or poorly trained staff
12. Failure to accurately assess the competition
13. Bad location
14. Inadequate cash flow
15. Insufficient sales or revenue
16. Poor inventory control
17. Insufficient working capital or too much capital invested in fixed assets
18. Inadequate plans to meet rapid growth or expansion
19. Inability to be flexible, improvise, or compromise as needed
20. Failure to follow professional advice—you think you know better

What Is Your Plan?

Awareness of these major pitfalls is the first step in avoiding them. In Chapter 1, the importance of having vision was emphasized. In fact, we know that a lack of real vision is one of the top reasons some businesses

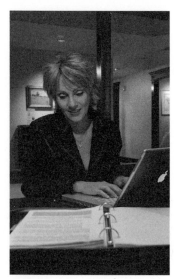

FIGURE 3-1 Careful planning is the key to implementing a successful business plan.

fail. But exactly how will you realize your vision? Here is where careful planning becomes critical to the success of your spa. Moving from your vision to the actual development stages of how you will operate your spa business requires thoughtful deliberation and a carefully drafted business plan (Figure 3-1).

While many associate the business plan with making a case for borrowing money, your business plan also functions as a practical guide to managing operations and handling finances. When used properly, a business plan should help you to define your goals and implement a plan of action for each facet of business development. Think of it as a road map to achieving success.

DEVELOPING A BUSINESS PLAN

Many business development consultants suggest that you begin working on your business by writing a solid business plan. This can be a significant source of stress for many new business owners, particularly those who have little or no experience in this area or those who are intimidated by the writing process. Although getting started can be difficult, it doesn't have to be overwhelming. Oftentimes, a little preliminary strategizing can help to ease the tension and eliminate much of the anxiety involved in creating a business plan.

Let's begin by establishing some simple ground rules for developing your plan. First, decide on a target date for opening your spa. This will give you a definite time frame for developing and writing your business plan. Many business plan protocols, books, and software systems can help you with the technical aspects of putting your plan together. Allow yourself enough time to research the "style" of plan that you are most comfortable with and will best suit your needs. As you do this, be sure to keep your goals in mind. What do you intend to accomplish with your business plan? Will you use it to seek financing, develop a plan of action, or both? Next, decide which parts of the business plan are most difficult for you and will require assistance from other professionals. Using this information, prioritize each section of your business plan in terms of difficulty and begin developing a list of resources. Other business owners and small business organizations in your community can be good resources for professional referrals. Finally, consider your business plan a working tool and use it to develop a definite plan of action for each section. This will help you to set and prioritize your goals as you move into the "writing" process.

Prioritize Your Goals

1. Set a desired date for opening your spa.

2. Establish a time frame for developing your business plan.

3. Decide on the style that is most comfortable for you and create an outline.

4. Determine which sections of your business plan will require professional assistance and begin developing a list of referrals.

5. Develop a plan of action for each section of your business plan.

The following outline highlights the typical sections of a business plan. You may decide to use other categories or add more specific subsections to your plan. There are many variations of the business plan; feel free to customize the outline according to your individual needs; however, it is important to note that lenders will want to have a clear understanding of your expenses and projected income, as well as how you intend to develop your business. This should include marketing and management strategies; be sure to incorporate these standards, especially if your goal is to obtain financing.

Each section of this business plan includes a to-do list that will help you develop the main categories of your business plan. Once you have defined all of these categories, you can begin to put your plan in writing or have someone else help you with the actual writing, if that is not your forte.

Business Plan Outline

I. Executive Summary

- Clearly identify the name and location of your business.
- State the nature of your business.
- Define your spa's mission.
- Give a brief history of your background and business history.
- Identify key management personnel.
- Describe your products and services.
- Explain your overall sales and marketing strategy.
- Identify your major competitors and describe your unique selling position.
- Identify the funds you will need.
- Explain the methods you will use to obtain financing for your spa business.

Plan for Success

Keep your readership in mind when determining the length of your executive summary. Banks generally want information that is clear, concise, and easy to read. Generally speaking, your executive summary could be a couple of paragraphs to several pages in length.

II. Marketing Plan

- Provide an overview of current economic conditions for the spa industry.
- Identify the resources you will use to support your statements.
- Identify your target market.
- Define your market in terms of *who, what, where, when,* and *how.*
- Perform a competitive analysis of other spas in your area. List their strengths and weaknesses.
- Describe your *unique selling position,* or how your spa business will be better than or different from the competition.
- State the methods you will use to attract new business, including key marketing strategies such as public relations, advertising, publicity, sales promotions, direct marketing, and personal selling.

III. Strategic Design and Development

- State your goals and objectives for developing your spa business. (For example, do you want to earn a certain amount or become the most popular spa in your area?)
- Describe your facility.
- List the equipment and supplies you will use and/or need to operate your spa.
- Specify the products and services you will offer in terms of the *marketing mix,* also known as the *four Ps:* product, price, promotion, and place.
- Determine *who* will perform *what* services in your spa.
- Name the professionals (estheticians, massage therapists, etc.) you will employ to perform services in your spa.
- Determine the *value* your services provide in relation to consumer needs and wants.
- Define your method of distribution. (For example, how many locations will you have, and will you retail any products via the Internet?)
- Define your sales strategy. How will you implement it?
- Determine key alliances and methods for cross-merchandising to promote your spa.
- Identify the key suppliers and vendors with whom you will do business.

- Calculate the cost of materials needed to perform individual spa treatments.

- Calculate the number of services you will need to perform and/or products you will need to sell to break even and maintain a positive cash flow.

- Identify your methods for maintaining quality control.

- Analyze your spa in terms of its strengths, weaknesses, opportunities, and threats (SWOT). This will help you to pinpoint your spa's internal strengths and weaknesses and to assess its external threats and opportunities.

- Discuss your plans for managing growth and expansion.

IV. Operations Plan

- Explain the procedures you will employ to operate your spa on a day-to-day basis. (For example, what methods of accounting and record keeping will you use?)

- List the resources and technology you will use to expedite your plan.

- List key management personnel and define their duties.

- Describe the qualifications of key personnel.

- Provide an organizational chart clearly demonstrating who is responsible for what and who reports to whom.

- Explain how your employees will add value to your operational strategy.

- Explain the policies and procedures you will use to manage your employees.

- Create job descriptions for each position in your spa, including service providers and administrative staff.

- Decide on a method of compensation and salary levels for your employees.

- Determine methods for employee training and development.

- Determine an employee schedule.

- Identify key resources for protecting and maintaining your business, such as legal counsel, insurance agents, accountants, human resource and marketing or public relations consultants.

Plan for Success

Developing a manual to address company policies and procedures will help you to run your business smoothly and efficiently. If you are unfamiliar with employee laws, it is wise to consult with a professional in human resources.

Plan for Success

Finances are often a source of difficulty for the small businessperson. It is always a good idea to seek the counsel of a qualified accountant when setting up your finances and financial management systems.

Plan for Success

Although writing a conclusion may seem like an unnecessary step, keep in mind that it will help to put your overall strategy into a broader perspective and will also demonstrate an attention to detail that most finance and loan managers will appreciate.

V. Financial Plan

- Identify initial start-up costs.
- Provide an estimate of your expenditures for the first three years of operation.
- Include a projected month-by-month income statement for the first year of operation.
- Include quarterly income projections for years two and three of operation.
- Supply an initial balance sheet listing the assets, liabilities, and net worth of your business.
- Create a projected balance sheet for year two of your business.
- Determine a cash budget.
- Determine your tax schedule.
- Identify resources for capital.
- Calculate a break-even analysis for your spa business.
- If you are seeking funding for your spa, be sure to:

  State how you will use the funds.

  State how you intend to repay loans.

  Describe the collateral you will use as a basis for loans.

  Calculate the anticipated return on your investment.

VI. Conclusion

- Provide a summary of your goals and objectives highlighting the key strengths of your *plan for success.*

Financial Planning

A solid financial plan is absolutely critical to the success of your spa business. The lack of one is at the top of the list of reasons for business failure.

During the planning stages, it is important to be aware of all the necessary costs associated with opening your business; however, if you are like most spa business owners, crunching numbers is probably not the reason you get up in the morning. If you are not well versed in accounting methods, it is in your best interest to sit down with someone who is. A good accountant can be invaluable in helping you to understand basic accounting principles such as assets, liabilities, cash flow, profit and loss, and break-even analysis. That person can also help you to determine your capital outlay and develop a system for controlling your finances.

GATHERING FINANCIAL INFORMATION

Before you schedule a meeting with an accountant, you should gather as much information as possible. Initially, your accountant will require financial data to establish the start-up costs associated with opening your spa. Start-up costs are those expenses that you can expect to incur before your business opens its doors. While these may vary slightly, they typically include the following:

- Initial investment in fixed assets (furniture, equipment, fixtures, tools, and professional supplies)
- Remodeling, construction, and decorating
- Starting retail inventory
- Cost of hiring and training personnel
- Salaries
- Fees for licenses and permits
- Professional fees for legal, incorporating, and accounting services
- Deposits for rent and utilities
- Marketing and advertising costs for logo design, business cards, brochures, a website, announcements, flyers, signs, etc.
- Office supplies
- Technology and related technical services
- Cleaning supplies and service
- Miscellaneous expenses

After you have established the start-up costs for your spa business, you will need to develop other important financial documents such as a *balance sheet, income statement,* and *cash flow statement.* Be prepared to supply your accountant with ongoing information, such as pricing, the cost of supplies and materials, and interest and loan payments, to assist in developing this vital business data.

THE BALANCE SHEET

The *balance sheet* provides an overview of your financial status at a certain point in time (Table 3-1). For example, it tells you whether your business is in good or poor financial condition. The key components of the balance

TABLE 3-1	SAMPLE BALANCE SHEET
ASSETS	**LIABILITIES & OWNER'S EQUITY**
CURRENT ASSETS	**CURRENT LIABILITIES**
Cash $_____	Accounts Payable $_____
Accounts Receivable $_____	Short-Term Notes Payable $_____
Inventory $_____	Other $_____
Prepaid Rent $_____	
Total Current Assets $_____	Total Current Liabilities $_____
FIXED ASSETS	**LONG-TERM LIABILITIES OR DEBT**
Fixtures $_____	Notes Payable $_____
Equipment $_____	Bank Loans $_____
Land $_____	Other Loans $_____
Buildings $_____	
Total Fixed Assets $_____	Total Long-Term Liabilities $_____
TOTAL ASSETS $_____	TOTAL LIABILITIES $_____
	Owner's Equity or Net Worth $_____
	Retained Earnings $_____
	Total Equity or Net Worth $_____
	TOTAL LIABILITIES & NET WORTH $_____

sheet as set forth in the system of *generally accepted accounting principles* are assets, liabilities, and capital. *Assets* refer to anything your business owns. *Liabilities* are any debts your business owes to creditors. *Capital* refers to the monetary investment you or others have made in your business. This is also referred to as **owner's equity**, or what the owner's interest is in the assets of the company after all of the business's liabilities have been deducted and is often addressed as the *net worth* of a business.

A simple equation is used to determine your financial status at any fixed point in time:

$$\text{Assets} = \text{Liabilities} + \text{Capital}$$

Using this standard, your assets should always equal your liabilities plus your capital investment. Businesses in good standing have assets greater than their liabilities, or a positive value. If your liabilities are greater than your assets, your business has a negative value. Continuing to operate at a negative value or deficit places your business in jeopardy.

THE INCOME STATEMENT

The *income* or *profit and loss statement* is used to calculate revenues or sales and expenses for a specific time period. *Revenue* refers to the amount of money your business takes in from the sale of products and services. The *cost of goods sold* refers to what it costs you to manufacture or produce the products your business sells. In the spa business, this means the cost of manufacturing any products made specifically for your resale, such as a signature scrub or private label products that you resell to your customers. It can also indicate the cost of purchasing retail products from another manufacturer for resale. Your *gross profit* is your profit minus the cost of goods sold. *Operating expenses* are all of the costs required to run your business. These include the general expenses associated with conducting business, such as salaries, supplies, repairs, maintenance, and insurance. Your profit is calculated by subtracting from your revenues all the expenses associated with manufacturing and selling your products and services and operating your business. Your *net profit* refers to your income after taxes have been paid. Income statements (see Table 3-2) are generated for a fixed time period, typically on a monthly, quarterly, or yearly basis. This provides a standard of comparison that will help you to determine more productive or slow time periods and make the appropriate adjustments necessary to stimulate sales and allocate funds accordingly.

TABLE 3-2	SAMPLE INCOME STATEMENT			
	1st Qtr	**2nd Qtr**	**3rd Qtr**	**4th Qtr**
Net Sales or Revenues:				
Less the Cost of Goods Sold				
Gross Profit:				
Operating Expenses				
Salaries, Wages, & Commissions				
Operating Supplies				
Repairs & Maintenance				
Laundry				
Advertising & Promotion				
Loan Interest				
Rent				
Utilities				
Telephone				
Insurance				
Payroll Taxes				
Benefit Costs				
Administrative Costs				
Legal Fees				
Licenses				
Training & Development				
Depreciation				
Total Operating Expenses:				
Profit [or Loss] Before Taxes:				
Taxes:				
Net Profit [or Loss] After Taxes:				

CASH FLOW

Having enough cash on hand to cover everyday expenses is a primary concern for business owners since any business simply cannot afford to continually run at a deficit.

Preparing a *cash flow budget or statement* is a good way to determine how much money is flowing in and out of your business on a regular basis. This budget is usually calculated on a yearly or quarterly basis; however, it is recommended that new spa owners track their cash flow on a monthly basis during that all-important first year.

Now, if you are like most small business owners, you are probably asking yourself: Why do I need to create yet another financial document to know how much cash I have on hand? Shouldn't my income statement and balance sheet suffice? Not exactly. While the income statement and balance sheet provide a useful summary of your assets, liabilities, and net worth, they do not indicate the amount of cash that is readily available on a month-to-month basis, information that is critical when it comes to understanding how much money is available to meet your expenses.

In much the same way you would manage your personal finances, scheduling the payment of bills and weighing major purchasing decisions against your income, knowing where your money is coming from and where it is going will help you to allocate your funds wisely and plan accordingly for those times when you anticipate shortfalls. For new business owners the cash flow statement also provides a reality check on projected sales revenues, a significant factor that will help you to make better business decisions over time.

The cash flow statement reports on cash activity in three areas: *operating, investing, and financial* activities. These three categories cover all aspects of cash inflows and outflows, including receipts from spa services and retail products, the purchase and sale of equity instruments, stock proceeds, the payment of interest, dividends, etc. (Table 3.3). As a new business owner, calculating these activities is likely to be an involved process that requires professional help. If you decide to tackle this task on your own, there are many worksheets and resources available to assist you in creating a cash flow statement. The SBA is a good place to start and offers several worksheets with guided instruction to accomplish this task. But be aware that the bottom line will point to one of either of two situations: a positive or negative cash flow. A positive cash flow typically indicates that your business can sustain itself. If your cash flow is negative, outside funds will be needed to finance your business operations.

Plan for Success

Taking the time to prepare and review a cash flow statement during that all-important first year of business will help you to determine if your revenue projections are on target and assist you in making the necessary adjustments to keep your business on the positive side.

TABLE 3-3	EXAMPLE OF A CASH FLOW STATEMENT	
Cash Flows from Operating Activities		
Cash received from sale of client services	$_____	
Cash received from sale of retail goods	$_____	
Interest received	$_____	
Dividends received	$_____	
Total Cash Provided by Operating Activities		$_____
Cash Paid to Suppliers for Inventory	$_____	
Cash Paid to Employees	$_____	
Cash Paid for Operating Expenses	$_____	
Cash Interest Paid	$_____	
Cash Paid for Taxes	$_____	
Total Cash Used by Operating Expenses		$(_____)
Net Cash Flow provided by Operating Activities		$_____
Cash Flows from Investing Activities		
Purchase of property, plant, & equipment (acquisition of assets)	$ (_____)	
Sale of property, plant, & equipment (disposition of assets)	$_____	
Sale of Other Investments	$_____	
Purchase of Other Investments	$ (_____)	
Total Cash Provided/(Used) by Investing Activities		$_____
Cash Flows from Financing Activities		
Sale of common stock	$_____	
Increase in short- or long-term debt	$_____	
Reduction of short- or long-term debt	$ (_____)	
Dividend payments	$ (_____)	
Total Cash Provided/(Used) by Financing Activities		$_____
Net increase (or decrease) in cash and cash equivalents		$_____
Cash & cash equivalents at the beginning of the year		$_____
Cash & cash equivalents at the end of the year		$_____

BREAK-EVEN ANALYSIS

Most spa owners are keenly aware of the income or revenue they are generating and whether that translates to a profit or loss for their business. However, many times they have difficulty understanding the cost factors involved and the volume of treatment and product sales needed to make a profit. The break-even analysis is a useful tool designed to help business owners determine how much they need to sell on a monthly or yearly basis to cover their costs and be profitable. More specifically, it defines the point at which a business generates zero profit or breaks even—that is, the point at which all costs are covered and you can begin to make a profit. Starting out, these figures will be based on sales projections, or your anticipated revenues; as your business develops, you will want to replace these figures with actual data. This information is extremely useful in controlling the cost of doing business, for example, in decreasing overhead costs or developing price points for products and services, particularly if you are considering raising your prices to increase revenue.

There are several ways to calculate the break-even point, but whichever method you use, you will first need to identify both your fixed and variable costs. Fixed costs are those costs that are independent or constant in relation to sales volume. For example, the cost of your rent will not vary no matter how many products you sell. On the other hand, variable costs, such as the cost of the products you sell or the products required to conduct services, may fluctuate.

Once you have established these costs, you can calculate your *gross profit margin or gross profit percentage*, or the difference between the selling price and the variable costs associated with it. Ideally, your analysis should include every source of revenue. For example, because the spa business involves the sale of both services and retail products, you would want to know how many services you need to perform, as well as the number of products you must sell, to break even. This is especially important for spa owners since the number of services that can be performed is typically limited by the number of available practitioners, time, and space. Therefore, retail product sales will have a significant impact on your ability to realize a profit.

There is another important factor to consider. Because the spa business has varying price points for services and retail products, calculating the break-even point generally begins with determining a gross profit percentage for each service category (for example facials, advanced skin care treatments, body treatments, massage, hair, waxing and nail services, etc.) and retail product sales. So let's say that you have determined the average gross profit margin for all facials to be $20; you would then divide that average gross profit of $20 by the average sale price of $75, which gives you a gross profit margin of 26 percent for facial services.

Now let's compare that figure to retail sales where profits tend to run higher. If the average sale price of retail products is $40 and the average cost associated with selling that product is $15, then your average gross profit margin would be $25, which would give you a gross profit margin of 63 percent for retail sales. You can see that if you are dealing with numerous products and treatments, this can become a complex process. If you are not good with figures and calculations, it makes sense to seek professional assistance in this area.

Once you have obtained a detailed account of your fixed and variable costs and gross profit percentages for all of your products and services, you can then calculate the volume of sales needed to reach your break-even point. For example, if your fixed expenses total $8,000 per month and your average gross profit percentage is 25 percent, then you will need to generate $32,000 in sales revenue to break even.

The results of break-even calculations are often graphed. Graphs can be extremely useful in motivating sales and setting goals. If you prefer to work with visual tools, it might be helpful to create a break-even chart that you can enlarge to display in your office. Having this as a reminder can be helpful in sustaining your enthusiasm for meeting sales goals.

Determining Strategic Value

Another critical aspect of business planning involves strategic value. Before you write your business plan, it is important to have a basic understanding of what you bring to the world of commerce and the need it satisfies. This is known as determining *strategic value.* Assessing the value of what you do in terms of satisfying the consumer's need or desire for the products and services your spa offers is critical to understanding the viability of your business. Sound complicated? Actually, it is easier than you might think.

To simplify the process, let's begin with your menu of services, breaking down each service and/or product into its features and benefits (Table 3-4). This is also a great way to determine exactly what services and products you will offer. From here you can calculate who actually needs or wants your services. Once you have this on paper, it may suddenly become clear to you that a particular product or service has no real value to your target market and that you are likely to lose money rather than make money on a particular product or service.

SWOT Analysis

A clear understanding of the value of the services you offer will help you to perform another important function—how well you are performing those services. Just as you analyzed your personal strengths and weaknesses, it is equally important to take stock of your business situation from year to year.

TABLE 3-4	STRATEGIC VALUE ASSESSMENT
To determine the value of your spa business, make a list of all the services you will provide, specifying the value of each in words.	
What Do You Do? [Features]	**What Is the Value to the Customer? [Benefits]**
Some examples to begin with...	
1. Perform facials.	1. Cleanse, beautify, and maintain the health of the skin.
2. Perform skin-specific facials such as a Vitamin C facial.	2. Promote skin clarity, improve tone and texture, and brighten the complexion.
3. Perform body treatments.	3. Smooth, exfoliate, and rejuvenate the skin and promote relaxation.
4. Apply makeup.	4. Enhance and beautify the physical appearance.
5. Perform massage therapy.	5. Improve circulation, relieve stress and discomfort, and promote healing and relaxation.
Use the remaining blank spaces to assess those services that are unique to your spa business.	
6.	6.
7.	7.
8.	8.
9.	9.

A SWOT analysis will help you to measure your progress and assess your strategies, a process that is vital to maintaining a competitive edge.

SWOT is an acronym that refers to a business's *strengths* (S), *weaknesses* (W), *opportunities* (O), and *threats* (T). This format takes into account *internal* and *external* factors that will help you to assess your market position and apply strategies for building future business. Table 3-5 provides an example of internal strengths and weaknesses and external opportunities and threats as they might apply to the spa industry. Using these general categories as a guideline, be prepared to assess the *what, where, how,* and *when* of your spa business each year: what your current status is, where you would like your spa to be at the same time next year or in two years, what is needed to improve your current position, how you plan to make it happen, and when you will implement those strategies or the time frame you have established for achieving your goals.

TABLE 3-5	EXAMPLE OF POSSIBLE STRENGTHS, WEAKNESSES, OPPORTUNITIES, AND THREATS ASSOCIATED WITH A SPA SWOT ANALYSIS	
Internal Measures	**Strengths**	**Weaknesses**
Customer Base	Established clientele	Need to develop a larger clientele base
Customer Service	Manager dedicated to maintaining customer satisfaction	No customer service policy in place
Products & Services	Use and resale the best products available	Retail products lack brand-name recognition
Management	Experienced	No experience in spa industry
Staff	Low turnover rate	Inexperienced staff
Marketing Tactics	Solid marketing plan	Sporadic and immeasurable
Information Systems	Inclusive system that provides information on all aspects of business operation	Lack of computer technology
Financial Status	Positive cash flow	Limited financial resources
Facility	State-of-the-art facility with all amenities	In need of cosmetic repair and technological updates
Location	Highly visible location with ample parking	Isolated location with limited opportunities for exposure
Spa Atmosphere	Friendly, relaxed, and accommodating	Staff lacks managerial support for implementing spa policies
Spa Size	Able to accommodate large groups and private parties	Only two treatment rooms
Research & Development	Offer incentive for employees to participate in continuing education programs; work with manufacturers and vendors to test market products	Little or no interest in establishing funds for education or educational materials

TABLE 3-5	EXAMPLE OF POSSIBLE STRENGTHS, WEAKNESSES, OPPORTUNITIES, AND THREATS ASSOCIATED WITH A SPA SWOT ANALYSIS CONTINUED	
External Measures	**Opportunities**	**Threats**
Economic Conditions	Robust economy	High unemployment rate
Competition	No other full-service spas in the area	Larger, established spa controls 70 percent of market share in the area
Laws/Government/ Industry Regulations	Industry supports national standards for qualifying and licensing spa therapists; FDA adheres to strict standards for qualifying all product and equipment claims used in spas	Laws prohibit the performance of certain spa treatments; for example, certain treatments require a licensed physician on the premises
Technology	A number of new products and services available to increase the effectiveness of spa treatments	Small businesses are unable to afford newer technology
Consumer Trends	Growing acceptance of the value of spa services	Consumers seek to use home spa products in lieu of going to the spa, such as purchase of home Jacuzzis, body scrubs, and massage oils
Demographics	Professional population seeks more ways to relax from stressful jobs	General population views spa service as unaffordable/frivolous

THINK IT OVER

In this chapter, we have uncovered many of the basic business tools needed to survive those critical first few years of business. With your chance of succeeding beyond the first four years being less than 50 percent, you will have to work hard at implementing these strategies if you would like to achieve long-term success.

A carefully drafted business plan is vital to your overall strategic plan, but that alone will not ensure your spa's success. To be successful, you will need to assess your business's strengths and weaknesses on a regular basis and be willing to make adjustments where necessary.

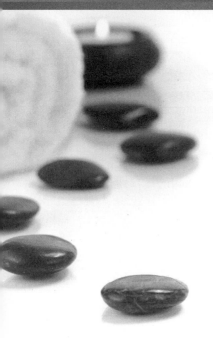

PURCHASING A DAY SPA

Numerous opportunities are available to those looking to purchase a day spa. Finding the situation that is right for you is a matter of identifying your priorities and carefully researching all of your business options. As you explore the many choices available, use your vision as a guide and keep an open mind. The perfect opportunity may not be out there, but you can find a perfectly workable option if you are willing to make a few concessions.

PRELIMINARY PURCHASING CONSIDERATIONS

Before you begin your search, it is important to think about how flexible you are willing to be. Would you consider relocating for the right opportunity, or are you interested in a particular geographic area? How much of a commute are you willing to endure? Do you have a family, children, spouse, or significant other whose needs you must consider? How does your target market factor into the equation? Is an urban or suburban setting more conducive to attracting the clientele you want? How does your particular spa concept fit; is it appropriate for the demographic and desired area?

Location is only one of the many business decisions you will need to make. You must also decide on the type of business structure that most appeals to you and how you will finance your spa. Are you interested in operating your business as a sole proprietor, or would you consider taking on a partner? Will you be looking for others to invest in your business? What about the actual facility? Are you interested in purchasing an existing spa, or would you rather build a spa from the ground up? Does that include owning or leasing the property that houses your spa? How large a space will you need to create the spa operation you envision?

As you contemplate these questions, make a list of the criteria that are most important to you and those where you would be willing to compromise (Table 4-1). If you do end up making some sacrifices, be sure you can live with them for awhile. A difficult commute will definitely wear thin quickly and is also likely to hurt business if you are the main person responsible for opening and closing each day. Likewise, having to negotiate every decision with a partner who lacks knowledge of the spa industry may ultimately be more stressful than it is helpful.

TABLE 4-1	EXAMPLE OF PRIMARY CONSIDERATIONS IN PURCHASING A SPA	
Criteria for My Day Spa	**Nonnegotiable**	**Negotiable**
Example:		
1. Location must be within 10 miles of home.	A commute time greater than a half hour	
2. Prefer an exclusive urban setting.		Would consider certain sections of town adjacent to my target area
3. Price range must be between $15 and $20 per sq. ft.		Would consider something slightly higher if option to renew in five years is written into the lease agreement
4. Facility must have enough space to house four treatment rooms of adequate size for facials and massage therapy.		Would be willing to sacrifice one treatment room to create ample retail space
5. Facility must have enough water pressure to accommodate basins in each treatment room, pedicure stations, a Swiss shower, and a Vichy shower.	Must be able to install plumbing in every room with at least one freestanding shower stall centrally located	Would be willing to substitute a steam shower for the Vichy shower

EXPLORING BUSINESS OPPORTUNITIES

Once you have identified your top priorities, you can begin networking; however, it is a good idea to be discreet, particularly if you are currently working for someone else. Finding the right location and space can take time. In the meantime, you will need a steady income. Be conscious of any existing contractual obligations. If you have a non-compete agreement with your current employer, you must be careful not to set off any red flags. Consider also that testing the limits of a contractual obligation is probably not in your best interest as you begin a new venture. On the other hand, if you have a good relationship with your boss and know he or she is seriously interested in selling, you should make your intentions known. Many businesses have been passed on to valued employees.

Industry associations and trade publications are typically good places to begin searching for spa business opportunities. Spa business consultants may also be knowledgeable about spas for sale and in some cases are engaged in real estate activities as well. Real estate classifieds and online business marts make it easy to view businesses for sale anonymously, but it is also important to network; attend professional functions, and seek out those in the know who might be willing to assist you in your search. Be sure to alert family and friends that you are actively looking as well, but caution them not to disclose any personally identifying information. Professionals outside the industry, such as accountants, attorneys, and bankers in the community, are other contacts who are often knowledgeable about businesses for sale in the community.

You might also consider using a business broker to act as your agent. In addition to scouting locations, a qualified broker can help negotiate a lease or purchase price, explore financing options, explain the laws that regulate business in the area, and know which permits are required to begin construction (Figure 4-1). Using a business broker can also give you added confidentiality protection. Even if you decide to work with a broker, it is a good idea to keep abreast of the cost of commercial retail space and square footage that is generally available. All of these efforts will help you to broaden your search and act as an informed consumer.

The Right Location

We often hear talk about finding just the right location, as if a certain spot will guarantee business success. Certainly, some locations are more advantageous than others, but in actuality, there are many great places to open a spa (Figure 4-2). Whether you prefer the urban scene or are more inclined to

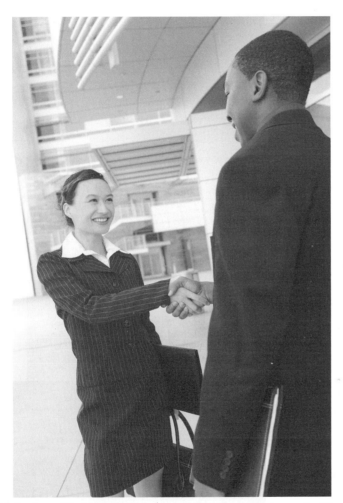

FIGURE 4-1   A qualified commercial real estate broker can help you find the right location for your spa.

appreciate the convenience of a suburban shopping mall, it is important to consider the physical and demographic constraints of any location carefully.

Where your spa is located will have a significant impact on the way you market your business. If you eventually decide on a remote setting because the rent is cheaper and it is close to home, remember that a more accessible and visible location is generally a lot easier and less expensive to market than one that is isolated and out of the way. You could easily make up the difference in marketing and advertising costs.

what prices? Who are their clients? Can the market sustain another spa, or has it reached the saturation point? These questions are crucial.

Although the spa business has become fiercely competitive in some areas, when it comes to learning more about what other spas are doing, many spa owners take a very defensive position, insulating themselves from the rigors of competition with an "I don't care what anyone else is doing" attitude or naively bank on the loyalty of their clientele. If you are one of those who ascribe to this philosophy, take another look at the top 20 reasons businesses fail listed in Chapter 3. Denying the competition could be the biggest mistake you make.

Even if you recognize that investigating the competition is a matter of business, it is perfectly natural to feel somewhat uncomfortable with the process. For many, investigating other spa businesses feels too much like "spying." If you fall into this category, have someone you trust perform this task for you. Whichever method you choose to investigate your competitors, be sure to use proper etiquette. Your new business colleagues are bound to be suspicious if they are bombarded with a million questions. They are also not likely to appreciate your copying their menu and advertising or mimicking their promotions. Simply observe what you are up against and respond creatively using your own methods to attract new customers. In the end, understanding the competition is an important strategic tool that will help you to grow and develop a unique selling position.

Consider the Neighborhood

Image and safety are paramount when building a business. Take a good look around the neighborhood. Is the area conducive to your vision? This does not mean that you cannot turn a "fixer-upper" into a luxurious and profitable spa, but be attentive to your neighbors and the types of businesses located in the area. Will they help you to attract the type of clients you want? If you are considering an urban or busy suburban location, consider the effect that noise pollution and congestion will have on your business. Treatment rooms that back up to very noisy neighbors or heavily trafficked highways can be problematic.

Likewise, be aware of the crime rate and any safety issues that might keep clients away. Do not forget that people come to spas to relax, replenish, and rejuvenate. A well-lit area with convenient accessibility to public transportation or parking will help to promote the concept of a stress-free environment (Figure 4-3).

Determine the Potential for Profitability

In the final analysis, any location you choose should be one that has the potential to be financially successful. A feasibility study or comprehensive

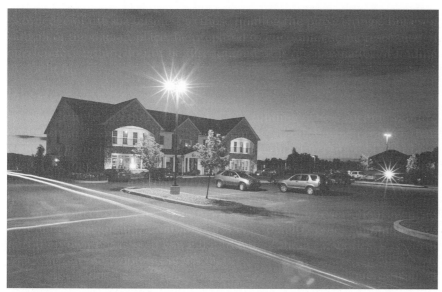

FIGURE 4-3   Ample parking in a well-lit area promotes the concept of a stress-free environment.

analysis of the proposed business concept is essential to determine the profitability of a location. This is best done by business professionals who are equipped to perform a complete marketing and demographic analysis and who are also able to determine the finances needed to build and sustain a successful spa operation in the desired area. This generally includes a pro forma or sales projections for the first three to five years of business.

If you decide to conduct your own feasibility study, you will need to assess all of the previously mentioned criteria and several additional components, such as the number of treatment rooms and/or workstations that can be accommodated, the volume of traffic in the area, the economic status of the community, and, most importantly, the amount of money required to finance your spa concept in terms of operations and design. As you work the numbers, pay special attention to the amount of available retail space and do not be fooled into thinking that you can sell lots of product from your dispensary or a mini-cabinet in your treatment room. While too much dead space is just that, a dedicated retail area will add to the value of your business and help to turn your spa into a profit center.

For many spa owners, starting out with a moderately priced space with room to expand is the best option until business is firmly established. Initially, this may mean sacrificing some of the more luxurious amenities you would like to include, such as a hydrotherapy tub or special couples

Plan for Success

A feasibility study should include a thorough assessment of the spa's potential for success in terms of the overall spa concept, location, area demographics, target market, the competition, demand for your services, operational requirements, space planning or build-out, and, most importantly, the finances needed to take the project from concept to design, construction, and business development. The sum total of these items along with a solid understanding of current economic conditions and sales projections should determine the overall financial profitability of the proposed spa venture.

accommodations. Do not confuse this with compromising your goals. Instead, use it as a stepping stone to leverage the next phase of your spa vision. We will talk more about the best way to handle architecture and design matters to accommodate future spa services in Chapter 5.

Negotiating a Lease

If you are renting property, you will need to negotiate a lease. A lease is a contract between you and the landlord, or owner of the property, which establishes the terms of using a specific area of space for a certain length of time. The lease price is typically based on dollars per square foot. Your lease may cover usable and unusable space along with repairs and maintenance, construction, common areas, and parking. All of these clauses should be reviewed carefully. Leases are typically drafted by the *lessor*, or landlord, who is renting the space. In the lease agreement, you will be known as the *lessee*.

Whether you are using a professional broker or intend to work out the terms of an agreement yourself, the most important thing to remember when it comes to leasing is that all terms are generally negotiable. To begin negotiations, create a list of those items that are most important to your business, but be realistic and expect to make some compromises. For example, if you cannot convince your landlord to lower the rent, you might be able to negotiate additional parking spaces, which could turn out to be just as valuable in the long run. Bear in mind that negotiations are more powerful in leaner economic times and wherever there are more vacancies. The length of a lease is another big factor that usually affords some latitude, but do not be surprised if you have less bargaining power in desirable areas.

Whatever agreement you come to with your landlord, be sure to get it in writing. It is also recommended that you have a qualified attorney review the fine print to ensure that your interests are protected. A lease is a legal document that you should understand clearly before signing.

Owning Property

Most start-ups simply cannot afford the luxury of owning their own space. Tying up valuable assets in property ownership can make it more difficult to break even and become profitable. On the other hand, if you can afford it, owning the building that houses your spa has the potential to increase your business value and gives you an additional investment in real estate. If you decide that owning property is the right business decision for you in the long run, you will want to take all of the same precautions you would in leasing space and then some.

A qualified business broker can be invaluable in helping you to assess fair market value and negotiate a *purchase and sale agreement*. Just as a lease specifies the agreement between landlord and tenant, the purchase and sale (P&S) agreement defines the terms of your real estate transaction. It should contain a complete description of the property you are buying, along with the purchase price and date of closing.

The P&S is a legal document that represents binding obligations, so it is advisable to seek legal counsel. A qualified real estate attorney can walk you through all the necessary requirements, such as conveying a clear deed and title and property inspection. As part of the process, you will want to have a complete investigation conducted to make sure the building is zoned for business and that there are no ordinances or restrictions related to conducting a spa business in the area. Your attorney can advise you as to what should be incorporated in the P&S to protect you in the event that the building or land does not comply with zoning, building, or health ordinances or if a breach of any part of the contract becomes an issue.

Assessing Market Value

Expect the cost of commercial real estate to vary according to the region and specific location of the property. For instance, the cost of owning or leasing real estate may be higher in the Northeast than it is in the Midwest.

A qualified commercial real estate broker can provide you with a comparative market analysis of specific locations, but in general, the cost of leasing or buying property tends to get higher as you move closer to metropolitan areas. This means that a spa in the city is likely to cost significantly more than a spa in the suburbs or a more rural area, although you may encounter certain exclusive or popular resort areas that match or even exceed top market prices. Economic conditions and the availability of space will also play an important role.

If you are leasing, the price will vary according to the amount of square footage you rent. Although it is generally understood that more space will cost more money, in some cases you may be pleasantly surprised to find out the price per square foot could actually come down if you opt to take more space. The condition of the facility will also affect the sale price. For example, a well-kept building in a prominent neighborhood is likely to cost more to rent or buy than a space that needs a facelift in a less desirable location. For a more precise analysis of the market in your area, seek the advice of a reputable commercial real estate broker.

FINANCING YOUR SPA

Understanding the cost of leasing or purchasing space is a major consideration in establishing capital outlay. To fully appreciate all of the expenses involved in operating your own spa, you will need to conduct a realistic estimate of all items outlined in the financial planning section of the business plan provided in Chapter 3. Once you have a handle on these financial requirements, think about where you will find the money you need to make your vision a reality. Although there may seem to be innumerable sources of capital, in reality there are only a few options. These include using your own savings, borrowing money, and accepting funds from investors.

Savings, Loans, or Investors?

Putting your own money on the table should be the first step in financing your spa. Before you consider any other options, sit down and take a good look at your personal finances. What are your current obligations? In addition to ordinary expenses, do you have any debt or loans that you will continue to be responsible for as you build your business? How much do you have in savings? Will you need to access this money for ordinary living expenses during this period? After you have determined what you need to live on, you will be able to make a more realistic assessment of what you can reasonably contribute to building your business from your personal funds. At the same time, you will need to project your business finances for that all-important first year of operation. Planning ahead will help you to avoid some of the more common mistakes start-up businesses make, such as relying on insufficient capital.

A solid understanding of the amount of money needed to maintain your personal and business interests will help you to answer an important question when it comes to financing: How much do you have in savings or equity that you are willing to invest in your own success? Keep in mind that even if you ultimately decide to borrow money, those investing in your business will want to have the confidence that comes from knowing you are serious enough to risk your own assets to make your dream a reality.

Benefactors

Many times relatives, friends, or even clients are willing to help with financing by offering relatively low-interest or interest-free loans. If these funds are available to you, you will want to take full advantage of them, but be sure to draft a legal document or *promissory note* that clearly defines the terms of your agreement.

Small Business Administration

If you are not so lucky, numerous other loan options are available. The Small Business Administration (SBA) is a good place to begin your search.

The SBA is an independent federal government agency set up to help small businesses succeed. It is a great resource for those looking to raise capital, acting primarily as a guarantor for loans from private investors and other institutions, such as banks and credit unions.

The SBA is also an excellent source of financial and business management advice with access to numerous other professionals and training facilities, such as the Service Core of Retired Executives (SCORE), Small Business Development Centers (SBDC) and the Small Business Training Network (SBTN), an online tutorial program. For more information on these programs, visit the SBA's Web site at *http://www.sba.gov.*

Loans

Banks, credit unions, and commercial loan companies are other viable sources of capital for entrepreneurs. However, be aware that there are many types of loans with varying interest rates and obligations. Most have qualifying restrictions or require a certain amount of owner equity or other collateral, such as equipment or inventory, to secure the loan. Payment schedules can vary with different requirements for short-term and long-term loans. If you be unfamiliar with the ins and outs of bank financing or are unsure of what type of loan would be best for your personal circumstances, seek the professional advice of a certified public accountant, business attorney, financial advisor, and/or business development consultant before meeting with a bank or loan officer. When you do, it is especially important that you be prepared. This is where your business plan will carry a great deal of weight. A carefully prepared business plan is a tremendous asset when it comes to filling out loan applications and demonstrating your knowledge of the spa business to those holding the purse strings. But even with all of the data in place, be prepared to encounter some resistance. If one lender says no, do not be discouraged. It is often a matter of finding the right fit.

Investors

Investors can be another viable source of funding. These include venture capitalists and small business investment companies, which, rather than loaning you money, will give you money in return for a share of your business. This may come in the form of stocks or other percentage-based dividends. If you decide to pursue this option, remember that part owners will have some control over how you manage your business.

In certain circumstances, money is available from government agencies or other private organizations whose goal is to help women and minorities start their own business. If you fall into one of these categories, it is worth checking out these options.

Debt-versus Equity-Based Capital

Before you commit to taking money from any outside source, it is important to have a complete understanding of debt-versus equity-based capital. Any loan that must be paid back, with or without interest, is known as *debt-based capital*. For example, a loan from your uncle, although it may have no interest fee attached to it, is still a debt that must be repaid. Loans from banks, commercial finance companies, credit unions, or credit card companies are also debt-based—that is, you are expected to repay them with varying degrees of interest and other obligations. If you do not, expect to be held liable to certain penalties.

On the other hand, *equity-based capital* is funding provided by others for a stake in or some form of ownership in your business. If you are incorporated, this generally occurs by selling shares of stock in your company. Although equity-based financing is rarely paid back, it does come with a price tag. That is, investors typically have some control over your business and receive some form of compensation. For example, venture capitalists or stockholders may contribute capital in return for a set percentage of your profits. In most cases, investors are "partners" for the life of your business, unless there is an option for you to buy back their stock at some point.

Other equity-based funding can come in the form of partnerships. For example, you might consider taking on partners who contribute a substantial amount of capital from their own savings. This might be someone who works alongside you in the same capacity or someone who contributes to a certain aspect of the business, such as managing the business functions. Some business owners have limited partnership relationships with several individuals who have little say in the day-to-day operations but exert certain controls over how the business or spa is to be run or managed.

BUSINESS OWNERSHIP

How you structure the ownership of your business will have significant consequences in terms of finance and liability. Before you set things into motion, you should review all options carefully with both your attorney and your accountant to determine which makes the most sense for your personal circumstances.

There are many ways to run a business but only a few choices when it comes to ownership. You can establish your business as a *sole proprietor*, engage in a *partnership,* set up a *corporation,* or form a *limited liability company.* Each of these legal structures has its pluses and minuses. The big decision for most small businesses, including day spas, is whether or not to incorporate.

Sole Proprietor

The sole proprietorship is the simplest form of business ownership. Under this format, the business is owned, operated, and managed by one person who takes full responsibility for all business decisions and obligations. If you choose this structure, that person is you! The good news is that you get to run your business pretty much any way you want to within certain legal boundaries. You write all policies and derive all income; however, it also means that you are personally responsible for paying all debts and assuming all liabilities.

In terms of tax obligations, the paperwork is fairly straightforward. Your business income and expenses can be reported on the same 1040 form that you use for your personal income tax with the addition of what is known as a *Schedule C.* On the plus side, if your spa incurs losses, these may be offset by any income you earn from other sources. This is not a bad deal; however, if your spa runs into problems, you will be held personably liable for any debt you accrue. This means that your personal funds could be subject to claims resulting from any legal disputes incurred as a result of doing business. You will also need to file a *Self-Employment* (SE) form that obligates you to make your own Social Security contribution to the federal government, and in most cases, you will be subject to quarterly tax payments. You should check with your accountant for a more detailed understanding of your personal obligations.

Partnerships

For many, a partnership provides the added confidence needed to start a business. Along with shared decision-making and management responsibilities, there is also the benefit of increased capital. This can be appealing to those who prefer to share tasks and enjoy working cooperatively with others. The downside is that partners also share in unlimited joint liability when it comes to debt. In a business partnership, this means that each partner assumes responsibility for the other's debts, and each partner can act on behalf of the other according to the terms of their agreement. They also divide all profits, which can significantly lower the amount of income each takes in, especially at start-up.

When it comes to structuring a partnership, there are two choices: a limited or general partnership. In a limited partnership, some of the

Plan for Success

How you structure the ownership of your business will have significant financial, tax, and liability consequences. A qualified business attorney can help you to weigh the pluses and minuses of each business structure and select the best one for your individual business needs.

partners act solely as investors, supplying capital without having any real decision-making power. In a general partnership, each person shares equally in all decision-making, liability, and financial obligations. Income is filtered through the partnership to the owners, who each file a K-1 for tax purposes. The paperwork involved in a partnership can be fairly complex and is best left to professionals who can attend to all the details without bias.

While there are certainly some drawbacks to running your spa as a partnership, many thrive in such a union. If you are considering taking on a partner, it is a good idea to make sure that your values are truly compatible and that you respect and trust your partner to make choices and act wisely on your behalf. Before signing on the dotted line, you should also be clear about the roles and expectations of both parties. As in any partnership, it is painful when a "perfect union" goes sour.

Corporations

A corporation is considered a separate and legal entity with its own rights, privileges, and responsibilities, and as such, it affords the owners liability protection; however, corporations must adhere to more complex rules and regulations, which are governed according to specific laws enforced by each state.

To establish a corporation, you must file what is known as a *charter* in the state in which your business resides. This identifies the owners of the corporation and contains a set of bylaws by which the corporation is governed. Corporations are managed by a board of directors who make all decisions according to the bylaws of the charter. They are also allowed to sell stock; however, these shares are not necessarily equally distributed among owners and can be bought and sold while the corporation continues on indefinitely.

Setting up a corporation is more complicated than other ownership options. As a result, many seek professional help to decide on a format, manage the paperwork, and adhere to the numerous laws that regulate corporations. There are several options available for establishing a corporation, including the *S corporation*. Each has its individual benefits and features. Tax obligations are often an important consideration in deciding which format is right for your company. Your attorney and tax accountant can provide detailed advice on which is best for you, but whichever corporate structure you choose, expect to spend more on legal and accounting services to maintain your business.

It is possible to incorporate on your own. Should you decide to do so, there are many books and computer programs available to walk you through the process. You can also access more information through the Internal Revenue Service and the Small Business Administration.

The Limited Liability Company

The *limited liability company (LLC)* and *limited liability partnership (LLP)* are two relatively new business structures that have become more appealing to a growing number of small businesses. The main reason for this is that they provide many of the same benefits as a corporation, including liability protection and tax benefits. Earnings and losses pass through the business owners, who have the option to be taxed as a sole proprietor, partnership, or a corporation. Owners are also protected against loss. If you are interested in adopting this business structure, seek professional guidance. Laws continue to change around these new structures. Owners are also required to file articles of organization.

Franchises

Franchises like Dunkin Donuts and McDonald's are a familiar business entity. Spa franchises, while less commonplace, are also available to those who would rather follow a distinct method of operation than create one of their own. In a franchise relationship, the *franchisee* purchases the right to use the *franchisor's* name along with a specified business plan and set protocols in exchange for ongoing royalties.

Advantages of Franchise Ownership

There are several advantages to purchasing a franchise from a well-managed organization. First, you are gaining a system that is proven to be successfully duplicated with every detail of operation worked out for you. This means you do not have to think about which products you will use, what your menu of services will be, what methods of treatment you will perform, how you will manage your employees, what computer system you will use for scheduling or accounting, or from which vendors you will buy. These business decisions have all been made for you. In addition, you can expect ongoing training and support in managing all of the tasks associated with using these systems. You also gain the credibility of a recognized brand name that provides consumers with a certain level of quality assurance. This can save you a great deal of money in terms of marketing, advertising, and promotion.

In most cases, you can also expect other important business decisions such as the size of the spa, its location, and physical layout to be planned out for you by the parent company. Before signing on another franchisee, the franchisor typically researches the best location and conducts a competitive analysis to ensure the success of its individual operations. This can be extremely helpful to those intimidated by market analysis and lease negotiations. Attractive employee benefit packages and national advertising campaigns are other perks generally associated with becoming a franchise.

Disadvantages of Franchise Ownership

Of course, there are also some drawbacks to owning a franchise. If you are an independent thinker, you are likely to have trouble with a system that controls all aspects of spa operations. With business management and treatment protocols dictated, there is little room for creativity in franchising. Under these conditions, those who thrive on the creative process can feel stifled or unfulfilled.

In terms of finances, the payment of franchise fees and ongoing royalties to the parent company can be expensive, cutting into a spa's profitability. If you decide that a franchise is right for you, hopefully yours will be a lucrative venture, but it is important to note that whether or not your spa is profitable, you will still have to pay out additional monies in franchise fees to maintain your business.

Investigating Franchise Opportunities

Franchises have become more popular in the spa industry, but buyers should beware that not all franchises are equal. Before entering any franchise agreement, it is in your best interest to gather as much background information as possible. A good place to begin your investigation is the Internet. Trade organizations and magazine publications are other good resources for industry-specific information. If you are serious about pursuing a particular opportunity, always insist on a complete financial history and make it a point to speak directly with other franchise owners to get a more precise reality check.

Franchise Regulations

Unfortunately, when it comes to franchising, there have been numerous incidents of fraud and broken promises. This has prompted government officials to adopt laws that enforce better business practices. The Federal Trade Commission is the government agency responsible for overseeing franchise regulations. By law, the FTC requires franchisors to supply specific detailed information about the franchise, which must be included in an *offering circular*. Most states use what is known as the *Uniform Franchise Offering Circular (UFOC)*. According to FTC regulations, the franchisor must deliver the offering circular to prospective franchisees at the initial face-to-face meeting or within 10 business days before any agreement is signed or money changes hands. You should also be aware that certain states have explicit regulations regarding business franchises; so be sure to investigate what the requirements are in your state as well. Again, it is always best to obtain qualified legal counsel before signing any agreements or contracts.

Buying An Existing Spa Business

Buying an existing spa business is often more appealing to the entrepreneur or novice looking to become a spa owner. An established business has many benefits. First of all, most of the difficult tasks associated with setting up a spa have already been done for you: finding the right location; carrying out renovations; purchasing equipment, supplies, and furnishings; hiring employees; and establishing operating systems. Unlike a franchise, you gain the added benefit of having complete control over your own operation. Of course, this does not mean that all spa facilities are in good working order. If you decide to purchase an existing spa, you will want to have a clear understanding of why the owner is selling, exactly what it is you are buying, and how to go about valuing the real worth of the business.

Assessing the Real Value of a Business

Simply relying on an owner's opinion of what their spa business is worth is rarely in the buyer's best interest. Owners tend to have an inflated opinion of the real value of their business and are likely to put a good deal of emphasis on the transfer of goodwill, or the intangible assets associated with an established business, such as its reputation, its relationships with clients, employees, and vendors, its standing in the community, management and marketing strategies associated with the spa, etc. So how do you come up with a fair and equitable price? Many cringe at the idea of negotiating a purchase price, and while it is fair to say that it is often an involved and lengthy process, it is fairly straightforward. As you navigate your way, keep in mind that all of the generally accepted methods for valuing an existing business are somewhat negotiable.

Evaluation Methods

There are numerous ways to value a business. More popular methods include an assessment of the business's market value, earnings, and cash flow.

To begin the process, a business is typically evaluated according to the market value of its assets, which includes the net worth of its inventory

Plan for Success

When shopping for an existing spa business, prospective buyers should expect to sign a confidentiality agreement. This is standard practice and helps to protect both the buyer and the seller from any potential damage to the business, for example, the loss of clients and/or employees, before the final deal is negotiated.

Plan for Success

There are numerous ways to value a business. Those with limited experience should seek the help of a professional appraiser. Ideally, that person will have experience in the spa industry; Certified Public Accountant (CPA) and Certified Value Analyst (CVA) credentials; and be listed as a member of a reputable appraisal organization. While there are many variables to consider, in general buyers should look for :

- A reasonable explanation for why the business is being sold.
- Accurately detailed financial records and computerized operating systems that demonstrate solid growth and good business practices for several years
- Tangible evidence that supports the seller's assessment of goodwill
- A facility that is well maintained with properly functioning equipment, furnishings, and fixtures.
- A business that is free from any legal encumbrances or debt.
- If the space is rented, a long-term transferable lease

and equipment. Less-tangible assets, which are generally more difficult to measure, such as the spa's name recognition and customer base, are also factored into the asset equation. A review of the spa's earnings comes next, with special attention to the owner's income and cash flow. To get a true picture of the overall financial health of the business, your investigation should go back a few years and include a thorough review of all of the spa's financial documents, for example, income statements, balance sheets, cash flow statements, the seller's or owner's discretionary cash flow statement, tax returns, etc. Once you have all of the data in hand, you can begin to negotiate a price.

Owner's Discretionary Cash Flow

The owner's earnings are an important consideration in establishing the value of a business. These are assessed by using what is commonly referred to as either the Seller's or Owner's Discretionary Cash Flow Statement.

This financial document reports on a number of financial factors, such as the owner's salary and the salaries of any additional family members, payroll taxes for the owner's salary, any personal benefits such as a company vehicle, travel and entertainment, and other benefits such as health insurance that are attributed to the owner. These items are combined with any pre tax profit (or loss) and then weighed against other financial items, such as depreciation, amortization, or interest expense, to arrive at the *seller's discretionary cash flow*, or what is available to a potential new owner as income benefit. The bottom line is an important economic indicator that is sometimes multiplied to estimate the worth of a spa business. For example, a spa may be valued at approximately two to three times the amount of the income benefit received by the owner; however, when it comes to valuing a spa business this approach is generally viewed as an oversimplification of what is typically a more involved process that should include a detailed valuation of all of the previously mentioned data.

Hire a Professional Appraiser

While the process of assessing the real value of a business is seemingly straightforward, many prospective business owners find it overwhelming. If you are unsure about how to properly evaluate all of the necessary documents, tangible and intangible assets, it is wise to hire a professional appraiser to value the business for you. Ideally, that person will be someone who has experience in the spa industry, is a Certified Public Accountant (CPA), and Certified Value Analyst (CVA). Such a person is trained to evaluate the viability of a business and can also give you a good idea of what similar businesses typically earn. If you are not sure of a person's credentials, there are several organizations, such as the American Society of Appraisers, the National Association of Certified Valuation Analysts, the American Institute of Certified Public Accountants, and the American Business Brokers Association, available to help you in your search.

Whether or not you decide to use a professional appraiser, you should work closely with your attorney and accountant. Other professionals, such as financial planners and business brokers, are usually part of the acquisitions team. These professionals will help you sort through all of the necessary legal documents and financial statements, including purchase and sales agreements, loan documents, leases, titles, balance sheets, cash flow statements, tax returns, and accounts receivable. There are other considerations, such as changes in zoning laws or ordinances, which could possibly prevent a new owner from performing certain aspects of business. On the positive side, these factors may ultimately give you some bargaining power.

Do not overlook analyzing the spa's relationships with vendors, customers, and employees. You will want to be fully aware of any litigation proceedings, such as contractual obligations, labor disputes, lawsuits, or other claims against the spa. Your final purchase and sale agreement should also include a non-compete clause that protects you against the owner directly competing with you for a reasonable period of time.

Transferring Ownership

Once you have a complete understanding of the spa's business status, proceed cautiously. There is generally some fluctuation in revenues and operations upon the transfer of ownership. Do not count on business as usual, particularly if the owner has not agreed to stay on during the transition to help you maintain business. Employees may decide to leave, or customers may seize the opportunity to try another spa.

On the other hand, if the seller is interested in staying on to ensure a smooth transition, it is worth exploring this option, especially if you are relatively inexperienced in the spa business. Most sellers perform this duty in a consulting capacity; however, those who are also service providers may be interested in staying on as employees. This may or may not be in your best interest. Be sure to evaluate any impact such an arrangement might have on your effectiveness as a new manager. There are also legal and tax requirements mandated by the IRS and the SBA which may apply and should be addressed with your attorney and tax advisor before traveling down this path.

UNDERSTANDING BUSINESS LAW

The saying goes that "ignorance is no defense against the law." When it comes to managing a new business, this goes double. Being unfamiliar with local, state, and federal laws or forgetting to pay your taxes is not likely to keep the Internal Revenue Service or any other government agency from knocking at your door. If you are clueless when it comes to the laws that govern the spa business, it is simply and unequivocally your responsibility to find out what you need to know.

Spa owners should be aware of four general areas of law: trade or licensing regulations, labor laws, tax laws, and health and safety regulations.

Licensing Regulations

Whether you are a licensed spa professional, such as a licensed esthetician or cosmetologist, or a prospective business developer looking to open a spa, the first place you should go for answers regarding operating a spa business is your state licensing board. For day spas, this is typically the State Board of Cosmetology; however, there is a good chance that you will need to review the standards of other licensing boards. With so many new products and protocols being developed in the health and beauty industry, many states are adopting new measures to regulate practitioners and the type of beauty treatments they can perform in spas today. It is also important to note that laws vary from state to state. Before you purchase equipment or hire staff, be sure you understand exactly which individual licenses and permits are necessary for opening a spa in your state, the limits of those licenses, and your responsibility when it comes to having other professionals, such as medical personnel, to perform services on your premises.

Local, State, and Federal Regulations

Spas must also be aware of local, state, and federal agencies when it comes to operating a business, managing employees, adhering to health and safety standards, and paying taxes. Starting at the local level, you will want to begin by finding out what business permits or licenses are necessary for operating a spa in your community. Local government officials are typically responsible for enforcing zoning laws, building codes, and safety and sanitation requirements. Before beginning any new construction or renovations—even hanging a sign—you should be aware of these regulations.

Spas must also abide by state and federal laws pertaining to sales tax, labor laws such as workers' compensation, and unemployment insurance. The federal government administers laws relative to public health and safety, fair labor practices, and environmental protection. It also levies taxes. A good accountant and lawyer can be extremely helpful in sorting out the requirements of many of these issues; however, even if you hire an accountant, lawyer, or other consultants to handle these matters for you, as a business owner it is a good idea to become familiar with the state and federal laws that govern your business and the agencies that regulate and supervise them. These are easily accessible via the Internet and local and regional directories. Do not be afraid to pick up the telephone and ask questions if you need clarification.

Health and Safety Regulations

As a spa owner, you will want to pay special attention to matters related to health and consumer protection. Because spas perform personal services, they must be careful to comply with the standards of the Occupational Safety and Health Administration (OSHA). This federal agency oversees safety in the workplace. OSHA supplies those in the health care and personal care industries with specific guidelines to prevent the transmission of disease. Under its guidance, spas are required to implement an educational program to make all employees aware of safety issues, such as those involved in handling waste and blood-borne pathogens.

The state licensing board and the local board of health in your community will also have criteria for controlling public health and hygiene with which you must comply. As you process these regulations, keep in mind that violations are often made public. A negative image in this area can have an extremely detrimental impact on a spa's reputation. It could ruin your business. Other federally mandated regulations, for example, those set forth by the Americans with Disabilities Act (ADA), should be scrutinized carefully.

Spa owners should also be aware of their responsibility when it comes to products used and sold in the spa. Although the Food and Drug Administration does not require cosmetic products or their ingredients to undergo approval before being sold to the public, they do have regulations regarding packaging and labeling. This is particularly important to those spa owners who carry private label products made expressly for their use, a topic that will be discussed further in Chapter 6. To learn more about these topics and other issues relating to the sale and use of cosmetics, visit the FDA's Web site. The FDA publishes a *Cosmetic Handbook* and offers numerous other resources that can help spa owners understand their responsibilities and liabilities.

U.S. GOVERNMENT AGENCIES YOU SHOULD KNOW

CDC	Centers for Disease Control
CPSC	Consumer Product Safety Commission
DOC	Department of Commerce
DOJ	Department of Justice
DOL	Department of Labor
EEOC	Equal Employment Opportunity Commission
EPA	Environmental Protection Agency
FDA	Food and Drug Administration
FTC	Federal Trade Commission
HHS	Health and Human Services
INS	Immigration and Naturalization Service
IRS	Internal Revenue Service
OSHA	Occupational Safety and Health Administration
SBA	Small Business Administration

NAMING YOUR BUSINESS

Before you decide on a name for your spa, there are a few legalities to consider. Make sure your business name is not already in use by some other business or spa. Not only would you not want to be confused with another business, but you will want to make sure you are not infringing on a trademark that someone else owns. However, even if a business has not registered a trademark, a name that is too closely identified with another business could be construed as interfering with its ability to conduct business, a situation that could have legal ramifications.

If you have a definite name in mind, it is a good idea to begin your search by looking through local directories. Local and state government officials, such as the town or county clerk's office and the corporation division in your state, should be able to supply you with a list of registered business names. These offices can also help you to determine the necessary steps required to establish or register a business name. This often depends on the type of business structure used. For example, if your business is a sole proprietorship, you may only be required to register your business locally. But registering your business at the state and local levels is often two separate issues; so it is important to research both. Finally, it is a good idea to check with the U.S. Patent and Trademark Office to make sure you are not infringing upon any trademark rights.

Trademark and Service Marks

The words *trademark* and *service mark* are legal terms that are often used interchangeably; however, each has a distinct meaning. The word *trademark* refers to a word, phrase, design, or symbol that is used to identify a product brand. A service mark is similar but refers to a word, phrase, or symbol that identifies the provider of a service. Some companies use both service and trademarks to designate each facet of their operation.

Understanding the legalities of trademarks can be confusing. In general, if your spa business is not incorporated and you do not intend to do business across state lines, you need not worry about registering a trademark; however, you should be aware that just because your spa is incorporated does not automatically give your business rights to a trademark or service mark. Increased use of the Internet for e-commerce has raised additional concerns for businesses that may find they are inadvertently infringing upon the trademark rights of another business. To gain a better understanding of your individual circumstances, it is best to seek qualified legal advice on these important issues.

If you are interested in registering a trademark or service mark, you can contact the National Trademark Office to learn more. Trademarks and service marks are registered with the U.S. Patent and Trademark Office (USPTO), an agency of the U.S. Department of Commerce. The USPTO also has a Web site that permits online searches of registered names.

PROTECTING YOUR SPA BUSINESS

Running a successful spa business requires a great deal of hard work and dedication. To ensure that your spa remains successful, you will need to develop a reliable risk management program that protects your business

Plan for Success

The transfer of risk to a third party via an insurance policy is a spa owner's best protection against business casualties. Your *business owner's policy* outlines the agreement between you, the *insured,* and the insurance company, or the *insurer.* The insurer is usually represented by an insurance agent who is trained in risk management and earns a commission for selling insurance to you. To safeguard your business, always read and review all of the information on your policy and seek clarification on any item which you are not clear about. It is your right to have the terms of your policy explained to you in a manner that is confidently understood.

against such unforeseen incidents as fire, theft, business interruption, lawsuits, and employee injury.

Insurance

Insurance, or the transfer of risk to a third party, is your best protection against the vulnerabilities associated with conducting business. It should be purchased wisely from a reputable and trusted source, preferably an insurance agent who is experienced in the spa business and knowledgeable about the many new treatment options.

Many types of insurance are available to protect your business. Some, such as workers' compensation, are mandated by law, while others, such as travel insurance, although they provide peace of mind, may or may not be necessary for your business. Most coverage begins with a basic *business owner's policy,* commonly referred to as a *BOP.* This generally includes items such as property or casualty, general liability, and business interruption insurance; however, spa owners typically require more than the broad coverage listed in a basic business policy, which ordinarily does not include items like professional liability, health, auto, disability, or workers' compensation insurance. Your insurance agent can help you sort through the "must haves," and should also be able to point out those additional items that are warranted for your particular circumstance.

How Insurance Works

Under the terms of your business owner's policy, you, the spa owner, agree to pay a certain amount of money to transfer the risk associated with conducting certain activities; the insurer agrees to pay certain amounts to cover any damages that may occur as a consequence of those activities, *within certain limits.* These limits are typically written in terms of the dollar amounts per occurrence per person. Be sure you have a complete understanding of the limitations of these terms, and if you do not, be sure to ask for clarification. Learning that you are responsible for hundreds of thousands of dollars in damages after the fact, should an accident occur, is not the time to begin questioning your agent. The risks involved in spa business ownership are high and in some cases could exceed the limits of your coverage. It is your right to have all of the items in your policy carefully explained to you in a way that is confidently understood and to seek other options as needed to safeguard your business.

Before sitting down with your insurance agent, it is a good idea to become familiar with the many types of business insurance that are available to you. The SBA is a valuable resource and provides an excellent overview of the common types of insurance in its *Small Business Insurance and Risk Management Guide.* This free publication, available online, provides an overview of the risks associated with business ownership and the various options available to protect your business against them.

Another organization that may be helpful to spa owners is the Insurance Information Institute (III), whose mission is to improve the public's understanding of insurance. The Insurance Information Institute provides information on a wide variety of insurance topics, including answers to many of the typical questions that prospective business owners have about business insurance. III also publishes a guide for small business owners which may be purchased in print format. More information is available on their Web site (*www.iii.org*).

BASIC TYPES OF INSURANCE COVERAGE

1. *Property or casualty insurance:* protects your business from physical property damage, as in the event of fire, theft, or other disasters

2. *Liability insurance:* protects your business from damages associated with negligence, accidents, or injuries

3. *Malpractice insurance:* also referred to as *professional liability insurance,* protects you in the event of a lawsuit resulting from alleged negligence or errors and omissions that result in harm or injury to your clients

4. *Life, health, and disability insurance:* provides direct benefits as a result of death, illness, or injury

5. *Workers' compensation:* covers employee medical and rehabilitation expenses as a result of injuries on the job. This type of insurance is mandatory and required by law in all states

Please note that these are general descriptions of common types of insurance and are not meant to be inclusive. For more specific information and an assessment of your individual needs, you should seek the professional advice of a qualified insurance agent.

Plan for Success

Expensive equipment, increasingly complex treatments, and a high-profile industry that is now widely associated with generating billions of dollars has made it critical for spa owners to do everything within their power to avoid potential harm or injury and the possibility of costly litigation. Establishing a risk management program that ensures best business practices should be a vital part of any spa business owner's business plan.

Insurance Regulations

Insurance is another facet of business that is regulated by state law. Prior to purchasing a policy, it is a good idea to contact the office of the insurance commissioner for specific guidelines as they relate to conducting business in your state. It is also wise to seek references from other professional sources, such as your accountant, lawyer, business associates, or professional trade organizations, before contacting an agent to help you set up a business policy. In some cases, trade associations may recommend agencies that are well versed in the specific insurance needs of the spa industry. These organizations may offer special rates or discounts for members. Still, it is always wise to check out their track record.

Hopefully, you will never have to recover from a disaster or mishap. Unfortunately, accidents do happen, and lawsuits have become altogether too commonplace in our litigious society. While no amount of insurance coverage can prevent certain occurrences, it is important for the spa owner to take responsibility for encouraging the highest professional standards and implementing good business practices. If situations beyond your control occur, you will be glad that you took the time to be prepared by protecting your business as much as possible.

THINK IT OVER

Purchasing a spa is a major undertaking that requires a great deal of practical knowledge and business acumen. Many of the situations that you will have to deal with will require far greater expertise than you may have at your disposal. When in doubt, always seek competent professional advice.

ARCHITECTURE AND DESIGN OF YOUR SPA

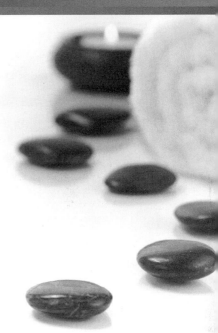

In recent years, spa design has taken the forefront, with highly stylized interior and exterior features that have some people comparing spas to theme parks. For many spa-goers looking for a way to escape the stresses of everyday life, the ambiance is an important part of the spa package that contributes greatly to the overall pleasure or "experience." This trend has encouraged many day spa owners to indulge their fantasies in creating environments that are typically found in destination or resort spas. It has also raised the bar for spa designers who are working hard to generate that all-important "aah" response, sometimes within the constraints of limited budgets and restricted spaces.

DEVELOPING A PLAN

Designing your spa is likely to be one of the more exciting tasks you will encounter in developing your spa business. Choosing colors, materials, furnishings, and accessories is typically a fun and exhilarating experience. But it is important to understand that your spa design will have a direct effect on your profitability, the way you conduct business, and the type of clients you are able to attract. A quality design calls for expert knowledge in the areas of architecture, construction, interior design, marketing, products, and equipment. If you lack experience in these areas, you can easily get in over your head, spending more than you can afford or making costly construction mistakes that could become a significant nuisance down the road. Before you engage an architect, designer, or contractor, you will want to be clear about your goals and objectives, the costs involved, and, most importantly, your budget.

STRATEGIC DESIGN

Planning the physical space of your spa begins with the right location and a good business plan. If you have worked through the exercises in Chapters 1 and 4, you should have a clear vision of the type of spa you would like to build and the amenities you would like to include, as well as the cost of leasing space or purchasing property. This information is critical to the strategic design and development section of your business plan, discussed in Chapter 3. It is also an important step in the design phase that will bring you closer to determining the physical layout of your spa and the cost factors involved.

Preliminary Step 1

The first order of business is to create a detailed description of the services and products you intend to offer. Many find it easy to begin with a general outline of each service category, such as face, body, massage, hair removal, nail, and makeup services. Your individual philosophy or spa concept is likely to dictate others that should be included here. It will also affect the type of products and equipment you decide to incorporate, which will be discussed further in Chapter 6.

Preliminary Step 2

Next, you will want to name the professionals who will provide the services you intend to offer. Make sure you understand the spatial and mechanical requirements of all the treatments they will perform and the equipment that will be used to conduct them. For example, a massage therapist may be able to work comfortably in an 8' × 10' room to perform a massage that requires little more than lotions, stones, and oils; however, an esthetician or bodywork professional working with specialized equipment is likely to need more space when performing services. A list of all the service providers who will operate in your spa and the equipment they will use will come in handy when meeting with spa consultants and designers.

Calculating Cost

The question on every spa owner's mind is how much it will cost to build a space that accommodates all the service providers they intend to use and the equipment they need to perform those services. The answer to this question depends on a number of factors, including the size and focus of your spa; whether you are working with an existing space or building from the ground up; the building materials, furnishings, and decorating accessories you select, etc. A small- to medium-sized day spa will, of course, differ significantly in comparison to the capital required to build a large resort, destination spa, or medical practice. The type of products and technology your spa uses will also affect the cost. Sophisticated equipment such as laser and light technology, hydrotherapy tubs, and showers will increase your initial investment and may dictate certain building requirements, such as reinforcement beams, sound- and water proofing materials, special mechanical and electrical engineering, etc., that will add to the overall cost.

Whatever your focus is, the design of your spa should ultimately be one that generates financial success. If you haven't already done so, this is a good time to begin to crunch the numbers. The cost of purchasing or leasing property, construction, furnishings, equipment, professional services, and supplies will be important factors in determining the type of spa you can afford to design and build. The business plan and financial worksheets in Chapter 3 will help you to get started. We will take a more detailed look at product and equipment in the next chapter. Establishing costs at the outset is the best way to stay within your budget.

Seek Professional Advice

Once you have decided upon a location and have a clear understanding of the type of amenities you would like to offer, you are ready for the next phase of development: engaging building and design professionals.

If you are like most prospective spa owners, chances are you have an idea of the ambiance and style you would like your spa to exude. Still, you may be feeling somewhat intimidated by the many choices you will have to make and by the cost involved. Building a spa is an enormous undertaking, and it is perfectly normal to feel a few pangs of apprehension. Even if you are confident that you could negotiate a basic spa plan and select the appropriate products and equipment with the support of a qualified vendor, it is likely that you will need some assistance when it comes to the actual layout, construction, and mechanical requirements involved in building your spa, such as plumbing and electrical work. Your spa plans will also need to comply with a number of local, state, and federal health safety and building regulations, including Occupational Safety and Health Administration (OSHA) and Americans with Disability Act (ADA) requirements. Experienced architects, designers, general contractors, and spa consultants can offer invaluable advice in these areas that can actually save you time and money in the long run.

Plan for Success

Whether your spa project falls under the category of new construction or renovation, the architecture and design of your spa must comply with all local, state, and federal health, safety and building regulations. This typically involves a number of government agencies, such as the Department of Health, State Board of Cosmetology (and/or other professional licensing board as they apply), local Building Department, Occupational Safety and Health Administration (OSHA), and Americans with Disability Act (ADA) requirements. Experienced architects, general contractors, and spa consultants can offer invaluable advice on these topics that is likely to save you a great deal of time and money in the long run.

ARCHITECTS

A skilled architect will help you to turn your spa dream into a physical reality (Figure 5-1). To inspire your vision, that person must have a good understanding of your total spa concept, the atmosphere you would like to create, the size of the space, the equipment that will be used, and the functional requirements of your business. You are ultimately responsible for supplying a great deal of that information. However, a good architect will be attuned to your vision, the mechanical requirements, and business goals of your spa and will include all of these components in developing a set of plans or blueprints.

Finding the right architect for your project usually involves a little scouting. Trade associations like the American Institute of Architects (AIA), local builders, suppliers, and vendors are often good resources for recommendations. Trade publications and consumer magazines that feature photographs and stories about spas are another way to "shop" for designers and architects. It is also a good idea to visit as many spas as possible. If you see a spa design that appeals to you, inquire about the architect.

It is always a plus to hire someone who specializes in spas or has some experience in designing a spa; however, this does not mean that

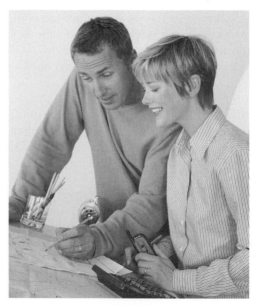

FIGURE 5-1 A skilled architect can turn your vision into a reality.

an experienced architect could not provide an adequate plan with the help of a qualified spa consultant. Whichever way you decide to go, be sure that the architect is aware of the zoning, building, and construction codes in your area since your plans must be inspected and approved by the local building commission. In many cases, an architect will need to consult with an engineer to determine the feasibility of a plan or its structural requirements. This is especially important when it comes to spas since there are often concerns about weight-bearing walls and floors, particularly when it comes to heavy equipment, such as that required for hydrotherapies.

Architectural and Design Fees

What should you expect to pay for architecture and design services? There are no hard-and-fast rules when it comes to architecture and design fees. Some architects and designers work on a percentage basis; others work according to an hourly rate, or calculate a set fee. You can also expect prices to vary according to the architect's level of expertise, experience, reputation, and the size of the firm. All of this is complicated further by the fact that each project and every budget is different.

To avoid spending more than you have, it is very important to find professionals who are first and foremost willing to work within your budget; however, determining that budget, as we discussed in Chapter 3, will take more than a cursory glance at the capital and credit lines available to you. There are several important variables to consider, such as the cost of building from the ground up versus renovating an existing building or negotiating a lease-hold or rental space. While this may require hiring professionals to assist you in crunching the numbers, it is important to have some preliminary cost projections that will allow you to measure the merits of one versus the other.

A carefully drafted business plan that defines the spa concept and includes a three-to-five-year cost projection is the best place to start. Design firms that specialize in the spa industry may have financial experts on staff to assist you with this; others may work closely with spa consultants. If the architect you decide to work with has no experience in the spa industry, it is wise to seek the advice of a spa consultant who has experience working with architects and designers. Some architectural firms and spa consultants get involved in market analysis and feasibility studies before tackling any project. This may turn out to be the best money you spend. Nixing a project before you get in over your head, while disappointing, ultimately makes good business sense.

ARCHITECTURAL CHECKLIST

The architecture, design, and building of your spa requires a significant outlay of capital and is a critical component of your budget and business plan. Before signing a contract, the spa owner should have an in-depth proposal that outlines the entire scope of the project.

This should include an itemized accounting of all of the deliverables along with the responsible parties, for example, a certified architect, structural engineer, general contractor, interior designer, spa consultant, landscape designer, lighting designer, etc.

The following questions will help you to begin working with a design team.

☐ Are you building from the ground up, starting from a shell, or renovating an existing spa space?

☐ Will you own the space or lease it?

☐ Can you make use of any existing utilities? To what extent?

☐ Are there any improvements, such as mechanical, plumbing, or construction costs, that can be negotiated in the lease or lease-hold agreement?

☐ What is the level of luxury you wish to achieve, and more importantly can afford: a basic, moderate, or luxurious spa design?

☐ What experience designing spas does the firm have?

☐ Does the firm have professional spa consulting, engineering, and design services on staff, or will some or all of these have to be out sourced?

☐ Will you need a site evaluation to determine zoning and building requirements?

☐ Are there any additional services such as landscaping design that are required? Who will be responsible for hiring and paying for these services?

☐ Will the architect stay on through construction to protect your interests? If so, are there a limited number of meetings, on-site visits built into the proposal? Are these adequate for the size and scope of the project?

☐ Does the architect's fee include the cost of construction? Will there be a general contractor? An additional project manager?

Is there a separate fee for these services or are they incorporated into the architect's fee? The cost of construction?

☐ Do construction costs include labor and materials? Painting? Are all materials specified? Does the budget reflect the level of luxury you anticipate for your spa concept? Include important spa-specific materials such as sound- and waterproofing?

☐ Who will be responsible for obtaining and paying for all of the necessary building and zoning permits?

☐ What additional expenses can you expect in terms of furniture, fixtures, equipment, and supplies?

☐ Will you need to hire a spa consultant to work with the architect? What services will they provide? Do they have previous experience working together on similar projects?

☐ Has the firm worked on any comparatively sized projects? If so, what data or research can they supply? How did they arrive at this data? Is the information based on current market rates? Does it take into account any unique geographic, building, or structural limitations that may apply to your project?

☐ How will the feasibility of the project be determined? Will this include a demographic analysis that evaluates the compatibility of your target market and spa concept? An on-site evaluation? A competitive market analysis? A financial profitability factor? Current economic conditions?

☐ What is the cost of a feasibility study? Is this incorporated in the architect's fee? Can some of this data be derived from other sources, such as financial documents you have invested in from other professionals? Applied to the total cost of the project?

☐ Are you comfortable with the architect's, designer's, and spa consultant's method of negotiating fees?

☐ Have you seen the firm's work on other projects? Spoken with the owners? Visited the site? Does the firm come well recommended?

☐ Do you have a good rapport with all of the professionals you will need to interact with?

☐ Has an allowance been made for soft operating expenses and other professional services?

☐ What is the time frame for the project? Is this reasonable?

Plan for Success

CAUTION: There are many cost variables when building a spa, but even a small spa can easily hit the million-dollar mark. This is where many get into trouble. Establishing a firm budget for architecture and design is critical to the success of your spa business plan. Be sure you have calculated all of the additional pre-opening and operating expenses, such as marketing, hiring and training staff, needed to open your doors and begin generating revenue before splurging on additional interior design features. Certain items can always be added once you have a quality infrastructure.

Blueprints

Before you can begin the construction of your spa, you will need a set of plans. In some cases, builders or general contractors are able to supply simple sketches or drawings, but ordinarily blueprints are supplied by an architect. Your architect will develop a plan that displays the physical layout of your spa (Figures 5-2, 5-3, and 5-4). This should include detailed specifications, or blueprints, of the entire facility noting the mechanical, plumbing, and electrical functions required. Your blueprint may also include the stylized details that portray the ambience of your spa, such as decorative columns, cabinets, fixtures, window boxes, stone walls, handrails, and placement of the furniture. When designing a building from the ground up, you will need plans for both the interior and exterior design.

Spa Consultants

Spa consultants offer a variety of services and often have a certain niche or specialty. For example, some are focused on space acquisition and feasibility studies, while others may specialize in concept development, architecture and design, menu planning, product and equipment selection, or education and training for different product lines, treatment protocols, and equipment. Many spa consultants incorporate all facets of spa development by outsourcing or collaborating with others as part of a team. If you are unclear about what a consultant does, ask!

SPA CONSULTANTS MAY ASSUME SEVERAL ROLES AND RESPONSIBILITIES INCLUDING:

- Concept development
- Architecture and design
- Facility or space acquisition
- Feasibility studies and market analysis
- Project management for spa development
- Menu planning
- Product and equipment selection
- Education and training

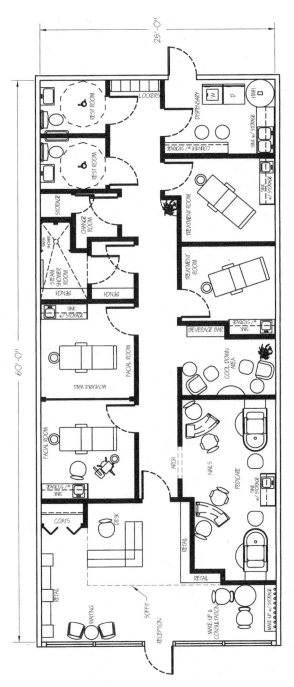

FIGURE 5-2 Blueprint for 1,500-square-foot day spa.

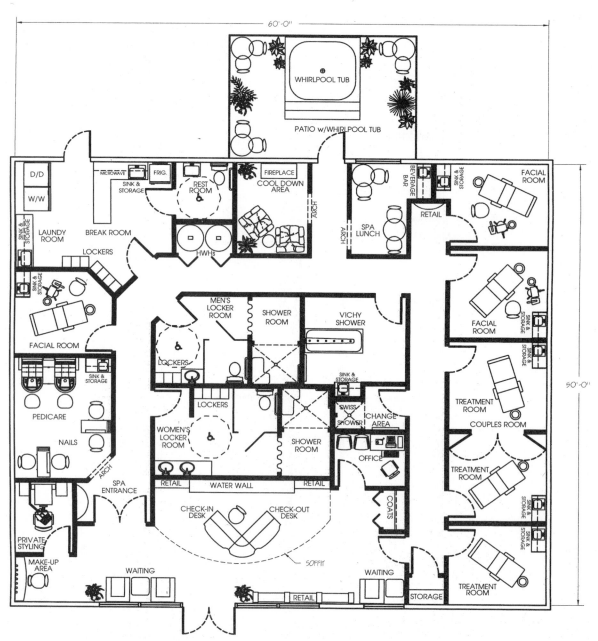

FIGURE 5-3 Blueprint for 3,000-square-foot day spa.

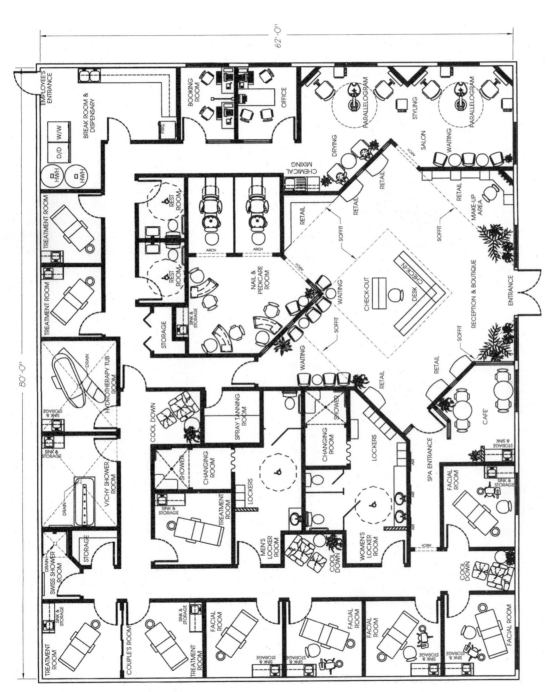

FIGURE 5-4 Blueprint for 5,000-square-foot day spa.

Plan for Success

Pay careful attention to the following details as you enter the construction phase:

- **Energy sources**—You will need ample electric power and a generous water supply.
- **Plumbing**—Sufficient heat and hot water are vital to the client's comfort in a spa.
- **Drainage**—Waste management can be problematic, particularly when dealing with multiple hydrotherapies; be sure your facility has adequate drainage.
- **Structural capacity**—Be aware of the weight load for all equipment, especially hydrotherapy equipment.
- **Technology requirements**—Telephone, computer systems, video, television screens, and sound systems are critical to day-to-day operations; wiring these correctly is vital to the success of your spa.
- **Equipment requirements**—Be aware of the specifications for operating all types of spa equipment.
- **Lighting**—Sets the mood or tone of your spa and has a direct effect on employee performance; it is also instrumental in creating a profitable retail sales area.

What you want to know before you hire a spa consultant is where the bulk of their expertise lies. After you determine their niche, find out if they have experience planning small- to medium-sized day spas, medical spas, larger destination spas, or amenity-type spas. Although consultants may have tons of experience in the hotel or resort industry, they may not be the right firm for you if your goal is to open a smaller day spa. It is also wise to cover fees and payment schedules up front. If you are concerned about costs, present your budget and find out if the consultant can work within it.

It may also be important to engage a consultant who is physically available throughout the planning and building stages. If the consultant is unable to visit your spa or meet with you on a schedule that makes you feel comfortable, find out if they have relationships with people in your area who can provide on-site interaction as needed. In some cases, several strategic visits combined with regularly scheduled telephone conferences are sufficient. Computer software and technology can transcend many miles; so do not rule out a consultant that you otherwise find suitable because of distance.

One last word of advice: spa consultants that also serve as vendors may have a vested interest in selling certain equipment. They may also represent a varied number of suppliers from which to compare and contrast your options. If after researching similar equipment you feel confident in the brand, it makes sense to use it. Otherwise, do not. Compromising quality for the sake of a good deal generally isn't worth it in the long run.

Construction

General contractors work closely with architects, engineers, and spa consultants to build the physical space. These are the people who take the blueprint and turn it into a spa. General contractors supervise and hire subcontractors, such as electricians, carpenters, plumbers, and communications technicians, to put the physical and mechanical requirements in place, including the heating, ventilation, and air-conditioning systems, sinks, showers, tubs, windows, walls, doors, electric panels, lighting, and wiring for telephone and computer systems. Spa owners looking to save money may decide to act as their own general contractor, hiring the individual technicians themselves. If you are so inclined, keep in mind that supervising subcontractors often turns out to be a full-time job and requires a level of expertise that many ultimately do not have. This can actually end up costing more and is not recommended.

Contractors generally charge a set fee per square foot for supervising a project. This fee may or may not cover the cost of subcontractors' labor charges or materials. When hiring a contractor to carry out your plans, ask for an itemized account of all expenses—and always get at least three bids to assess whether or not you are being charged fairly. The Better Business

Bureau and Attorney General's office can be helpful in identifying any past problems or unethical business practices that you should be aware of before engaging a contractor. It is also wise to speak to other customers and take a look at the contractor's finished work.

Another crucial consideration in construction is time. The longer it takes to put a project together, the more money it requires. To avoid additional costs, you will want to be up and running as quickly as possible; so it is important to be aware of time frames and make informed decisions well in advance. Wasting time with indecisiveness at critical moments will not help you to stay on schedule or within your budget. Generally, you can expect construction to take about nine months, but it is wise to expect some delays and bureaucratic dilemmas. A last-minute notice that an item has been back-ordered for several months, difficulties in acquiring the appropriate building permits, or inspection setbacks are unfortunately all too common.

LEAVE ROOM FOR EXPANSION

Spa owners who are also practitioners tend to have a certain focus. This often lays the foundation for an economically sound spa program. However, in today's competitive spa environment, it is wise to explore all marketing possibilities.

Many times I hear, "We are not really a spa—we are focused on skin care; so I don't have any interest in plumbing for water therapies." Later, that same spa owner will sigh, "I wish I had given more thought to including a Vichy shower." Even if you do not plan to offer a certain service immediately, consider plumbing or allocating space to accommodate other services down the road. Once construction is complete, it may be possible to add or renovate, but it certainly will come at a higher price.

TREATMENT ROOMS

The size of your facility will ultimately determine the number of treatment rooms, equipment, and type of services that can be accommodated. For example, if you are renting 1,000 square feet of space, you will certainly be limited in the number of treatment rooms and hydrotherapy options you can incorporate comfortably. The situation will differ significantly if your spa contains 3,000 to 5,000 square feet of space or more. Additional space will naturally allow you to build larger, more comfortable treatment rooms that can accommodate more amenities.

Plan for Success (continued)

- **Temperature control**— Maintaining the appropriate temperature is a significant factor in efficiency and comfort.

- **Air quality**—Efficient ventilation systems are essential in creating a healthful spa environment and are particularly important if your spa provides such services as nail tips, wraps, or acrylic nails.

- **Noise control**—Soundproof rooms will help to maintain the serenity of your spa and avoid outside distractions.

- **Housekeeping facilities**—Laundry and maintenance are an essential part of day-to-day operations in the spa industry; however, to maintain an aesthetically pleasing atmosphere, you will want to hide these from view.

- **Ease of transition**—Consider function and flow when connecting treatment rooms so that you can transition clients from one service to another easily.

- **Safety**—Minimize risk exposure with adequate safety measures and strict compliance with health and sanitation codes, non hazardous building materials, and an ergonomically correct set up in all treatment rooms.

Plan for Success (continued)

- **Expansion possibilities—**
  Consider your long-term goals and leave room for expansion; install plumbing even if you are not ready to purchase a major hydrotherapy piece just yet.

A standard-size treatment room is approximately 10 × 10 feet. Larger treatment rooms will vary in size depending upon the type of facility (Figure 5-5). Some treatment rooms may contain folding or pocket doors for the purpose of expanding to accommodate couple services and other treatments that require more space. As you plan the size of your treatment rooms, allow for some flexibility.

Consider the Needs of Clients and Service Providers

When planning the layout of your treatment rooms, the needs of clients and service providers should be a top priority. Pay attention to the practical aspect of operations as well as the psychological components. If a room is jam-packed with apparatus, it can have a claustrophobic effect on clients, making them feel ill at ease rather than relaxed and comfortable. Tight spaces also affect the mood of your service providers and are likely to make them feel confined and restrained. More spacious surroundings, on the other hand, encourage a free flow of energy.

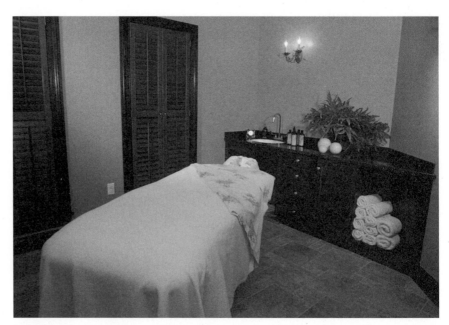

FIGURE 5-5 A spacious treatment room.

Treatment rooms should be functional with cabinets, shelves, and sinks strategically placed for the convenience of the therapist. Furniture should be comfortable for clients and ergonomically correct to prevent injury to service providers. Electrical outlets and lighting should be readily available and the latter easily controlled. Ideally, you should be able to control the temperature in each room or area of your spa to maintain individual comfort levels and protect and prolong the life of equipment.

Client and practitioner safety is a must at all times. Make sure your treatment rooms include stools and rails to assist clients on and off facial beds and bulky equipment. Provide a chair to assist clients in changing comfortably. This is particularly important if your clientele is older. Each treatment room should also have a place for clients to hang clothing and rest personal belongings, especially if your spa does not have designated locker space. To ensure everyone's safety, keep all pathways clear and avoid slippery surfaces. Proper disposal of waste, sharps, and other blood-borne pathogens should comply with OSHA standards.

DRY ROOMS

Spa treatment rooms are generally divided into two categories: dry rooms and wet rooms. *Dry rooms* are those that do not contain water services or hydrotherapy equipment, with the exception of a sink basin. These rooms are primarily used to perform facial and massage services and are often used interchangeably to conduct both. Other services, such as those that are adversely affected by moisture, such as waxing and microdermabrasion treatments, may also be performed in dry treatment rooms.

WET ROOMS

Hydrotherapy or water-based treatment rooms deserve careful consideration. Equipment for *wet rooms* is expensive, and safety precautions are imperative. An adequate water supply, sufficient drainage, and a solid structural foundation are primary concerns that should be thoroughly investigated before installing any plumbing and purchasing or leasing equipment. Remember that hydrotherapy tubs, whirlpools, Jacuzzis, and relaxation pools carry considerably more weight with water and bodies in them. Be aware of the maximum weight load and review these specifications carefully with your architect, engineer, and builder.

Standard water therapies, such as hydrotherapy tubs and Vichy, Swiss, and steam showers, are typically housed in rooms that are constructed of tile or stone for ease of maintenance. However, where indoor space is limited, there may be opportunities to use outdoor space creatively. Placing a sauna or hot tub in a patio or garden area can be a delightful experience even in colder climates (Figure 5-6). Think about how good it feels to enjoy a warm Jacuzzi or whirlpool tub outdoors in the middle of winter; however, even when placing hydrotherapy equipment outdoors, you should be aware of structural and waste drainage requirements. Privacy, climate, and noise control are other factors to consider to ensure gaining the maximum return on your investment.

Indoors, all materials used in wet rooms, including wall coverings, paint, and furnishings, must be able to withstand moisture. Adequate ventilation and temperature control must be perfectly calibrated to ensure the comfort of clients. To avoid the toxic buildup of mold and mildew and maintain proper sanitation, wet rooms must be hosed down on a regular basis. Nonporous materials, such as tile and certain types of stone that can

Plan for Success

Outdoor patios and courtyards are an excellent way to expand treatment options for those with limited square footage. However, such space should be planned carefully. Privacy issues, climate, and noise control are just a few things to consider, especially for spas located in crowded areas and/or subject to extreme temperature variations. The cost of additional structures, such as porticos, outdoor change rooms and cafés, patio furnishings that can stand up to the elements, landscape features, and maintenance should be weighed carefully before investing in expensive equipment and elaborate construction plans. The bottom line for any spa owner is: *Is it worth the additional expenditure and, as always, is it something that clients want?*

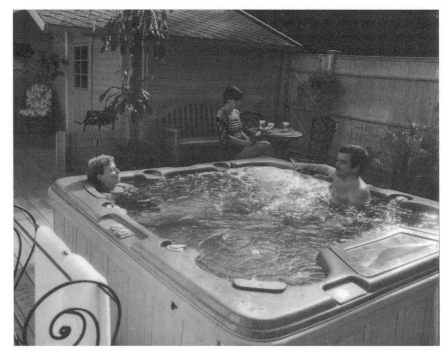

FIGURE 5-6   Outdoor Jacuzzi at Essential Therapies Day Spa in Bolton, Massachusetts.

withstand water and continuous cleanings, are imperative. Proper electrical wiring is paramount to safety in these rooms. Be sure your builder understands these requirements before installation.

RETAIL, ADMINISTRATIVE, AND COMMUNITY SPACE

It is easy to get caught up in the detailed requirements of treatment rooms and the more luxurious aspects of spa design, but do not overlook those areas that provide important business functions. Your retail and administrative areas are as vital to business as the areas in which services are performed. Likewise, community space can enhance the flow of business and turn dead space into a premium spa asset.

Retail Space

Merchandising is an important function in the spa business, with many ascribing to the philosophy that retail sales should account for at least 30 percent of a spa's profits. Be sure your designer understands this critical spa business concept and allows for ample retail space. I have seen more than one gorgeously decorated spa miss the mark completely by hiding retail products behind counters or tucking them into corners that are virtually inaccessible.

While you should always take precautions to prevent slippage, your retail area should be a place where clients can browse leisurely or relax with a cup of tea while they review literature or watch a video that explains the benefits and features of your products and services. Shelving and counter space should be arranged in a warm and inviting way so that clients are free to walk through aisles without bumping into things and feel comfortable lingering over sample products (Figure 5-7). If possible, leave enough room for an inviting table display and comfy chairs. As a general rule, there should be enough space in your retail area for clients to sniff, sample, and enjoy the process.

Administrative Areas

Your front desk, check-in, checkout, and scheduling rooms are critical to the flow of business. Make sure these areas are user-friendly.

Administrative areas are definitely places where you don't want employees to feel strained (Figure 5-8). A relaxed and happy staff will

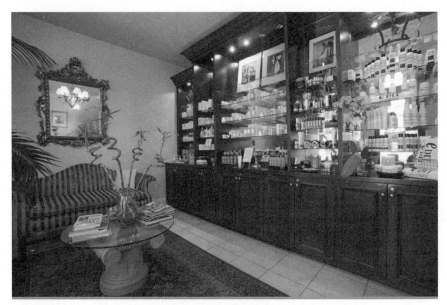

FIGURE 5-7   An inviting retail display encourages spa guests to linger.

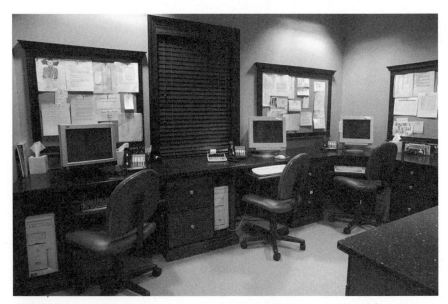

FIGURE 5-8   Administrative areas should be functional and comfortable.

be more inclined to provide your clients with excellent customer service. Comfortable chairs and workstations with adequate lighting are in order here. Working all day at a computer can cause eye and muscle strain. Make sure furniture is ergonomically correct and include accessories such as telephone headsets to make administrative staff more comfortable. Avoid any type of lighting or fixtures that might cause a glare on computer screens, and keep all necessary office equipment within easy reach. If you have a busy spa with several staff members taking calls simultaneously, consider a separate call center with soundproof panels between workstations and designate a quiet area for service providers to make follow-up calls to clients.

Electrical wiring is critical to operations in administrative areas. Be sure to install cable lines that supply immediate Internet accessibility and plenty of outlets to accommodate the simultaneous use of office equipment, such as a fax machine, copier, and credit card processors. It is frustrating for employees to be waiting for technology access, and even more frustrating for clients in a hurry.

Clients should be able to move in and out in as little time as possible. A simple design will help to orchestrate your check-in and checkout areas with minimal confusion (Figure 5-9). After receiving an excellent service,

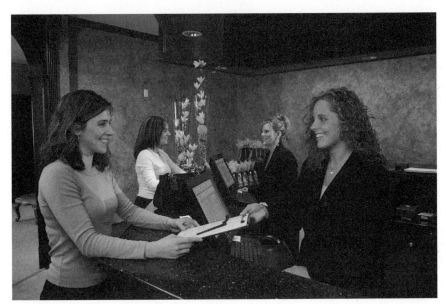

FIGURE 5-9   The check-in and checkout areas are critical to business operations.

you do not want a client's parting memory to be that "it took me longer to get out of here than it did to have my nails manicured." That, unfortunately, is an all-too-frequent scenario in busier spas. Privacy can be a concern as well, particularly if your spa offers services that clients prefer to keep under wraps. If clients are leaving in a less-than-flattering state, provide them with access to a secluded exit.

Community Space

Small and medium-sized day spas may not be able to offer some of the more luxurious amenities seen in lavish resort and destination spas, such as a relaxation pool, whirlpool, or sauna, but they can certainly compete in terms of efficiency, hospitality, and an outstanding experience (Figure 5-10).

The entrance to your spa will set the tone for the entire guest experience. This is where a good designer attuned to your philosophy and goals can help you to make that all-important first impression an exquisite one.

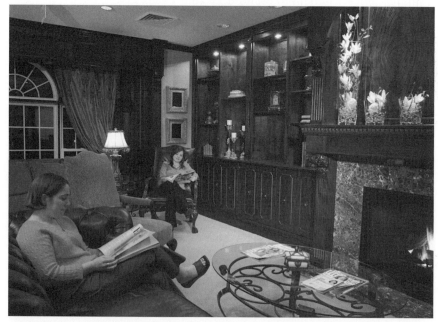

FIGURE 5-10   The waiting area at Kimberly's Day Spa in Latham, New York, has all of the ambience of a luxurious destination spa.

Take extra care to ensure that this area is attractive and welcoming. If space is limited, consider a minimalist approach rather than cramming too much into a small space. A simple water fountain or an exquisite vase of flowers can provide just the right impact.

A spa's entrance typically flows into the reception area, where again you will want to send a warm and inviting message. Your receptionist or front desk manager should be facing guests in a welcoming position. Walking into a room where the first view is the back of the receptionist's head sends the wrong message and may be interpreted as your guests are not important.

Clients are likely to be ushered from your reception area to a changing room. Consider the details in making storage and locker facilities here neat, attractive, and user-friendly. Once clients have donned robes, you will also want to make it easy for them to transition from the changing area to treatment rooms. Clients receiving multiple services should be ushered from one service to another with a minimum of inconvenience or disruption to the relaxation benefit. It is also important for clients to feel comfortable if they have to step out into a more public area. Modesty is a huge concern for some; so be sure the shower is strategically located as well. Adjoining spaces and interconnecting treatment rooms, arranged to go with the logical flow of services, not only increase customer service, they save time. In the end this will also increase profits.

Manicure-Pedicure Stations and Makeup Areas

Certain services, such as manicures and pedicures, should be placed away from quiet zones. These services are often noisy and are best situated in areas that will not disturb other guests (Figures 5-11). Sanitation and drainage are a critical part of the design here that should not be overlooked, so be sure that your architect, contractor, and plumber understand the hygiene requirements. We will talk more about choosing equipment in Chapter 6; however, it is important to have furnishings that are easily sanitized and equipment that can be drained and disinfected quickly in between clients in this area to prevent the spread of bacteria. Makeup is another service that can require a good deal of conversation, especially if your spa offers makeup instruction (Figure 5-12). Protecting the privacy of individuals who may not want to be seen without makeup is another factor to consider when arranging makeup stations.

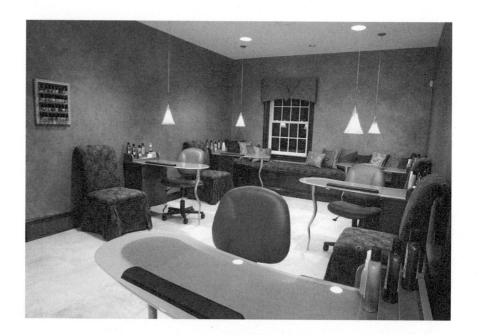

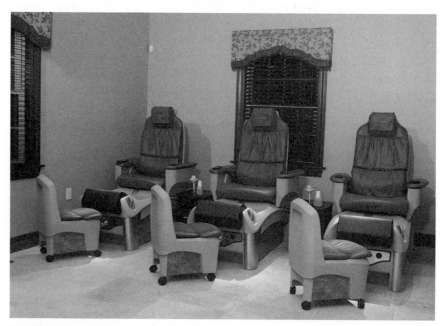

FIGURE 5-11   Manicure and pedicure stations should be placed away from quiet zones.

SPA OPERATIONS

Two areas that deserve more attention than they sometimes get are housekeeping stations and the dispensary. While these areas are not front and center, they are essential to spa operations.

Housekeeping

Airing your dirty laundry is definitely a no-no in the spa world, where beauty and tranquility reign. Washers, dryers, and housekeeping supplies should be kept hidden from the client's view and treatment rooms should contain hampers that are unobtrusive and large enough to prevent overflow between treatments (Figure 5-13); however, there should be ample evidence that your spa is clean, sanitized, and properly maintained. This can

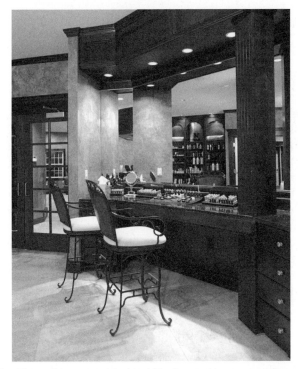

FIGURE 5-12   The makeup counter should be located in an area where conversation can take place comfortably.

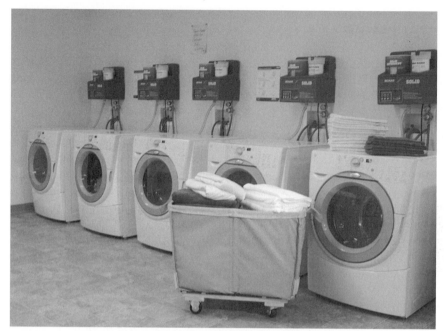

FIGURE 5-13   Housekeeping facilities should be hidden from guest view.

be accomplished by keeping linens, sanitizing agents, and other supplies well stocked and within easy reach and by installing surfaces that are easy to keep sparkling clean.

In designing your spa, pay special attention to bathroom and change areas where towels, cleansers, shampoo, conditioners, blow-dryers, lotions, and tissues should be readily available to guests in convenient cubbies, attractive canisters, and baskets or customized shelves. Don't forget to leave extra cabinet space to accommodate disinfectants and waste receptacles. Cleanliness is indeed next to godliness in the spa business.

Product Dispensary

Your spa's dispensary may not be the highlight of your interior design, but it is critical to maintaining an efficient and profitable operation. This room should be strategically located to allow for easy access (Figure 5-14). Walking across an entire facility to replenish supplies is counterproductive.

Ideally, each treatment room or area, such as manicure and pedicure stations, should have enough space to accommodate a day's supply of

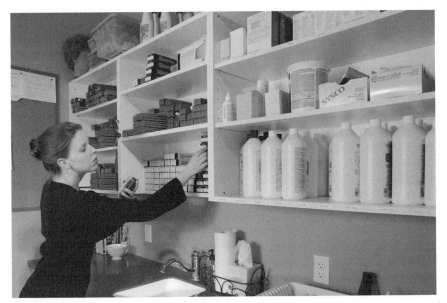

FIGURE 5-14   The dispensary should be strategically located.

materials and linens. Where space is limited, you will need to implement a foolproof system that is conducive to maintaining inventory control, yet allows support staff and service providers to replenish provisions from the dispensary as needed.

Employee Areas

Ideally, your employees should have a separate entrance and a private rest area to eat or take a break (Figure 5-15). This serves two purposes: it establishes boundaries between clients and practitioners, and it says that you value the comfort and professionalism of your staff. Segregated eating areas, locker rooms, and consultation areas go a long way in establishing positive employee relations.

Interior Design

A well-designed spa should be aesthetically pleasing, functional, and comfortable. It should add value to your business, enhance your profitability, and provide a safe environment for all who use and perform services in it. In these competitive times, it must also wow your guests (Figure 5-16).

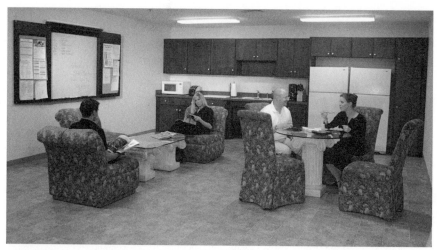

FIGURE 5-15   Employee break room.

A great design starts with good architectural planning. This is enhanced by color, lighting, fabrics, floor and wall coverings, furnishings, and accessories. These elements generally fall under the realm of interior designers; however, in some cases, an architect may be qualified to perform both services.

Finding a designer whose style you are comfortable with is important. Many of the same considerations we discussed in choosing an architect hold true here. That person should be someone who can inspire your vision. They should also understand the concept of retail space, flow of treatments, current spa trends, structural requirements, and equipment needs and any cultural themes you would like to incorporate. Again, whenever possible, it is wise to choose professionals with experience in the spa industry. If you decide to go with a designer who lacks experience in the spa business, you may want to use a spa consultant to oversee the project or work with your designer. Be sure the two are compatible.

When we talk about interior design, we are talking about furniture, cabinetry, shelving, wall coverings, floor and ceiling materials, fabrics for draperies and seating, lighting, paint, and other accessories. Interior design does not encompass the equipment used to perform services. Before selecting any of these items, it is a good idea to specify a design budget and stick to it. Lavish fabrics and furnishings can be enticing, and it is easy to go overboard without too much strain. If your finances

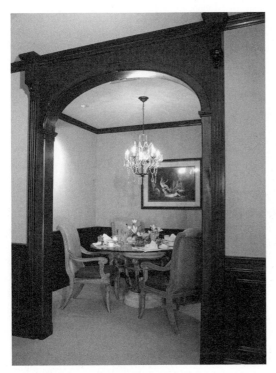

FIGURE 5-16   An exquisitely decorated dining area.

are limited, remember that a good interior design does not have to be expensive to be pleasing.

AMBIENCE

The ambience, or style of your spa, is typically a matter of personal taste, but it should reflect your spa's philosophy. If your treatments are tied to the latest industry trends and you enjoy whimsy, bold colors and a funky décor might be appropriate. On the other hand, if you are a naturalist, you would probably be more comfortable with the serene colors of sand, sea, and plant life and rather subdued furnishings.

Before sitting down with an interior designer, take time to review the basic principles of your spa philosophy. For example, are your treatments heavily influenced by Native American, Indian, or Eastern practices, such as ayurveda, yoga, or tai chi? Do they incorporate organic healing elements? Or are they mainly focused on results-oriented procedures? Look closely at the symbols that reflect your ideology. What colors are most often associated with these techniques? A good designer can help you incorporate these elements in a way that integrates your personal style with your business goals to create a theme that truly reflects your vision.

COLOR

It used to be that soft feminine colors ruled in spa environments. Today, we are seeing richer, bolder colors that in some cases are just as capable of creating a tranquil environment as are their less-dramatic counterparts. The new neutrals go beyond shades of white, beige, and taupe to include a variety of intense colors, with many vivid shades of red, orange, blue, and green now taking center stage in spas.

Color can transform an ordinary room into one that is sleek, sophisticated, warm, relaxing, earthy, fun, or festive; however, it is important to note that color, like music, has an emotional effect on people and can trigger a wide range of reactions. As a general rule, light colors and pastels tend to be calming and soothing, whereas bright colors are stimulating or energizing.

While many are willing to take greater risks with color today, it is still important to be aware of socio-emotional or cultural differences. For example, in Western cultures, yellow often takes on a bright, cheerful, and optimistic character, but it is also known to stimulate mental activity, something that is not likely to promote relaxation in the spa. Yellow can also be associated with sympathy or longing; note that yellow ribbons are often wrapped around the trees of those with loved ones who are missing or at war. In Eastern cultures, yellow takes on a different character. In some instances, it represents aristocracy, but it may also indicate a confrontational or malicious nature.

If you like the idea of using bolder colors, many good interior design books provide illustrations and discuss the effects of color in depth. To get the full impact, seek out real settings where you can experience the color firsthand. How do walls of intense color make you feel? A good designer can help you to create harmonious themes by combining strong, bold colors with more muted tones or by softening a look with natural lighting, special effects, or textures. When selecting colors, it is also important to keep your clientele in mind. Strong color can put some on edge, causing feelings of anxiety, and many still prefer more sedative color schemes when they want to relax. If you are in doubt, get feedback from your target market and be sure that the colors you choose instill a sense of calm, serenity, and pampering (Table 5-1).

TABLE 5-1	COMMON COLOR ASSOCIATIONS
RED	high energy; passion; excitement; warning; danger; sensuality
ORANGE	stimulating; invigorating; cheerful
BLUE	tends to evoke peace and calm; healing; trust; but can also be equated with depression or "feeling blue"
GREEN	soothing; rejuvenating; natural; refreshing
YELLOW	evokes mental stimulation; compassion; sympathy, happiness
BROWN	stable; dependable; organic
PURPLE	royalty; power; richness; spirituality
BLACK	grief; mourning; sophistication
WHITE	purity; safety; cleanliness

MATERIALS

We've come a long way from the natural steam baths and hot springs of our spa ancestry, with innovations in design and technology that withstand the rigors of a more sophisticated spa environment. Still, many of the materials used in spas today come from natural and man-made substances that are environmentally friendly.

Ecologically sound, nontoxic, non hazardous materials that can stand up to mold and mildew have infiltrated spa design in a big way with durable products such as tile, concrete, natural stone, epoxy grouting, and biodegradable resins showing up on spa ceilings, floors, and walls around the globe (Figure 5-17). These materials are able to withstand moisture and are cleaned easily; however, it is always wise to confirm the extent to which all materials can be disinfected when making your selections.

The increased focus on sustainability has also influenced spa furnishings, which are being made from naturally textured woods, such as bamboo and cork, which are easily propagated without harm to precious trees. Other materials such as glass and wood products are being produced from recyclable materials and harvested from local sources whenever possible.

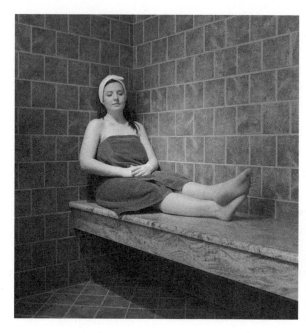

FIGURE 5-17 The natural stone used in this steam room is easily cleaned and able to withstand moisture, mold, and mildew.

Simple elements like earth, air, water, and fire are also playing a major role as naturally available waterways, open skies, clay, rock, and other landscape features become the focal point in many spa designs. Those subject to more confined spaces and limited budgets are taking advantage of fireplaces, wood stoves, candles, and natural scents to give spa-goers the sensation of communing with nature.

Luxurious stain-resistant and natural fabrics, textured walls, cultural artifacts, sandblasted glass, copper, and other metals that can stand up to high-traffic areas add another dimension to spa décor. Other less noticeable materials, such as soundproofing wallboards and rubber door seals, while not at the forefront of design, show the attention to detail that creates the ultimate spa experience.

LIGHTING

Lighting is an important component of interior design that serves two major purposes in the spa: it enhances the ambience and supports operations.

Light fixtures can provide just the right touch to spa décor, emphasizing period details or promoting a theme. For example, natural light can turn an otherwise claustrophobic environment into one that feels connected to nature no matter how small the window, an amenity that has been shown to have a soothing effect on clients. Natural light also brings out the beauty in colors, textures, and wall coverings and has the added benefit of conserving energy, another bonus for the ecologically conscious spa.

Lighting can also be used to accent or highlight prominent features, such as artwork, certificates, diplomas, and awards. In the retail area, the right lighting can actually encourage shoppers to linger longer and buy more.

In work areas, lighting should support the task at hand. Dimmer switches, soft accent lights, and candles are good choices in spa treatment rooms where lighting is an important part of setting the mood for a relaxing massage. The use of colored lights has become another popular choice in spas for its healing benefits. Lighting often needs to be changed to perform detailed tasks, such as those required for facials and hair removal. Makeup and nail stations are special areas of concern in the spa since the wrong lighting can cast shadows or significantly alter the true color. It is equally important to be attentive to the needs of administrative staff, who will appreciate replacing harsh fluorescent lighting with glare-resistant options.

When developing a list of all of your lighting needs, do not overlook outside lighting. Well-lit parking areas and walkways are imperative to safety. And be sure to explore energy-efficient options such as LED, compact fluorescent lighting, low-voltage and solar-powered landscape lighting.

DESIGN TRENDS

A number of trends are currently influencing spa design. A prominent theme is one that integrates various aspects of the local culture. Many spa designers are finding ways to bring the outdoors in by taking advantage of breathtaking views, flowers, plants, artwork, and other elements indigenous to the native habitat. Others are focusing on the historical aspect, ethnicity, or cultural heritage of an area, particularly in those instances where older homes are being renovated and refurbished into spas that reflect true period style.

With demographics at the forefront, designers are also making an effort to have spa décor reflect the target market by studying the color and style likes and dislikes of a spa's preferred clientele. The male market is one that has been studied carefully in an effort to attract more men to spas. This has resulted in less feminine environments that can cross the gender boundary and in spas that are designed solely with men in mind.

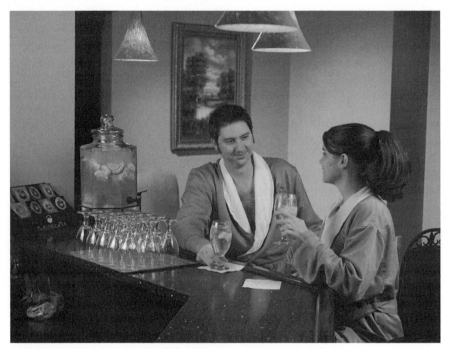

FIGURE 5-18   Café at Kimberly's Day Spa in Latham, New York.

Some spas are designing special rooms for exercise, yoga, meditation, movement, or dance therapy and other forms of energy work. Others are integrating cafés or tea lounges as an adjunct to diet and nutrition programs and coaching or consulting services (Figure 5-18). As spas begin to play a greater role in connecting people and raising awareness on a variety of health, beauty, and wellness topics, function or conference rooms that can accommodate social, business, and networking groups are also popular. If you have the space, this can enhance your profitability; however, it is wise to conduct a feasibility study before committing valuable square footage for this use.

The Environmentally Conscious Spa

In keeping with the whole health experience, we are witnessing an increasingly growing trend toward breeding ecologically conscious spas. Special-interest groups, local, state, and federal environmental organizations looking to protect the earth, consumer interests, and workers have a vested interest in conserving water, plant, and energy resources, eliminating waste, protecting the quality of our air, and promoting the safe use of chemicals. When planning your spa, be aware of any environmental standards that exist within the community or your state, since these could have a significant impact on the mechanical systems you choose to control air quality and ventilation. At the same time, you would be wise to investigate wind- and solar-powered resources that might be available to you.

The Environmental Protection Agency, the federal government agency responsible for developing national standards and enforcing government regulations and laws to protect the environment, is an excellent resource for best practices in environmental controls and offers several partnership programs for small-business owners, educators, and industry leaders. For more information, visit *www.epa.gov*. The Green Spa Network, a nonprofit organization dedicated to bringing sustainable practices to the spa industry, is another spa-specific resource that offers a number of practical tips on how to begin going green. For more information, visit the Green Spa Network Web site at *www.greenspanetwork.org*.

Maintaining Your Spa's Allure

A beautiful spa design deserves impeccable care. Engage your service providers and administrative staff by instilling clean work habits and enlist housekeeping in reporting signs of wear and tear. A monthly inspection will keep everyone focused on maintaining your spa's allure and can also help to prevent accidents.

The beauty of your spa can be further enhanced by paying attention to the many details that are so critical to creating a pampered effect. Surprise clients with simple amenities, such as fresh flowers that reflect the season, refreshments served on handsome trays, and delightfully scented soaps and candles. If your budget is tight, solicit local artists to display their artwork and embellish your waiting room with beautifully bound books purchased from resellers. Lush gardens, potted plants, and soothing waterfalls are other ways to instill a sense of beauty.

THINK IT OVER

The choices are endless when it comes to creating a beautiful spa design, but in the final analysis, it is important to remember that the most spacious or lavishly decorated spas are not always the most successful. It is not necessarily the number of treatment rooms you have, but rather how well they are used, that will make your spa a success. You can have the most beautiful interior design with expensive furnishings, but if it does not flow well,

---

Plan for Success

Some tips for designing an earth-friendly spa:

- Use naturally powered energy resources such as wind and solar power.
- Use locally harvested and/or reclaimed building materials.
- Install the most energy-efficient heating and air-conditioning systems available.
- Zone space for maximum climate control and efficiency.
- Select spa furnishings made from sustainable resources.
- Use easy-to-clean, nontoxic building materials.
- Make use of natural light and ventilation.
- Use LED and compact fluorescent lighting.
- Incorporate indigenous plants and the natural landscape in your spa design.
- Install low-flow fixtures in showers and basins.
- Incorporate a water-softening laundry system to reduce the use of water, detergent, and other chemicals.

is not managed properly, lacks attention to retail, or employs a staff that does not provide quality customer service, you have nothing more than an expensive showpiece.

A good design is one that incorporates a spa's philosophy, addresses its business goals, and immediately puts guests at ease. It is also one that never loses sight of the main reasons that people go to spas: to relax and rejuvenate.

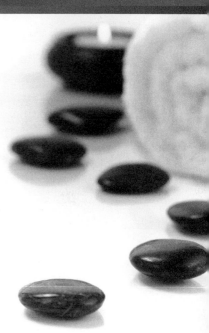

PURCHASING PROFESSIONAL PRODUCTS AND EQUIPMENT

Literally thousands of product and equipment manufacturers and vendors are vying for your spa's dollar in this fast-growing market. The good news is that a large number of them are working hard to provide spa owners with the tools they need to run a successful business by offering education, training, technical support, marketing materials, special incentives, and, in some cases, financing. How will you choose? Determining which products and equipment are right for your spa is a process that calls for careful examination of your spa concept and a great deal of investigation into the products and equipment that will produce the results you expect.

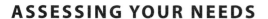

ASSESSING YOUR NEEDS

As you sort through various company literature, your primary concern should be: "What products and equipment best fit my business?"

Your spa concept or philosophy will be the biggest factor in the type of products and equipment you choose to incorporate in your spa treatments. If that philosophy is results-oriented, you will likely be searching for active ingredients and high-powered equipment. A spa that takes a more natural approach may be more interested in how the products they use are manufactured or the sources from which their ingredients are derived. Some spas attempt to integrate various methodologies, combining high-tech apparatus with relaxing spa therapies. Whatever your philosophy is, think about how the products and equipment you use will help you to establish a unique selling position. The right products and equipment are the main ingredients in setting your spa apart from the competition.

SETTING GOALS

Before making any spa purchase, you should be clear about two things: your budget and your target market. Budgeting should be at the top of your list. Remember that it is not hard to spend more money than you have, and overspending at the onset will definitely put you at a disadvantage. The best way to avoid this is to plan carefully and set limits. Go back to your business plan and look at your product and equipment allowance.

A solid financial plan will specify your initial investment in equipment, professional tools, treatment products and starting retail inventory. How did you arrive at this figure? Does it represent current market rates? Allow for top-of-the-line or more moderately priced equipment? Does it reflect high-end, moderately priced, or economical products? Incorporate all of the treatments you plan to offer? Cover accessories and incidentals, such as facial sponges, spatulas, linens, robes, waste receptacles, and other operating supplies?

If you have difficulty budgeting, sit down with your accountant or enlist the help of a spa consultant to assess viable options for your budget. You may need to make some sacrifices initially or postpone certain purchases until you are in a better financial position. Don't be too concerned about those items that do not affect your immediate business goals. There is usually more than one method to achieving a particular outcome. Perhaps you will decide to use certain products, such as enzymes and glycolic acid, and take some time to gauge client interest before investing in more expensive equipment, such as microdermabrasion, to perform exfoliation treatments.

CALCULATE THE RETURN ON YOUR INVESTMENT (ROI)

A clear understanding of your initial set-up costs is the best place to begin calculating the return on your investment. From this knowledge base you can begin to analyze the average costs and subsequent profit margins for each service and/or department, for example, the profitability of each facial, microdermabrasion treatment, chemical peel, or entire skin care, massage, hydrotherapy, nail care, etc. department. As an example, Table 6-1 outlines the equipment, products and supplies needed to set up a facial treatment room.

TABLE 6-1	COSTS FOR INITIAL SET-UP OF FACIAL TREATMENT ROOM
Equipment	**Cost per unit**
Bolsters (knee, head and neck cushions)	195.00
Boots & Mitts	70.00
Facial Bed or Table	2500.00
Facial System (high frequency, galvanic, vacuum, rotary brush, steamer, magnifying loupe)	1600.00
Hot Towel Cabinet	300.00
Hydroculator	325.00
Microcurrent Machine	6,800.00
Microdermabrasion	8,000.00
Oil/Lotion Warmer	130.00
Paraffin Kit (equipment and product starter kit)	190.00
Surge Protector	20.00
Swivel Stool	250.00
Trolley Cart	235.00
Utensil Sterilizer	170.00
Waste Receptacle	45.00
Wax Hair Removal Starter kit (includes wax heater & supplies)	150.00
Treatment Supplies	
Brushes	25.00
Comedone Extractors	20.00
Cotton Pads, Swabs, Gauze & Wipes	50.00
Disposable Apparel	75.00
Eye Pads	17.00
Facial Tissues	2.00
Fan for Facial Peels	5.00
Finger Cots	5.00

(continued)

TABLE 6-1	COSTS FOR INITIAL SET-UP OF FACIAL TREATMENT ROOM (CONTINUED)
Treatment Supplies (continued)	**Cost per unit**
Hair Clips	3.00
Hand mirror	4.00
Head wraps	15.00
Heat Packs	75.00
Lancets	6.00
Linens	675.00
Liners for Boots & Mitts	10.00
Paraffin Starter Kit	190.00
Plastic & Spray Bottles	5.00
Robes (robes, wraps & lounge pants)	800.00
Rubber Gloves	16.00
Scissors	9.00
Slippers	50.00
Sharps Box	4.00
Sponges	10.00
Stainless Steel Mixing Bowls	50.00
Table Paper with single roll dispenser	45.00
Tweezers	37.00
Utensils	45.00
Wooden Spatulas	5.00
Housekeeping Supplies	
Cleaning Supplies	10.00
Disinfectants	25.00
Laundry Bags & trolley	50.00
Paper Towels	1.00
Receptacle liners	4.00

TABLE 6-1	COSTS FOR INITIAL SET-UP OF FACIAL TREATMENT ROOM
Professional Skin Care Products (back bar size)	**Cost per unit**
Cleansers	220.00
Enzyme/Exfoliating Grains	150.00
Essential Oils	300.00
Eye Makeup Remover	52.00
Masks	500.00
Moisturizers & Lotions	875.00
Pre and Post Waxing Products	20.00
Professional Peels	1,000.00
Serums & Ampoules	850.00
Specialized Skin Care Products	1350.00
Sun Protection Lotion & Gels	300.00
Toners	275.00
Miscellaneous Items	
Ambience items, such as candles, etc.	150.00
Beeper/Pager	50.00
Client forms	16.00
Clipboard	5.00
Clock	15.00
Employee Uniforms [aprons, lab coats, pants, smocks]	55.00
Extension Cord	20.00
First Aid Kit	25.00
Estimated Total:	29,551.00

Please Note: These prices are meant to provide an example and should not be used to determine your cost basis. Individual prices will vary based on a variety of factors including current market rates for the type of product and equipment (basic, mid-grade, or high-end) you select, the manufacturer or vendor you purchase from, any discounts applied, package deals, etc.

Keep in mind that certain types of equipment will generate costs beyond the price of products or tools needed for operation that are not immediately obvious, such as the extra cost of linens and laundry services typically associated with hydrotherapies. Other factors, such as the method of compensation used for service providers will have a significant impact on your profitability. A detailed accounting of all of the direct and indirect expenses associated with performing each service is critical to calculating a realistic return on your investment.

Vendors can be an excellent resource when it comes to developing an understanding of profit margins. They are typically able to supply such information as the number of treatments that can be performed per quantity of product and the cost of using certain equipment. Remember that products used to perform services will be based on bulk product sizes, commonly referred to as *back bar*, or consumption supplies, not retail-size products.

Your vendor may also point out different equipment options, recommend multipurpose apparatus, or offer more economical package deals that allow you to save money. It is against the law for vendors to set prices; however, most companies will offer suggested retail product prices. Some provide guidelines for setting service charges. You will need to measure these prices against what the market will bear in your area.

Amortization

The rate of amortization, or depreciation, is an important factor in assessing the cost of equipment. According to the *Wiley GAAP 2004 Interpretation and Application of Generally Accepted Accounting Principles,* amortization is "the process of allocating an amount to expense over the periods benefited." When applied to tangible assets, such as equipment, amortization is generally discussed in terms of *depreciation,* or "the periodic charge to income that results from a systematic and rational allocation of cost over the life of a tangible asset." Calculating these deductions is a complex process with several tax consequences that should be reviewed carefully with your accountant prior to opening your spa.

Generally speaking the IRS allows you to recover, deduct, or amortize the cost of certain capital expenditures over a fixed period of time provided you have a valid business. To qualify for depreciation expenses property must first meet certain criteria, for example, the property must be something that wears out, or becomes obsolete, and has a determined useful life that extends beyond the tax year. Furniture and equipment are among those items that can be depreciated by a spa business; however, spa owners should be aware that the amortization allowance for start-up costs is limited and cannot be deducted all at once. Your tax accountant can help you to determine a set schedule for allocating the remaining expenses.

Amortization is a critical factor in the total cost of doing business; however, it does not minimize the need to make wise purchasing decisions. As a spa owner looking to get the most value for your dollar, you will want to ask: "What is the useful life of this product?" To put it more succinctly, "How many treatments can I expect to perform with this piece of equipment before it expires?" Purchasing the best quality possible at the onset of business will help you to get the most from your initial investment.

LEASE OR BUY?

Before signing a contract to purchase, it is wise to investigate any leasing opportunities that might be available. Initially, it may make more sense to "rent" equipment than to tie up a huge chunk of your capital. Don't forget that the amount of money you have invested in product and equipment will also have a significant effect on your cash flow. It is a good idea to review these items and the tax benefits of leasing versus owning with your accountant before making any purchases.

EVALUATE YOUR TARGET MARKET

Understanding the needs and wants of the consumer is the basis for a successful business. If you have done your homework, you should have a good understanding of your target market. What services and products do spa-goers in your area already use? Are there any other services or products they want or need? Is there a certain price range they are likely to accept? Which treatments do they tend to request most? If you do not have an established clientele or knowledge of the local market, you should conduct a thorough market analysis before investing in expensive products or hydrotherapy equipment that clients don't want and won't buy.

If you decide to introduce a new product to the market, don't underestimate client knowledge. The current media blitz has produced a new breed of spa-goers who are quite savvy about treatments and products. These clients are looking for proof that your treatments will achieve exactly what you say they will, and they may already have strong opinions on certain topics, such as animal testing, petrochemicals, and recyclable materials. Supply them with verifiable facts, articles, clinical studies, and before- and-after photos that can substantiate your claims whenever possible. It's up to you to select products that you can stand behind and to build confidence in those products and techniques.

Even with the most carefully calculated plan, the smart businessperson knows to anticipate a period when an expensive piece of equipment will not generate a profit. For example, hydrotherapy services, which require a substantial investment, can be a tough sell. Once again, consider the top 20 reasons that businesses fail, listed in Chapter 3, and plan ahead. Set goals that are achievable and implement a long-range marketing plan that will gradually increase business.

FEASIBILITY

Another important factor in selecting products or equipment is the size of your spa. Some spaces, no matter how well planned, will never be able to accommodate certain services. For example, if you are starting out with two or three 10' × 10' treatment rooms with little opportunity for expansion, it is unlikely that you will want to use this space for a hydrotherapy tub or go to the trouble of installing plumbing for it; however, you may be willing to convert one of these treatment rooms into a wet room that can also double as a massage room by installing a Vichy shower, steam, or Swiss shower.

Gathering Information

Knowledge is power; it is important to be well-informed before making any purchase. Although the Internet tends to be the first resource that people go to, I suggest that you do a little practical research before hitting the keyboard.

TRADE PUBLICATIONS

There are a number of ways to access information on products and equipment. It is often a good idea to begin your search by browsing through the most respected trade publications. This will give you some idea of the more prominent vendors within the industry. It will also give you a good indication of the company's philosophy and image. You can tell a lot about a company from its advertising campaign. You should be comfortable with the artwork, language, and overall style of the ad. Take note of those product manufacturers that are featured in articles, win awards, or are recognized for their contribution to education. Most trade publications also print directories that are helpful in narrowing the search. Look for a brief synopsis of the company's wares. With the number of personal care product and equipment manufacturers reaching unmanageable proportions, you could spend hours of your time needlessly qualifying companies.

TRADE SHOWS

Not all manufacturers and service providers advertise consistently in trade publications. Whenever possible, attend trade shows and engage with vendors face-to-face (Figure 6-1). A personal encounter is often a good indicator of the type of customer service you can expect. If the sales reps are knowledgeable and courteous, you can probably expect that company to be invested in educating and supporting their customers. Consider follow-up as well. If a company representative promises to contact you with more information but doesn't, how can you expect the vendor to deliver good service?

WORD OF MOUTH

Word of mouth is another important measure of a company's success. If those using the product speak highly of it and have had a good experience with the vendor or manufacturer, you are off to a good start. Whenever possible, find out more from them. Many companies supply a list of references or publish endorsements from satisfied customers. Don't hesitate to call or e-mail those people. Ask specific questions about the quality and effectiveness of the product as well as about the company's business ethic. Were they happy with the treatment they received from salespeople and support staff? On a scale of 1 to 10, what are the chances of their doing business with the company again?

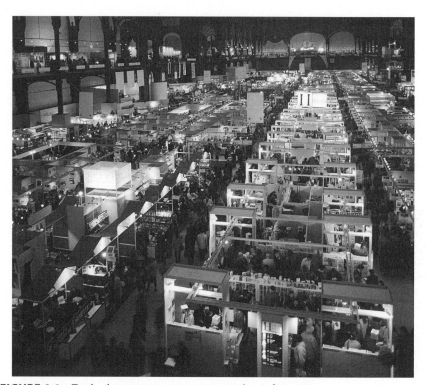

FIGURE 6-1   Trade shows are a great way to gather information.

COMPARATIVE ANALYSIS

You will also want to conduct cost and quality comparisons. For example, if you are interested in purchasing a Vichy shower, get information from at least three manufacturers. Carefully assess the benefits, features, and price of each model, and be sure you are comparing products of equal value. Products may appear similar but have distinctly different operating mechanisms.

Don't be too quick to buy, either. Acting hastily when you are presented with what seems to be a great deal may not be in your best interest. Take time to review all of your options carefully before making a selection, and always ask for documentation on the cost-effectiveness and life expectancy of the equipment, as well as claims about results or performance.

EXPERIENCE THE PRODUCT FIRSTHAND

You may find that a manufacturer does business with several distributors rather than interfacing directly with the consumer, in which case you may have the opportunity to visit a showroom in your area. If this is not possible, ask to be referred to someone in the area who is actually using the equipment you are interested in purchasing. Be up front about your mission and book an appointment to view the equipment and experience a treatment firsthand if possible.

OTHER RESOURCES

The best source of information is often the colleague sitting next to you at a seminar or trade show. Someone who has used the product or equipment or who has experience with a competitive product or technique can provide useful information. Professional organizations and product vendors are other viable resources and often conduct educational seminars. Of course, the latter will have a vested interest in promoting their wares.

Educational institutions are also good resources; however, as more schools become associated with or involved in distributing, manufacturing, and/or selling products and equipment, all information should be evaluated carefully. This does not mean that you cannot gain valuable information from an educator who is also a vendor, but it is important for you to substantiate any claims with scientific evidence and unbiased clinical studies. You must be comfortable with the credibility factor.

Finally, if all of this seems like too much work, consider hiring a professional. A spa consultant who is familiar with a multitude of products and equipment can help you to narrow your search by introducing products that are attuned to your philosophy, conscious of your target market, and respectful of your budget. This method could end up saving you valuable time and money.

Choosing a Product Line

It is rare that I meet a spa practitioner who does not have a strong opinion about the products they are currently using or those that they would prefer to be using. Whether the issue is quality, effectiveness, or ingredients, most service providers are passionate about their preferences.

BE AN INFORMED CONSUMER

- Attend trade shows.
- Read trade publications.
- Search industry directories.
- Request brochures.
- Compare cost and quality.
- Experience the product firsthand.
- Conduct your own testing.
- Join trade associations.
- Attend product seminars.
- Talk to others using the products.
- Seek expert opinions.
- Investigate the company's background and history.

Spa owners who are not licensed to perform spa services are often in a different position and may be forced to rely heavily on the expert opinion of their staff or spa consultants. If you are an unlicensed spa owner or one that is new to the spa industry, it is important to develop an unbiased and systematic approach to product selection. Taking advice from a loyal employee whose opinion you trust is one thing, but selecting products to accommodate an employee who has just begun to work for you can backfire if that person suddenly decides to leave without notice. The situation can intensify if no one else on your staff is familiar with the product.

Working with a spa consultant is often the answer for spa business owners with little experience in the industry. If you go this route it is important to ascertain the criteria the consultant will use to evaluate products for your spa and whether or not they receive a percentage for recommending certain products.

COSMETIC REGULATIONS

Spa owners, directors, and managers must be aware of regulatory standards when it comes to products used and sold in the spa. This has even greater importance if you intend to sell your own private label products. The Food & Drug Administration (FDA) is the federal government agency responsible for regulating the cosmetic industry. As we learned in Chapter 4, although the FDA does not require cosmetic products or their ingredients to undergo approval before being sold to the public, they do have regulations regarding packaging and labeling. If you decide to manufacture your own private label products you will be required to abide by those rules and list all of the ingredients contained in your products. Spa owners must also exercise caution in the way they describe cosmetic products which must avoid any reference to drug claims.

According to the FDA a cosmetic is "an article that is intended to be rubbed, poured, sprinkled, or sprayed on, introduced into, or otherwise applied to the human body or any part thereof for the purpose of cleansing, beautifying promoting attractiveness or altering the appearance." Drugs on the other hand are defined as "articles which are intended for use in the diagnosis, cure, mitigation, treatment or prevention of disease; and articles (other than food) intended to affect the structure or any function of the body of man or other animals." What is confusing is that certain products meet the definition of both. For legal purposes, the FDA determines the difference between the two by the intended use of the product; however, in today's sophisticated skin care market, the situation has become somewhat complicated with certain products commonly referred to as *cosmeceuticals* falling into what many cosmetic and health scientists perceive as a new category.

The term *cosmeceuticals* has been adopted by the beauty industry to denote the use of more active ingredients. Although these products may have a positive physiological effect on the skin; it is important to note the term cosmeceuticals is not recognized by the FDA. When marketing these products spa owners should be aware that cosmeceuticals are not drugs and should not be advertised as such. It is also important to train staff selling cosmeceuticals to steer clear of any reference that might imply altering the structure or function of the body (or skin). More information on this topic is available from the FDA's Center for Food Safety and Applied Nutrition, for those who wish to investigate further.

Plan for Success

There are several publications available through the FDA's online Cosmetic Industry Resource Center including a *Cosmetic Handbook* and *Cosmetic Labeling Manual* that can be helpful in navigating the *do's and don'ts* of cosmetic labeling and labeling claims. For more information, go to *www.fda.gov*, the official Web site of the Food & Drug Administration.

NARROW THE SEARCH

Fortunately, there is a way to make sound product choices and keep everyone happy. Begin by carefully researching only those products that fit your spa's philosophy. There will no doubt be numerous products that fit the bill, but the products you choose must also suit the wants, needs, and price range of your target market. This should help you to narrow the field significantly.

CHOOSE PRODUCTS THAT ENHANCE YOUR SPA'S IMAGE

Your final selections should be products that enhance your professional image. Before lining your retail shelves, take time to become familiar with the methodology behind the product and all facets of manufacturing. False claims, unethical advertising, poor working conditions, or the use of animal testing are some of the characteristics that can detract from a positive image.

ASSESS PRODUCT SAMPLES

When purchasing products, it is wise to sample them first, but don't expect samples to be automatically supplied. Small to mid-sized product manufacturers are often unable to provide free samples, so expect to pay a small fee to test their products. Some offer trial size packages that include a complete program for each skin type. In the long run, this is a cost-effective way to determine if a product line meets your criteria.

INCLUDE YOUR STAFF IN THE SELECTION PROCESS

It is important to include your service providers in the selection process. Your staff must be comfortable promoting the products you select. If the philosophy or methodology of a product is too difficult for them to understand or explain easily, it will come across poorly to clients. Without client confidence, those products are doomed to sit on your shelf, but the bottom line is that products not endorsed by your staff will not sell.

Engage your staff in the selection process by conducting your own studies with real subjects who are qualified to test the efficacy of a product. And keep in mind that asking someone with flawless skin to participate in a trial study of a product designed to improve wrinkles or correct hyperpigmentation is of no real value.

STUDY DISTRIBUTION IN YOUR AREA

Market saturation is another concern. Exclusivity is always a plus, but it is not always an option. Some distributors will claim to limit the number of accounts they maintain in an area, but it is still wise to check out the competition. Duplication drives prices down, and unfortunately, if you do not have a contract that guarantees your spa a certain share of the market, you have no recourse if the distributor suddenly decides to make the product available to your primary competitor. This practice has led many spa owners to develop private label lines.

GUIDELINES FOR CHOOSING A PRODUCT LINE

- Select only those products that fit your spa's philosophy.
- Be conscious of profit margins, wholesale price points and retail markup.
- Purchase products that your target market wants, needs, and can afford to buy.
- Make sure you are in agreement with the manufacturer's production standards.
- Have a good understanding of the manufacturer's methodology.
- Request product samples.
- Include your staff in the selection process.
- Assess product availability in your area carefully.

Philosophy + Client Satisfaction + Staff Endorsement
= Perfect Product for Your Spa

Brand Names versus Private Label

One of the biggest decisions spa owners face is whether to carry a recognized brand name or to custom-label products with their own identity. There are pluses and minuses to both.

BRAND NAME PRODUCTS

There are many high-quality brand name products on the market today. On the plus side, the right brand name, handsomely packaged at the right price point, will automatically enhance your spa's reputation. A well-established name brand offers instant name recognition and typically provides the spa owner with many valuable amenities, such as product education, training programs, and marketing materials that make it much easier to run a successful retail sales program. Larger brand name manufacturing companies are also in a position to use the newest technology to develop high-powered ingredients and methods that might otherwise be too expensive or complex to incorporate in a customized private label brand.

On the negative side, a brand name product may be readily available in too many places or priced too high to maintain profitable margins. This is not a reference to the brand name products sold on your grocery store shelf. There is a clear distinction between brand name products that are mass marketed and products that are distributed only through licensed professionals. Although it is important to note that occasionally, successful professional product lines have found it in their best interest to merge with larger conglomerations and "go retail," and spas end up in competition with products sold at the local mall or pharmacy. Another disadvantage to promoting a particular name brand is that it may be limited in its capacity to address all of the skin types and conditions on which your spa is focused, in which case you will be forced to carry several product lines to accommodate the needs of your clientele. Finally, the education and marketing a well-known brand typically supplies is usually built into the cost of the product. So although it may seem like a perk, it actually comes at a cost to you.

PRIVATE LABEL PRODUCTS

Private label manufacturers provide spa owners with an opportunity to place their logo or identity on a generic line of products. The major benefit to selling your own name brand is greater pricing flexibility. [Figure 6-2] Private label products are generally purchased at lower prices than brand names and then sold at much greater profit margins, with suggested retail prices often as high as three to six times the wholesale price. This profit potential, combined with the prestige of seeing your company name on the label, is often enticing.

On the negative side, private label products are sometimes associated with lesser quality. This is actually a fallacy since many high-quality private label companies offer a wide range of products for all skin types and conditions. What you should know is that research and development varies and may not be as current as you would like it to be and the selection of products may not include all of the latest ingredients and technology

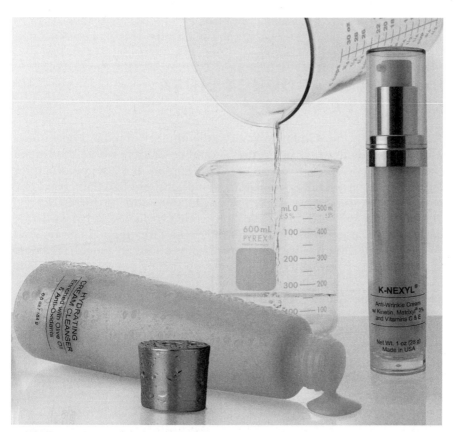

FIGURE 6-2 Private label products can enhance profitability.

your clients want. Unless you are developing a completely customized line and are involved in creating the formula, a process that could cost you considerably more money, you are really buying the philosophy of the manufacturer.

If you decide to put your name on a private label brand, keep in mind that you will still have to deal with the cost of label design and application, which generally includes additional plate fees and set-up charges. This could require more time and energy than you planned. Some private label companies will provide education and support, but it is not necessarily free. Marketing and promotional materials may also be available, but again, these will need to be customized for your use. If the private label company you choose does not produce camera-ready marketing materials, you will need to supply these on your own. All of these things can add considerable costs to what originally appeared to be a great way to stake your own claim in the marketplace.

HOW MANY PRODUCT LINES SHOULD I CARRY?

There are no set rules when it comes to the number of retail product lines your spa carries, however spa owners should be cautious not to overwhelm clients and service providers with too many options. It is also important for the products you sell to be in sync with your philosophy and the services you offer. Are your treatments mainly preventive, restorative, or corrective?

Many spas find that their philosophy is clearly aligned with a particular brand and will use this as the basis for their entire treatment program; however, frequently this practice does not encompass a broad enough selection. Supplementing your main product line with one or two other compatible lines, and/or targeted items from other collections, works for many spas. Keep in mind that there should be enough variety in terms of pricing and effectiveness to accommodate the needs and wants of all clients.

The location of your spa will also affect the number of product lines you can manage successfully. Generally, that number relates to the volume of customers you have and the size of your retail space. A spa situated in a busy shopping plaza or suburban mall is likely to have many more clients walk through its doors than one in a small village tucked on the outskirts of suburbia.

An important consideration is your staff. Juggling too many product lines can create confusion. Unless you have a dedicated sales staff, it is a good idea to limit the number of products you carry to a few quality lines with which your service providers are comfortable. Educating clients is an important part of building a successful retail sales department, and it is imperative that your staff appear confident in their knowledge. Maintaining relations with two or three vendors that can support your business with excellent training, marketing support and samples may ultimately be in the spa owner's best interest.

Skin Care Basics

You will need a variety of products to perform treatments and promote retail sales. For obvious reasons, not all professional products your practitioners use as back bar can be sold as retail items to customers. However, your back bar should support your retail efforts.

Back bar products include cleansers; toners; exfoliants such as chemical peels that contain alpha hydroxy, lactic, or salicylic acid; enzymes; scrubs; vitamin serums; ampoules, specialty masks; and other targeted skin solutions, lotions, oils, and creams for face and body treatments. These items should be supplemented with products that enhance the treatment benefit to the client at home. The following basic skin care products are the staples of a good retail program.

- **CLEANSERS** come in a variety of forms, such as cleansing milks, lotions, gels, and bars, and are typically categorized according to skin type. They may be further classified for deep cleansing or sensitive skin.

- **TONERS** complement the appropriate cleanser and are used to remove cleanser residue and balance the skin's pH level.

- **MOISTURIZERS** help to improve the skin's moisture balance and are typically designed for specific skin types and conditions, such as dry, oily, dehydrated, acne, or mature skin. They often have targeted ingredients to address specific skin care concerns, such as wrinkles or scarring.

- **EXFOLIANTS** are great for sloughing off dead skin cells between treatments. These come in several forms, including grains, scrubs, and lotions.

- **CORRECTIVE OR PREVENTIVE** treatments target specific skin conditions and body areas and include blemish lotions, anti-wrinkle creams and lotions, vitamin therapies, eye care, concentrated ampoules, serums, specialty masks, essential oils, body lotions, and cellulite treatments.

- **SUN PROTECTION** products should be a staple on every spa's retail shelf. These creams and lotions are typically formulated as either "chemical" or "physical" blocks to protect the skin against sun damage. They are often incorporated in everyday moisturizers and make-up products.

- **ACNE** products tend to be part of an all inclusive home care regime that includes cleansers, toners, blemish control lotions, and corrective treatments designed to work in unison.

- **AGE MANAGEMENT** products come in a wide variety of treatment forms such as serums, creams, lotions, and ampoules. They are typically part of a total skin care regime.

MakeUp

If your day spa offers makeup services, you will want to carry a line of professional makeup products for clients to purchase. Imagine how frustrated you would be if, after a 45-minute makeup session for a special occasion, you were not able to purchase the right shade of lipstick to touch up your look.

Many spa owners see makeup as an opportunity to sell their own line of cosmetics. For those who do not wish to carry a complete private label skin care line, this can be a less expensive way to invest in branding the spa's name; however, it may not be the most lucrative. If you cannot afford a high-quality, private label makeup line, you are probably better off with an established brand name. Makeup is an area where it is difficult to compete with well-known brands, and a poor quality product can leave clients disappointed after receiving an excellent service with luxurious products. If you can't compete here, the best advice is *don't.*

There are many good makeup lines to choose from. A number of spas are now opting to carry alternative makeup brands that are more in sync with a healthful spa image, such as mineral-based cosmetics. Mineral-based cosmetics may also be available from private label companies. This can be an excellent way to promote skin health, increase retail sales, and enhance your unique selling position.

Nail Care

Spas that offer manicure and pedicure services will certainly want to provide clients with their favorite polishes. Other hand and foot care items such as scrubs, body lotions, nail files, and pumice stones are an excellent way to promote maintenance between treatments. If you are concerned that supplying these items for sale will detract from repeat services, don't be. Manicure and pedicure services are two of the most popular spa amenities.

Clients purchasing these services are generally just as interested in the pampering aspect as they are in achieving a perfectly polished look.

Purchasing Equipment

Whether you are looking to wow clients with sophisticated technology and dramatic results or simply wish to procure the basics to provide therapeutic skin care and body treatments, you will need equipment.

Your spa concept is the most important factor when it comes to purchasing equipment, but there are other things to consider. Spa equipment is expensive and requires a substantial investment of capital.

GOVERNMENT REGULATIONS AND SAFETY STANDARDS

Technology is revolutionizing the spa landscape with new state-of-the-art apparatus, such as intense pulsed light, microdermabrasion, ultrasound, and photomodulation devices being marketed to spa professionals. This has generated a great deal of confusion and controversy over who is eligible to purchase and use such devices and how they are classified. To complicate matters further, laws vary from state to state. Before attempting to incorporate any equipment in a spa environment, it is extremely important to be well informed of the government regulations, safety standards, and liability issues involved. Always check with the governing boards in your state, as well as your insurance agent, when purchasing any piece of equipment to determine if it requires special licensing, medical supervision, or documentation of its use within your spa facility. Compliance with safety standards, such as those set forth by the US Department of Labor Occupational Safety and Health Administration [OSHA] for equipment usage in the spa is imperative.

FDA Classification

The Food and Drug Administration is the federal agency responsible for protecting the public's health and regulating controls on equipment use. It does so according to laws written under the Federal Food Drug and Cosmetic Act (FD&C Act) and what it assesses as the relative risk to the public. Under these laws, manufacturers of certain medical devices are required to obtain "marketing clearance" from the FDA before their equipment can be sold. To receive FDA clearance, a manufacturer submits

Plan for Success

Before purchasing any piece of equipment, the main questions for spa owners to ask are:

1. How will this equipment benefit my clients and improve my business?
2. Are there any regulations prohibiting this equipment's use in my spa?
3. Does my insurance company require any special training, licensing, supervision controls, or documentation to use this equipment in my spa?
4. Am I comfortable with the quality and safety standards of this product?
5. Is this piece of equipment worth the return on my investment?
6. What is the vendor's reputation for support, repairs and maintenance?

what is known as a 510k, or premarket notification (PMN) application. Other safeguards such as a premarket approval (PMA) may apply.

The FDA uses a three-tiered classification system to distinguish the level of risk involved in using medical devices. Class I indicates devices that present a minimum of risk or potential to be harmful. Class II devices are those that present a greater risk and subsequently require greater controls. Class III represents more complex medical devices that are used to sustain life, such as pacemakers, or those that have a far greater potential for unreasonable risk of illness or injury, such as breast implants, which require the strictest regulatory standards and controls.

What is confusing to many is that most Class I devices fall into a generic category of "exempted" devices. If a device meets the exemption criteria, its manufacturer is exempt from submitting a 510k application and does not need FDA clearance before marketing. However, it should be noted that the manufacturers of such products are still required to register and list their product with the FDA. It is also important to understand that any device that alters the skin can be construed as a medical device. Therefore, spa owners are wise to research the classification of each and every piece of spa equipment that is used in their spa carefully, including equipment that is used strictly for esthetic purposes.

Some equipment manufacturers are now issuing cautionary statements directly in their advertising to make spa owners and other consumers aware of the classification status of their equipment and to identify devices that must be purchased by a physician; however, not all are as conscientious. With laws changing so rapidly and some equipment falling into a "gray area," it will be up to you to research and determine how or if a particular device can be used in your spa and by whom. For more information on distinguishing medical devices and specific performance standards, visit the FDA's Web site.

STAFF TRAINING

It is a given that any new equipment you introduce to your staff will require some training; however, there is a difference between learning how to operate a certain piece of equipment and having a cognitive understanding of the theoretical principles involved. Before purchasing any new piece of equipment, especially those with high price tags, take time to assess your staff's capabilities. Are they familiar with the underlying theoretical principles and methodology, or will it require extensive training? This should be factored into the return on your investment.

BASIC SKIN CARE EQUIPMENT

Estheticians and skin care specialists use a variety of instruments to aid them in working more efficiently and productively. Basic skin care equipment typically includes a magnifying lamp, steamer, vacuum, spray and rotary brush, galvanic current, and high frequency machines (Figure 6-3). These items are often purchased in convenient multipurpose units. Your skin care philosophy is an important factor in determining whether or not this makes sense for your spa operation and budget. Purchasing these items separately may make more economic sense if you only intend to use a select few.

Magnifying Lamp

The magnifying lamp, typically referred to as a *loupe*, is one of the primary tools used by estheticians and skin care specialists to conduct skin analysis. These round-shaped lamps use cool fluorescent light bulbs and come in various powers of magnification, generally values of 3, 5, or 10, which are

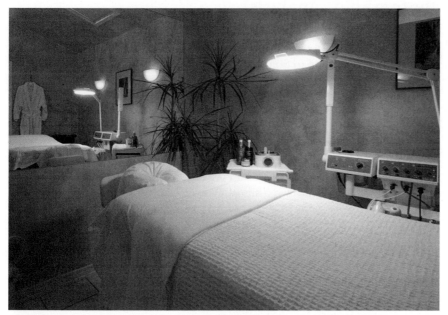

FIGURE 6-3 Treatment room with facial bed and basic skin care equipment.

known as *diopters*, that magnify an area to 3, 5, or 10 times of what the naked eye can see. This helps the practitioner to get a clear view of skin conditions. The magnifying lamp is particularly useful when working closely in the facial area, such as performing extractions to deep cleanse the pores.

Wood's Lamp

The Wood's lamp is a medically-based diagnostic tool that uses filtered black light (ultraviolet light) to illuminate certain skin disorders, such as fungi, bacterial disorders, pigmentation problems, and other skin irregularities. This lamp must be used in a dark room to reveal the different shades of color that are associated with various skin problems.

Skin Scope

This little "black box" creates a tent through which practitioner and client can simultaneously view the skin's condition via a two-way mirror. This setup is ideal for educating clients on their skin's condition. Various skin conditions are highlighted similar to the Wood's lamp.

Photographic Analysis

Advances in technology have introduced other more sophisticated complexion analysis tools that are capable of creating high quality, high resolution photos that can be used to quantify certain skin conditions (Figure 6-4). This has armed skin care specialists with a more objective approach to analyzing the skin.

Using ultraviolet light and white light photography client images can be manipulated to highlight various skin conditions, simulate the aging process and/or demonstrate the benefits of certain procedures. Sophisticated software archives photos and customizes individual client reports to aid the skin care specialist in client communication. Tracking client progress in this manner can have a significant effect on client compliance and the overall improvement of skin conditions, and lends credibility to many spa procedures that had previously been viewed as unquantified and subjective.

Steamer

The steamer acts as a mini-vaporizer to generate a fine mist of steam over the skin. Skin care specialists use it to oxygenate and stimulate the skin, improve circulation, and aid in unclogging pores. Many incorporate the

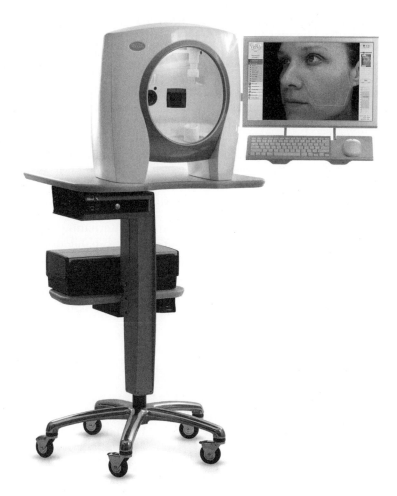

FIGURE 6-4 Photographic Analysis Equipment.

use of aromatherapy in steam sessions for added benefit and relaxation. Some steamers produce an antiseptic quality, which is beneficial in treating acne or blemish-prone skin types. Steamers come in several sizes and usually have a flexible nozzle for ease of use.

Rotary Brush

In recent years, rotary brushes have taken a backseat to more aggressive exfoliation products and treatments, but they are still used in many spas to gently cleanse and exfoliate the skin. When purchasing this type of equipment, make sure brush attachments can be removed easily for sanitization purposes.

Vacuum/Spray Machine

The vacuum is used to suction dirt and debris from the skin and promote circulation. Although its primary purpose is to aid in deep cleansing the pores, this type of stimulation is often conducted to "plump" the skin to give it a more youthful appearance. The vacuum is typically housed in a unit with a spray device that is used to scatter, or spray, a fine mist of product, such as a toner, over the facial area.

High Frequency

The high frequency machine makes use of an alternating or sinusoidal current to produce a mild heat effect, but it is not capable of penetrating products. This type of current helps to oxygenate the skin and promote circulation. High frequency also has an antiseptic effect on the skin, which is typically used post-extraction to coagulate open lesions. It is especially beneficial in the treatment of acne and blemish-prone skin.

Galvanic Current

Galvanic current is used by skin care specialists to perform two important functions: desincrustation and iontophoresis. *Desincrustation* is primarily used for deep pore cleansing, while *iontophoresis* is typically used to penetrate products into the skin. These techniques are extremely useful in treating a variety of skin conditions and have been used successfully in the skin care industry for decades.

The electricity in galvanic machines is typically measured in milliamperes (or one thousandth of an ampere). These machines supply a direct current of electricity (generally between 1-3 milliamperes or lower) that is regulated via a positive and negative pole to produce the desired chemical reaction. Newer models offer the practitioner greater control and a variety of safety features. As with any product or treatment, there are contraindications to its use which should be studied carefully and thoroughly reviewed with clients before administering any treatment.

ADVANCED SKIN CARE EQUIPMENT

Technological advancements have introduced several sophisticated new instruments to perform skin care and hair removal services in the spa.

Again, many of these newer technological tools are currently under a great deal of scrutiny by state regulatory agencies. As a reminder, before purchasing any advanced skin care equipment, always check the FDA classification and the regulatory standards that apply to its use in your state since these can vary. This should include a thorough investigation of the manufacturers' intended use and whether the state board that governs your spa business allows you to use it under the scope of your license. In addition, a careful review of the individual licensing regulations and scope of practice for each service provider who will be using the equipment is recommended. You will also want to be apprised of insurance

EQUIPMENT CHECKLIST

Spa equipment requires a substantial financial investment on the part of the spa owner with some of the newer technological tools, such as laser hair removal devices in the six-figure range; however, not all equipment is equal. Before purchasing any spa equipment review the following:

_____ Is the equipment registered with the FDA?

_____ What is the manufacturer's intended use?

_____ What safety checks are in place; does it have UL certification?

_____ Are there any contraindications to its use?

_____ What warranties and service contracts are available?

_____ What are the insurance requirements for liability and malpractice insurance?

_____ What are the laws and regulations for its use in spas in my state?

_____ What are the training and education requirements for service providers?

_____ Where and how can I receive training and education for this product?

_____ Is this equipment patented? By whom?

_____ Does the dealer/vendor have full authority to sell this equipment to me?

coverage for any piece of equipment you purchase. In some instances insurers may require proof of specialized training and education before issuing malpractice or liability coverage, or require other safety standards such as Underwriter's Laboratory (UL) Certification for equipment that poses a greater risk of harm.

The use of newer technological tools has also raised the bar in terms of education. Understanding the appropriate use of advanced technology in the spa including contraindications to its use is often a complex matter that requires increased education and training for all staff members. Today, many industry organizations are working hard to set standards and promote education. As a spa owner it is wise to investigate the political landscape and become familiar with the various groups sponsoring education. Attend trade shows and conferences and take as many unbiased educational classes as you can to understand the theory behind the technology, learn practical applications and become familiar with all contraindications to its use.

Additionally, if you are buying a product that is not manufactured in the U.S. you will need to take extra precautions. Be sure to investigate that the vendor has complete authority to sell and distribute the product or equipment you are considering, and is not infringing upon the patent rights of another, to avoid becoming involved in potential law suits.

Microdermabrasion

Since its introduction to the U.S. skin care market in the 1980s, microdermabrasion equipment has grown in popularity, evolving into a significant source of revenue for spa skin care departments.

Microdermabrasion machines perform a mechanical process that typically uses microcrystals made from aluminum oxide, or corundum to exfoliate or polish the skin (Figure 6-5). With little or no downtime and a wide range of treatment options that have demonstrated visible results over the years, many spa owners find this advanced treatment tool is easily integrated into the spa menu. The various models now available employ a variety of different features; including the use of various microcrystal substances, disposable tips and filters and diamond-encrusted tips; however, the basic design involves simultaneously spraying and vacuuming microcrystals across the face via a pressurized wand.

Specific licensing regulations and various education and training requirements for use of microdermabrasion in spas are in flux and continue to vary by state. Because microdermabrasion has the potential to do harm if used inappropriately, it is important that regardless of licensure

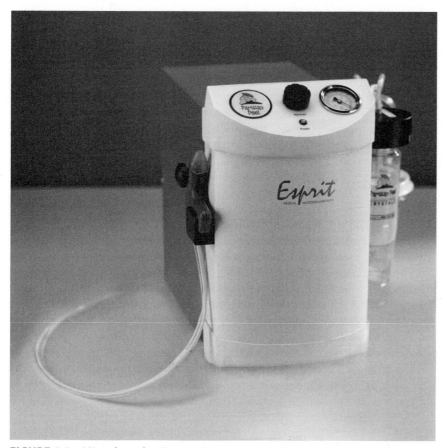

FIGURE 6-5 Microdermabrasion equipment.

anyone using this equipment have the proper training. This means more than a vendor-driven demonstration.

Microcurrent

Microcurrent is used to tone facial muscles, promote healing, stimulate lymphatic drainage, and penetrate products. Microcurrent machines use wave therapy, a minute level of energy (1,000 microamperes or less), similar to the body's natural energy system. They are commonly used to perform *electrical muscle stimulation*, a passive form of therapy that has been used to treat a variety of medical conditions.

In spas, treatments with these machines are commonly promoted as "nonsurgical face-lifts." Applications for body treatments, such as toning and firming the appearance of the skin are also popular. Microcurrent can have an immediate positive effect on the skin's appearance; however, it generally requires several treatments in succession to see longer-term results. If, you decide to purchase this type of equipment for your spa, be sure to appraise client expectations carefully and be cautious in marketing communications. This is not surgery, and you would be unwise to encourage clients to think they might achieve the same results.

Ultrasound

Ultrasound, or ultrasonic technology, uses a high frequency vibration or sound waves to warm the dermal layers of the skin. It is commonly used to penetrate products, a process known as *phonophoresis* (also referred to as *sonophoresis*), into the skin. Ultrasound frequency is measured in megahertz, with lower frequency levels producing greater depth of penetration of product. For example, machines used for esthetic purposes typically utilize an ultrasound frequency of 1 to 3 MHz, however equipment varies and should always be investigated for classification, intended usage and licensing requirements.

Ultrasonic machines for esthetic use are equipped with spatula and or blade-type hand pieces, that work through a water-based medium, such as a cleansing agent, specialized treatment serum or ampoule to produce high-frequency mechanical oscillations that can range anywhere from 20,000 to 28,000 vibrations per second. This action results in a process known as *cavitation*, which creates space between the layers of the skin allowing for greater product penetration and/or exfoliation of skin cells.

In addition to product penetration and the exfoliation of dead skin cells, ultrasonic waves are used to stimulate cells and increase circulation. Ultrasound also has a therapeutic cleansing effect, which can help heal certain skin conditions and reduce inflammation and edema. It is frequently used to treat cellulite and is often used in combination with other treatments such as microdermabrasion, microcurrent, or chemical peels to enhance its efficacy.

Lasers

The use of lasers has become a popular choice for the removal of unwanted hair, facial rejuvenation and other esthetic problems, for example, pigmented lesions, spider veins and varicose veins. Such treatments can be a significant source of revenue; however, the use of laser equipment requires a substantial financial investment and poses several safety, training, licensing, and liability concerns.

The term *laser* is an acronym for light amplification by the stimulated emission of radiation. This state-of-the-art technology uses a single colored light source that varies in strength and intensity and is capable of targeting a specific area of the face or body without damage to surrounding areas when used properly,.

Laser technology has come a long way since the inception of its use for esthetic purposes with several new models that are capable of producing excellent results on a variety of skin types with little or no downtime; however, lasers should not be thought of as generic devices with one model capable of performing all esthetic procedures. There are various types of lasers available for cosmetic purposes, each with specific uses that should be investigated carefully before purchasing.

Lasers are standard equipment in medical spas; however, there is currently a great deal of controversy surrounding their use in other settings. The potential for lasers to cause serious harm and bodily injury makes safety the primary concern. Although spa service providers, such as estheticians, may be allowed to use certain types of laser devices, for services such as hair removal, with proper medical supervision, spa owners should be aware that state laws for laser usage vary. Whatever the laws are in your state, highly specialized training and education is a must for all qualified technicians. Setup of your laser equipment requires strict adherence to laser equipment guidelines and special building and construction considerations, including adequate ventilation and electrical wiring. A thorough investigation of FDA, OSHA, and state requirements is imperative. Other safety standards such as those set forth by the American National Standard Institute [ANSI], a nonprofit, non-regulatory professional organization is recommended. Weigh the pros and cons of this equipment carefully before making any purchasing decisions.

Intense Pulsed Light (IPL)

Intense pulsed light, or IPL technology, is used for the purpose of removing unwanted hair and photorejuvenation. Photorejuvenation is a process that refers to the nonablative or nonvaporizing treatment of benign skin conditions such as vascular and pigmented lesions—more commonly referred to as age spots freckles, broken capillaries or telangiectasias, and spider veins. IPL treatments are also used to improve skin laxity by stimulating collagen production and are sometimes referred to as *photofacials*.

Similar to lasers, IPL devices use rapid pulses of light and heat energy to target specific areas of skin tissue, a process known as *selective photothermolysis*.

Variations in wavelengths allow the technician to gauge the effects of thermal penetration and avoid damage to surrounding tissue. IPL differs from laser in that, rather than using one color of light, it uses a broad spectrum of light. While the FDA limits the claim of permanent hair reduction to certain models and skin types, newer IPL technology allows for the effective treatment of a broader range of hair and skin colors and textures. There is generally no downtime and few side effects associated with IPL use; still it is important for spa owners to recognize that the use of IPL equipment can result in serious harm in untrained hands. As in the case of lasers highly specialized training and education and safety measures are crucial. All other general precautions for purchasing advanced equipment apply.

Light Therapy (LED)

Light emitting diode therapy, commonly referred to as LED, uses *photomodulation,* or light technology, to penetrate the dermal layer of the skin and is primarily used to stimulate collagen, reduce fine lines, and heal the skin. These devices use one or more individual wavelengths of light delivered at a low intensity, however model classifications do vary, so it is important to check the FDA classification and manufacturer's claims before purchasing.

LED is based on the premise that certain frequencies of light are capable of triggering a natural *photobiochemical* reaction to achieve specific results. For example, red light is commonly used for skin rejuvenation. In this case, the light is used to stimulate cellular activity that in turn prompts fibroblasts to produce collagen and elastin. Blue light is another popular treatment used to destroy the bacteria that causes acne.

Depending upon on its application, LED therapy may warrant a series of successive treatments to demonstrate visible results. These treatments may be used as adjunct or complementary therapies to other treatments such as microdermabrasion and chemical peels.

Hand-Held Devices

In much the same way that cell phones, laptops and PDAs have revolutionized the business world, the spa business boasts a number of convenient new treatment tools that are helping spa owners to maximize space and increase revenue.

Smaller battery-powered cordless devices, such as wearable visors for analyzing the skin, moisture-analyzation meters, hand-held ultrasonic exfoliation and mini-microcurrent devices are making their way into spas (Figure 6-6). These compact instruments can be conveniently carried to

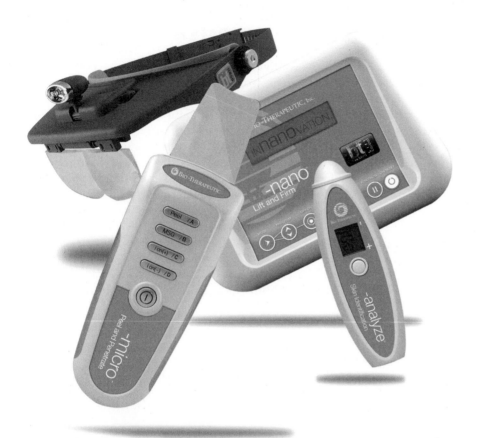

FIGURE 6-6 Compact treatment tools and hand-held devices offer convenience and versatility.

virtually any location making them ideal for combination treatments and promotions that can take place almost anywhere in the spa or may be used at off-site events, such as health and beauty fairs.

While not all equipment will be the right fit for your spa retail center, spa owners should be aware that other advanced mini treatment tools, such as microcurrent, microdermabrasion and LED technology, are now available to clients for at home use in treating acne, age management and conducting hair removal.

HYDROTHERAPY EQUIPMENT

Historically, the word *spa* is thought to be derived from the Latin phrase *salus per acqua*, meaning "health from water." Hence the notion of what is commonly referred to as "taking the waters." Before technology prevailed, *taking the waters* meant steeping the body in natural aquatic environments, such as mineral baths or hot springs. Today, the term *hydrotherapy* indicates the use of water or steam to perform a variety of therapeutic treatments that are conducted with different apparatus. If you take a traditional approach to spa therapy, you will want to include one of these options. In fact, by most standards a day spa is not considered a spa without some type of hydrotherapy equipment.

Hydrotherapy Tubs

Hydrotherapy tubs use pressurized air and water systems to mechanically alter the flow of water within (Figure 6-7). Newer technology allows

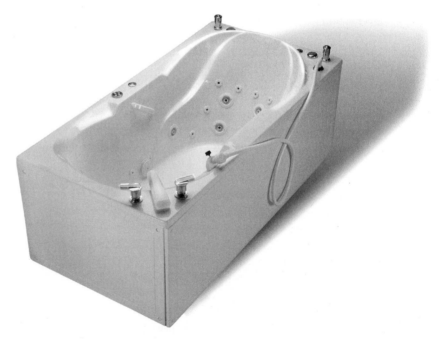

FIGURE 6-7 Waterford Hydrotherapy Tub.

therapists to choose from a number of programmable features that can be customized or coordinated with specific massage techniques while the client rests comfortably in the tub. A manual massage hose is often incorporated to increase the benefit of these treatments.

Hydrotherapy treatments are primarily used for detoxification, deep tissue massage, and relaxation purposes. They are typically used in conjunction with body scrubs, seaweed, and mud wraps. They are a favorite of athletes and can help to alleviate muscle aches and pains associated with many ailments. The hydrotherapy tub is also used for cosmetic purposes, such as in the treatment of cellulite.

When purchasing a hydrotherapy tub, pay careful attention to the size of the tub and water capacity. Water weighs approximately 8.35 pounds per gallon, so if your tub has a 66-gallon capacity, this means that it will be holding about 550 pounds of water. When you add the weight of the tub to body weight, you have a heavy-duty piece of equipment. The drainage system is another concern. Tubs must be emptied quickly, and it is imperative that they are sanitized with a hospital-grade disinfectant between each and every treatment to prevent the spread of harmful contaminants. Look for models that are ergonomically structured and make draining and sanitizing easy on the therapist. Check energy requirements and noise levels on these machines as well. Quiet, energy-saving devices will help to keep costs down and the relaxation benefit high.

Scotch Hose

This simple yet effective hydrotherapy treatment uses a long hose to direct hot and cold water pressure to precise areas of the body. The Scotch hose is ordinarily mounted on a wall and has two separate hose extensions with attached nozzles and temperature and pressure gauges to regulate the force of treatment (Figure 6-8).

This apparatus requires enough space for the therapist and client to be positioned approximately three centimeters away from one another but is easily incorporated in most wet rooms. Treatment is conducted by the therapist who guides the hose to deliver a small stream of water aimed at specific body areas. This treatment produces an invigorating yet relaxing massage and is often used to enhance athletic performance. It is also used to treat a variety of muscle and skeletal conditions and circulatory problems.

Vichy Shower

At first glance, the Vichy shower appears to be a complex instrument. However, with careful planning this popular hydrotherapy shower is easily

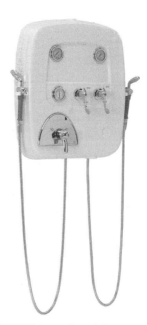

FIGURE 6-8   Scotch hose.

controlled and provides the spa therapist with substantial convenience when performing those treatments that incorporate messy exfoliating scrubs, mud, or seaweed-type body masks.

The Vichy shower is comprised of multiple shower heads placed above a waterproof table or bed and arranged to cover the entire body (Figure 6-9). Treatment is performed with the client lying in a relaxed position on the bed as a steady stream of water, similar to a gentle rainfall, cascades atop the body.

Vichy showers typically incorporate five to seven shower heads and vary in price accordingly. Shower heads can be plumbed directly into the ceiling or extended outward from a control panel placed on the wall. Beds are often sold separately and may be ergonomically designed to allow for flexibility in treatments. This is an important factor, as you will want beds that can be used for dry massage therapies or body treatments when not in use for hydrotherapy.

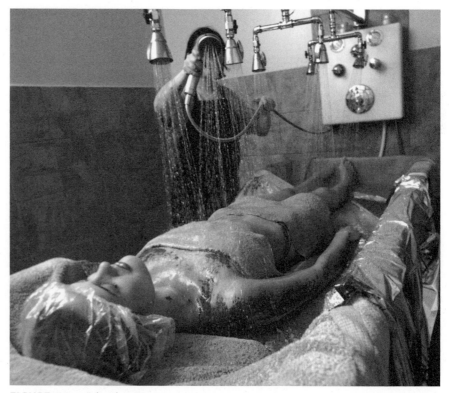

FIGURE 6-9   Vichy shower.

When purchasing a Vichy shower, look for materials that can withstand vigorous disinfecting agents and are also rustproof. These rooms require constant and impeccable sanitation standards to prevent the build up of harmful mold, mildew, and other bacteria that can cause cross contamination. Again, drainage is a primary concern. Mud, scrubs, and seaweed can clog drains and present significant waste disposal problems. However, with all of these under control, the Vichy shower is an excellent form of hydrotherapy massage that can be beneficial to many clients.

Swiss Shower

The Swiss shower is one of the most convenient hydrotherapies available and takes up considerably less space than the hydrotherapy tub or Vichy shower. This hydrotherapeutic shower uses nine or more high-powered spray jets positioned in each corner of the shower to surround the body (Figure 6-10). Some of these showers also include a Scotch hose or hand-held spray. The force of the sprays can be adjusted according to the purpose of the treatment and client preference.

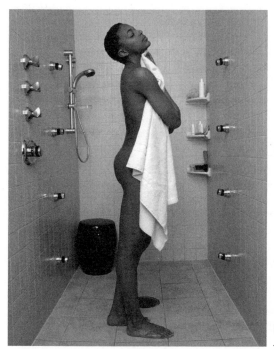

FIGURE 6-10 Swiss shower.

Swiss shower heads can be plumbed directly into the walls of a regular shower or purchased as a separate unit or module. The Swiss shower is often used in conjunction with body treatments and massage therapies for the purpose of relaxation and deep cleansing.

Steam Shower

Steam showers produce a fine mist of warm moist heat that is ideal for detoxifying, cleansing, and hydrating the entire body. This hydrotherapy treatment is often used in conjunction with aromatherapy and has a relaxing and therapeutic effect that is ideal for the muscle strain and pain associated with many ailments. Steam sessions are easily incorporated into body and massage treatments and are an ideal way to generate additional revenue. Units can be built in or purchased as prefabricated modular units. Again, when using this type of apparatus, sanitation is a primary concern. Make sure walls and floors can be easily sanitized to prevent the spread of harmful bacteria.

Foot Spas

Foot spas or pedicure stations are a great profit center for spas and have become extremely popular even with those who do not ascribe to other forms of hydrotherapy. The numerous models and styles range from simple, portable, foot spas that can roll in front of any chair to luxurious "throne-types" that require specialized plumbing (Figure 6-11). In addition to the standard whirlpool system, many of the luxury models incorporate features such as reclining and heated chairs with motorized massage functions, thermostatically controlled water basins, cushioned headrests, and cup-holders that contribute greatly to the pampering experience.

Because foot spas tend to generate a high turnover throughout the day, the danger of cross-contamination is again a primary concern for spa owners. It is imperative that all equipment and instruments associated with this spa service are completely disinfected in between clients. When purchasing a foot spa, look for one that provides quality sanitization assurance. Many of the newer models are incorporating power drains and automatic disinfecting systems, or what is known as *pipeless* technology. This eliminates the use of internal pipes that can harbor and spread bacteria. Whichever technology you choose, always ask for information to support the theory behind recommended sanitation methods. Follow up with your own research, investigating reports of any cross-contamination incidents associated with using the equipment.

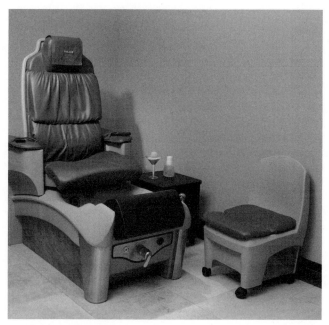

FIGURE 6-11 Pedicure throne.

The safety of the technician is another concern so keep the needs of the service provider in mind when purchasing a foot spa and pedicure station. Look for ergonomically correct models with adjustable stools to accommodate the needs of individual technicians. Otherwise, sitting in an awkward position without back support can turn into an occupational hazard.

Saunas

Saunas are self-contained rooms constructed entirely of wood. These rooms are set at high, but tolerable, dry heat temperatures that encourage the body to perspire profusely. Many incorporate the use of aromatherapy to help rid the body of toxins, relax aching joints or stiff muscles, and promote relaxation. The most popular is the Finnish sauna (Figure 6-12).

TREATMENT FURNISHINGS

Facial beds or chairs, therapist stools, massage tables, and workstations are basic tools of the spa trade. Over the years, these furnishings have

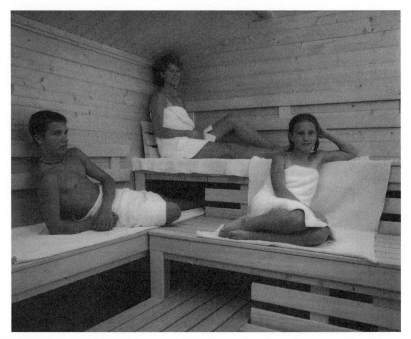

FIGURE 6-12   Finnish sauna.

become increasingly more sophisticated, incorporating a variety of high-tech features.

Facial Beds

Consider your facial bed (also referred to as a facial table), or chair, the main ingredient in any treatment you perform because how comfortable a client feels in it will affect everything else you do.

Three factors should be at the top of your list when purchasing a facial bed: (1) versatility, (2) comfort, and (3) durability. Many beds are designed for dual purposes, such as facials and massage or facials and pedicures. The type of services your spa offers will be the deciding factor in your selection. But whether you prefer a chair or bed, it should be ergonomically correct for both clients and service providers. Some beds come with electric or hydraulic lifts and swivel action that make it easier for clients to get on and off and for service providers to adjust the height of the bed to a comfortable working level. These great features will help to increase both client and employee satisfaction.

The size of your spa will affect your decision as well. If you are pressed for space, a facial bed that offers the most versatility is a good choice. Think about the other services you will need to perform, such as waxing and body treatments. Will your selection lend well to these types of treatments?

Durability is always a factor in high traffic spas. If your spa is open six days a week, 52 weeks a year, and your facial bed is used for a variety of treatments, this one piece of furniture will undergo tremendous use. Hopefully, it will be able to withstand the volume over several years. To increase the return on your investment, look for high-quality pieces made from durable materials that can be cleaned easily. Other amenities, such as storage cabinets, towel warmers, pedicure basins, and manicure arms, may also add to the appeal of your selection.

Stools

Many spa treatments are best performed sitting down. But sitting for long periods of time can create pressure in the legs and the back that cause fatigue. The right stool can help to eliminate many of these symptoms. You will want your service providers to be as comfortable as possible when performing treatments; so look for ergonomically correct stools that can be adjusted to support a range of heights. Seats should have ample padding made of quality vinyl or other material that is easily cleaned, and durable castors to allow for ease of mobility.

Trolleys

Most treatment rooms have built-in cabinet space for storage, but some items like towels, cotton pads, tweezers, and lancets are best kept close by to maintain the flow of services. Certain spa equipment will at times need to be moved to accommodate treatment procedures, and some equipment will need to be shared, in which case moving it from one treatment room to another is an issue.

Trolleys and carts are ideal for those items that require mobility or when having certain supplies nearby makes work more efficient. There are many styles to choose from depending on your needs. For example, heavy equipment will require a sturdier cart, while the simultaneous use of machines can require extra electrical outlets. Certain accessories may call for extra storage or drawers for supplies. Trolleys take a lot of wear and tear, so you will want to consider maintenance as well. Stainless steel carts cost more, but they can be cleaned easily and are extremely durable.

Manicure Tables

Manicure tables are often in a highly visible section of the spa, so they should be both attractive and functional. Choose ones that blend well with the theme of your spa's décor and can accommodate the type of nail services you provide. The height of your tables, accompanying technician stools, and client seating are important considerations in maintaining ergonomic viability. Tables with castors can also make it easy to provide simultaneous services or accommodate services in another location should the situation arise. If space is an issue, look for tables that have extra storage built in for paraffin heaters, polishes, and other supplies.

Wet Treatment Tables

Tables or beds used for hydrotherapy treatments must be safe, durable, and practical. The extreme conditions associated with the continuous application of water and other spa solutions call for tables made of high-quality, rustproof, and noncorrosive materials. Those with built-in drainage systems are ideal for body treatments that require the use of dense and grittier products, such as mud packs, seaweed wraps, salt scrubs, and other exfoliating agents (Figure 6-13).

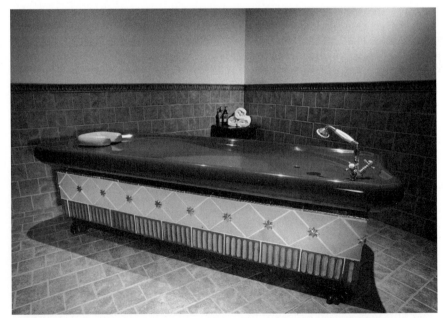

FIGURE 6-13   The Hamam Table at Kimberly's Day Spa in Latham, New York, incorporates a heating element that keeps the client warm during hydrotherapy treatments and is ideal for wet body treatments, such as mud or seaweed wraps.

Massage Tables

Many spa owners complain about the quick turnover rate in massage therapists, which often leaves me wondering about the quality of working conditions in this labor intensive field. An uncomfortable massage table is definitely out of the question for spa-goers looking to relax or relieve aches and pains. But it is just as important to recognize that a poorly designed massage table will have a negative impact on employee performance.

Investing in solid massage tables with sufficient padding, flexible armrests, and hydraulic lifts is money well spent. Some tables are now being designed with additional conveniences, such as storage space for equipment and towels or hot cabbies and lotion warmers to keep everything within the therapist's easy reach (Figure 6-14).

Tables that allow massage therapists to work on clients in either a face up or face down position will provide a greater range of motion and better work conditions. Any table you purchase should also have an adequate range of height and be able to accommodate variations in body size and weight. Those with hydraulic lifts will help to take the pressure off your massage therapists and prevent injuries. Tables that are compliant with the Americans with Disabilities Act (ADA), may also qualify for a tax deduction.

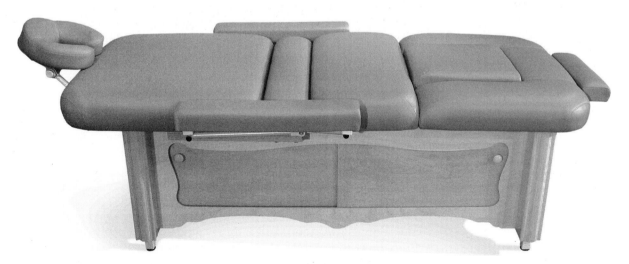

FIGURE 6-14 Massage table. The Grand Versailles by Golden Ratio. Woodworks, Inc.

If your massage therapists have adequate training, you might consider investing in a special table for pregnancy massages. Other more compact massage chairs can be ideal for quick stress-relief treatments or mini massages and have the added bonus of being easily transported to special events or on-site visits which can help to boost public relations and enhance your unique selling position. No matter how expensive or how many amenities a massage table has, it is likely that you will need to use other specialty pillows, bolsters, or head supports to make clients more comfortable.

Any massage table you select should ultimately be one that is within your budget, but it is also wise to employ your massage therapists in the selection process. A table that meets their standards will help you to pay it off more quickly.

PERMANENT MAKEUP

Permanent makeup, or cosmetic tattooing, has become a popular treatment on many spa menus. If you are interested in incorporating this procedure in your spa, be cautious. Equipment is expensive, and there is always a danger of infection, which makes it a high-risk procedure. Hire competent people or train only those with excellent makeup and fine motor skills.

Regulations for permanent makeup have several layers. The technique used to perform permanent makeup, sometimes referred to as *micropigmentation*, is conducted with a needle that applies colored inks. The inks that are used in permanent make-up application are subject to FDA regulation as cosmetics. The pigments used in these inks are considered color additives and require pre-market approval under the Federal Food, Drug and Cosmetic Act. Although the FDA has the authority to enforce this practice historically it has not acted upon it.

Procedural regulations are governed by the individual state and local municipalities in which they are performed. These vary widely, so it is important to check with all governing boards including city or town, county, and state offices that apply, as well as your insurance agent, before purchasing equipment. For a more detailed explanation of the FDA's current position and related research contact the U.S. Food and Drug Administration Center for Food Safety and Applied Nutrition at *www.cfsan.fda.gov*. The Society for Permanent Cosmetic Professionals (SPCP) is another nonprofit organization that can be helpful to those seeking guidance on education, certification, and industry guidelines. The SPCP also provides direct links to individual state legislative bodies. For more information, visit *www.spcp.org*.

There are other important factors to consider when consulting with clients. Although the goal should be to create a natural look, it is important to remember that permanent make-up can alter a person's appearance significantly. This technique is commonly used to treat the lips, brows, under eye, and areola, or nipple areas. To achieve satisfactory results, train staff to carefully assess each client's goals and expectations and take care to inform the client of any contraindications and/or risk involved.

AIRBRUSHING EQUIPMENT

This mechanical device is an excellent tool for spas that want to provide clients with the look of a tan without sun damage. Treatment is performed with a gentle air compressor that propels a fine mist of tanning solution across the body. It is also used to apply face makeup and is popular with those performing makeup services for weddings, film and television.

A variety of models are available; some more effective than others. Airbrushing "booths" are far more expensive than simple compressors, but all require adequate ventilation and diligent maintenance to deal with overspray, which can be a nuisance. If possible, conduct a trial run of the various types before making a selection, and research all safety precautions carefully to prevent inhalation of the mist, which is prohibited. You will also want to assess the return on your investment. In recent years, the number of "tanning salons" performing this technique as their primary service has increased. It is a good idea to survey client interest and determine whether or not this service will add any real value to your spa business before investing the time, space, and money.

ACCESSORIES

Your spa will need several other accessories to sanitize, sterilize and maintain the correct temperature of products and lotions used to perform services. Sterilizers, autoclaves, sanitizers, wax heaters, hydrocollators, hot towel cabbies, hot stone warmers, lotion warmers, heated mitts and booties, and thermal blankets are just some of the essential tools of the trade. Expenses associated with these smaller items can add up, so shop wisely. Anticipate a lot of wear and tear, and buy quality products that can stand up to what you hope will be rigorous daily use. Above all, don't skimp on important disinfection and sanitization tools. These items provide clients with the quality assurance and confidence they need to rebook your spa services.

SUPPLIES

Cotton, gloves, finger cots, lancets, sharps boxes, mixing bowls, shammies, facial sponges, cotton swabs, tweezers, cuticle sticks, nail files, buffing blocks, polish remover, oils, makeup brushes, mask brushes, clippers, wax strips, wax applicators, disposable spa apparel, headbands, tissues, towels and linens, head wraps, robes, slippers, alcohol preps, disinfectants, cleansers, and laundry detergent—the list of supplies needed to perform services may appear endless when setting up your spa for business. Your best bet when purchasing spa supplies is a vendor who is knowledgeable about the spa business and invested in providing you with excellent customer service. Shop before you buy, but don't base your decision on price alone. Look for quality products and the opportunity to build a working relationship with a vendor you can trust (Figure 6-15).

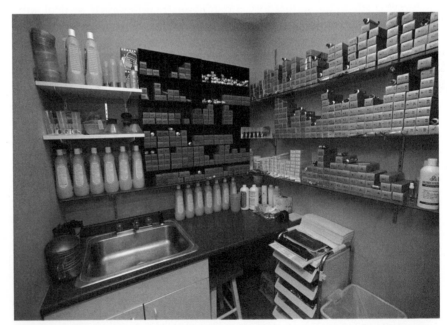

FIGURE 6-15   Purchase spa supplies from a credible vendor who is knowledgeable about the spa business and is willing to work with you to build a mutually satisfying relationship.

Qualifying Vendors

You know what you need to buy, but before you place your credit card or cash on the table, you should assess the reputation and business ethics of the supplier. Credible companies understand that their success comes from empowering you, and they will work hard to build a mutually satisfying business relationship.

CREDIBILITY

To find out if the company you are dealing with is credible, you will need to conduct a little research. First, find out how long the company has been in business. Is it a subsidiary or a distributor for a larger company? If not, will you deal with the manufacturer directly, or does the company have a sales representative in your area? If possible, sit down with that person for a face-to-face conversation. It is often helpful to create a list of questions before meeting. Some of the things you will want to know are: Is a minimum purchase order required? What warranties or guarantees do they offer on their products or equipment? How long does it take to process orders? Receive a shipment? What is the policy on returns or damaged merchandise? Can you expect a loaner if your equipment needs service or repairs? Will you be charged for this service, and what is the turnaround time? What type of training and education is offered? How many times a year is this available? What is the protocol for educating staff on new products and treatments that may become available? When you have completed interviewing potential vendors, rate the service you received. On a scale of 1 to 10, how knowledgeable did the company representative appear to be?

FINANCING

Financing and payment policies should be at the top of your list. Make sure you understand these policies prior to opening an account. Some of the things you will want to know are: Will you need to prepay for your first purchase? After that can you expect to be billed on a regular basis for additional orders? What terms are applied to invoices, net 10 or 30 days, or are all payments due upon receipt? If payments are late, will finance charges be applied? What forms of payment does the company accept? Will you be limited to the use of certain credit cards or need to supply cash or checks only? If you are purchasing expensive equipment, are there any circumstances under which the company will extend credit or offer a payment plan? Whatever information you are presented with, be sure to check the fine print. Although policy information and contracts can be lengthy and tedious to read, it is ultimately your responsibility to understand the terms of your agreement. If you do not understand the terminology, it is always best to seek professional advice.

CUSTOMER SERVICE

Spa owners and managers are busy people. Make sure the people you purchase the tools of your trade from understand the spa industry and can provide competent, reliable, and consistent quality service before you give them your business.

How well a company manages telephone calls is often a good indication of its customer service policy. Conduct a quick test before you sign on and note how easy it is to get through to the supplier by telephone. Are you left lingering for several minutes? Prompted through lengthy computerized messages? Does the messaging system refer you to a Web site rather than a real person? If you are referred to a Web site, is it user friendly and does it provide adequate information and support? Does it supply a means of contacting a company representative? Try contacting the company via telephone and the Web, and gauge how long it takes to get a response.

Once you get through to a company, perform a careful assessment of the sales staff. Are customer service and sales representatives knowledgeable and courteous? Do they return calls promptly? Do they answer your questions in a timely manner, or does every question need to be referred to a higher authority? A qualified staff can be the deciding factor in who gets your business.

TRAINING AND EDUCATION

Knowledgeable service providers are the key to selling any spa service or product. Therefore, you will want to do business with a company that takes education seriously. A manufacturer or distributor that supplies comprehensive instructional manuals and training is one that is invested in your success.

Whenever possible, examine the quality of the training manuals that will be supplied to you. Are they thorough, well organized, and well written? Does the company provide additional pamphlets, charts, or tables that make it easy for technicians to use as a quick reference or guide? Training videos can be another excellent resource for those who are visual learners. All of these tools can make a big difference in your staff's confidence.

Training methods vary among suppliers. Although it is typically the most advantageous to the spa owner, not all vendors provide on-site instruction. Many companies simply cannot afford the expense involved in sending educational staff to each and every account. A popular approach is one that involves educational seminars in several key geographic locations throughout the year. Many companies also offer classes and seminars at trade shows. Online tutorials may also be available. Whatever method is used, find out what the costs are to you. Some vendors charge a minimal fee to cover expenses or to provide lunch. Others offer complementary training seminars and arrange for discounts on travel and hotel accommodations. In certain situations, the cost of a seminar can be applied to an opening order.

MARKETING SUPPORT

Marketing is the driving force behind sales. Manufacturers and vendors that understand this concept will provide you with the marketing and promotional materials you need to be successful. These can include consumer brochures, posters, product displays, or direct-mail postcards that help you to promote their products and equipment throughout the year. Many vendors have cooperative advertising programs or are willing to supply you with the materials or artwork needed to launch your own ad campaign. This can cut down on the cost of advertising considerably. Others will supply photos and text that can be used in developing your spa's brochure.

One of the most important marketing tools supplied by vendors comes in the form of sales training. Teaching service providers and administrative staff how to sell is one of the biggest challenges spa owners face. Companies that are willing to support spa professionals in developing the skills needed to increase retail sales and promote services create a win-win situation for all.

THINK IT OVER

A great deal of effort goes into choosing products and equipment. Your spa's philosophy and the needs and wants of your target market are two of the biggest factors in the selection process. The amount of money you can afford to invest is another primary factor. Licensing restrictions and government regulations will also have a significant impact. But in the final analysis, it is often a vendor's business and customer service policies that are the deciding factor. Conducting business with a supportive team of knowledgeable professionals can make all the difference in which products and equipment you decide to use.

TECHNO-SAVVY: USING COMMUNICATION SYSTEMS IN THE SPA

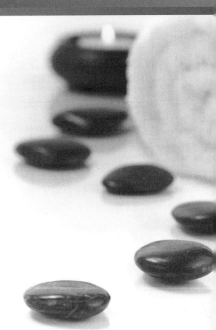

Those who can remember the days when financial record-keeping consisted of a general ledger on graph paper and client files on index cards are in an excellent position to marvel at the incredible progress in technology in the last few decades.

Younger generations have grown accustomed to the wonders of modern technology, but not long ago, business owners spent hours shuffling paper to arrive at the bottom line. This was unavoidably one of the more tedious tasks that went along with owning your own business. Fortunately, times have changed, and newer technology has replaced paper and pencil with more efficient and time-saving devices.

USING INFORMATION TECHNOLOGY IN THE SPA

Although some smaller spa business owners have been hesitant to jump on the technology bandwagon, studies indicate that more spa businesses are now using computerized systems to schedule appointments and manage day-to-day operations.

The truth is you could operate your spa business in a fairly productive way without the use of technology, but why would you want to? Computer software programs have made it easy for the spa owner to manage many of the tasks that must be performed on a daily basis, such as scheduling appointments, processing sales, bookkeeping, client record-keeping, sales analysis, inventory control, payroll, etc., far more proficiently. *E-commerce*

Plan for Success

In this techno-savvy age newer, more-efficient software has made it easy for spa owners to take full advantage of computerized business operations and online marketing opportunities. Learning to use the many technological tools available to you as a small business owner will help you to grow your business, and can ultimately make every difference in today's highly competitive spa market.

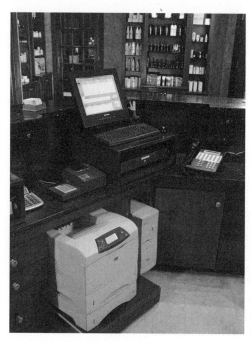

FIGURE 7-1 Technology has made it easy for spa owners to conduct business.

has also expanded marketing options, making it easy for spa owners to sell spa services, gift certificates and retail products online.

In today's competitive spa market, the smart spa business owner knows that computerization can make every difference in maintaining a competitive edge and is learning to take full advantage of all of the marvelous tools that are available to them (Figure 7-1).

COMPUTERS

There is no question that computers have become a significant part of our daily lives, replacing the way we perform many ordinary tasks. They enable us to write, calculate, organize, create, design, and manage our thoughts more efficiently than ever before. They have also opened us up to the fantastic world of cyberspace, a vast new frontier that has broadened communication capabilities in a way that few dreamed possible just decades ago.

Computers linked to the World Wide Web via the Internet allow us to shop, bank, schedule a flight, buy theater tickets, and book a day at the spa online. The Internet also provides almost instantaneous access to a wealth of information on numerous topics that used to take hours of time on the telephone or in the library. We can even communicate with people around the globe in a matter of seconds with little more than a few keystrokes. Amazing! But unless you have a degree in computer science, installing these systems can pose a significant challenge (See Figures 7-2 through 7-7).

Appointment Schedule

Detail	Tuesday August 9, 2010					
	Tom Jones	Mary Anne Miller	Barb White	Mike Miller	Jacquilyn Smith	Julie Thompson
Waiting List						
8:30 Am	Team Meeting	"	"	"	"	"
8:45 Am	"	"	"	"	"	"
9:00 Am	Williams, Cindy	Water, Shelly		Johns, Michelle		Thomas, Ann
9:15 Am	Massage	Manicure		Body Treatment	Manicure	Facial
9:30 Am	"	"	Female	"	Meyer, Natalie	Manicure
9:45 Am	Hanson, Kelly	Lake, Jill	Manicure	"	Massage (1 hr.)	Pedicure
10:00 Am	Massage	Pedicure	Smith, Bonnie	Jones, Ruth	"	"
10:15 Am	"	Manicure	Pedicure	Facial	"	"
10:30 Am	"	"	"	"	Johnson, Carrie	"
10:45 Am		"	"	"	Facial	"
11:00 Am	David, Tara	"	Ball, Kathy	Jackson, Donna	Brow/Lip Wax	Anderson, Patty
11:15 Am	Massage	Hefel, Lauren	Fleege, Linda	Facial	"	Pedicure
11:30 Am	"	Manicure	Manicure	Brown, Cheryl	"	"
11:45 Am	"	Runde, Josh	Pedicure	Body Treatment	"	"
12:00 Pm	Leibold, Emily	Manicure	"	Brow/Lip Wax	"	Taylor, Janice
12:15 Pm	Massage	"	"	Wilson, John	Moore, Jackie	Manicure
12:30 Pm	"	"	"	Body Treatment	Facial	Pedicure
12:45 Pm	"	Peters, Rick	"	"	Massage	"
1:00 Pm	"	Manicure	"	"	"	"
1:15 Pm	"				"	"

Confirmation | Schedules | Tech Tix | Appt. Log | Week View

FIGURE 7-2 Computerized appointment schedule.

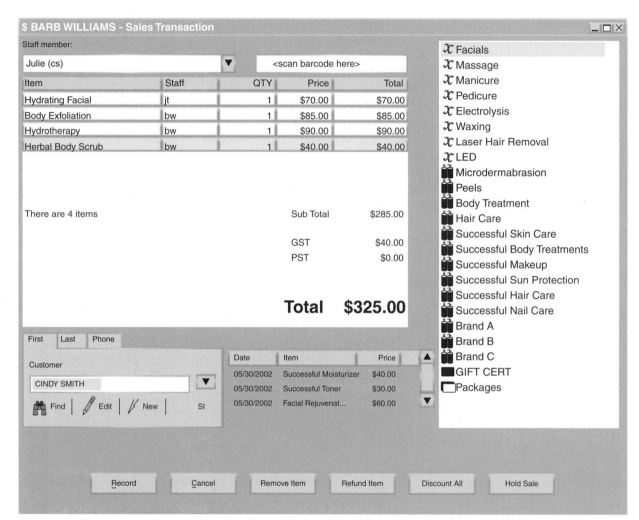

FIGURE 7-3   Computerized sales processing.

Working with Information Technology Consultants

Before purchasing any high-tech equipment, it pays to seek expert advice. However, if you are like many small independent spa business owners, you are probably concerned that you cannot afford to keep an information technology guru on the payroll. Don't despair. Many independent information

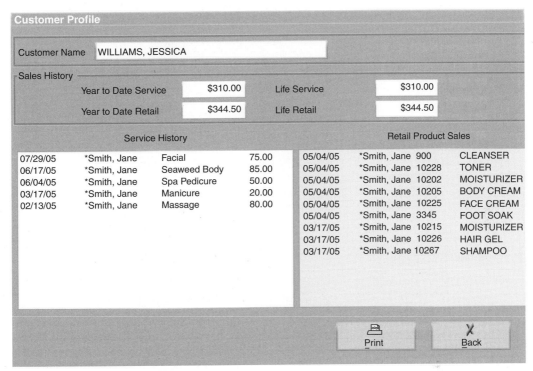

Customer Profile

Customer Name   WILLIAMS, JESSICA

Sales History

Year to Date Service	$310.00	Life Service	$310.00
Year to Date Retail	$344.50	Life Retail	$344.50

Service History				Retail Product Sales			
07/29/05	*Smith, Jane	Facial	75.00	05/04/05	*Smith, Jane	900	CLEANSER
06/17/05	*Smith, Jane	Seaweed Body	85.00	05/04/05	*Smith, Jane	10228	TONER
06/04/05	*Smith, Jane	Spa Pedicure	50.00	05/04/05	*Smith, Jane	10202	MOISTURIZER
03/17/05	*Smith, Jane	Manicure	20.00	05/04/05	*Smith, Jane	10205	BODY CREAM
02/13/05	*Smith, Jane	Massage	80.00	05/04/05	*Smith, Jane	10225	FACE CREAM
				05/04/05	*Smith, Jane	3345	FOOT SOAK
				03/17/05	*Smith, Jane	10215	MOISTURIZER
				03/17/05	*Smith, Jane	10226	HAIR GEL
				03/17/05	*Smith, Jane	10267	SHAMPOO

Print   Back

FIGURE 7-4   Computerized customer profile.

technology solutions providers, or *IT specialists*, will guide you through the process and help you to set up your business systems on a consulting basis.

To find a qualified IT specialist, follow the same principles that you would use in hiring any business advisor, such as an accountant or spa consultant. Begin by networking with other spa business owners. This will connect you to IT specialists who already have some experience in the spa industry. Once you have found someone who appears to be qualified for the job, ask for several references. If you are satisfied, define the terms of your agreement carefully.

A word of caution is in order here. Many times, small spa business owners rely on the services of family, friends, or clients who have some knowledge of technology or moonlight as consultants. These spa owners are sadly disappointed when they are unable to bring the project to fruition in a timely manner or respond to a crisis. If you should decide to trade services with a client or rely on your best friend, be up front about your expectations and outline the terms of your agreement in a contract.

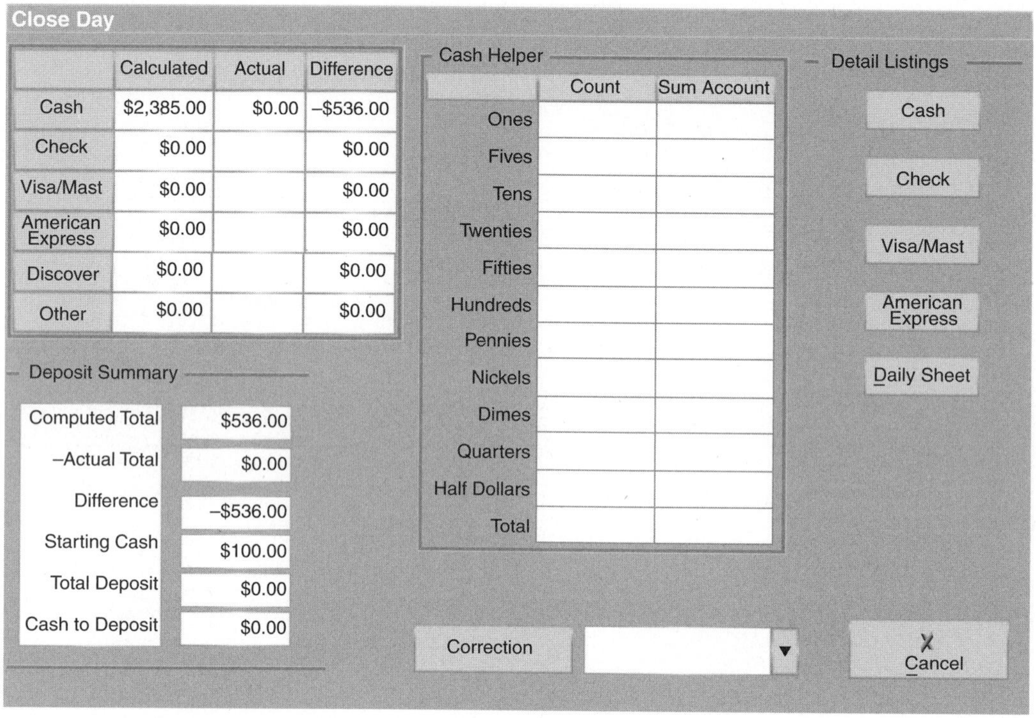

Close Day

	Calculated	Actual	Difference
Cash	$2,385.00	$0.00	–$536.00
Check	$0.00		$0.00
Visa/Mast	$0.00		$0.00
American Express	$0.00		$0.00
Discover	$0.00		$0.00
Other	$0.00		$0.00

Deposit Summary

Computed Total	$536.00
–Actual Total	$0.00
Difference	–$536.00
Starting Cash	$100.00
Total Deposit	$0.00
Cash to Deposit	$0.00

Cash Helper

	Count	Sum Account
Ones		
Fives		
Tens		
Twenties		
Fifties		
Hundreds		
Pennies		
Nickels		
Dimes		
Quarters		
Half Dollars		
Total		

Detail Listings

Cash
Check
Visa/Mast
American Express
Daily Sheet

Correction Cancel

FIGURE 7-5   Computerized bookkeeping.

ASSESSING YOUR TECHNOLOGY NEEDS

Before meeting with a consultant, it is wise to have some idea of how you would like to use technology and familiarize yourself with the growing number of software programs that have been developed specifically for the spa industry.

Again, many find it helpful to get feedback from other spa business owners. How are they using computer technology? Do they have more than one computer? Are these networked or routed to an off-site facility? What kind of computers are they using? Which software program would they recommend? How did they purchase their technology—online, at a retail or discount store, or through a consultant? Are they leasing, or do they own their hardware and software? If you are in the market for used equipment, find out if your colleagues know of any reputable pre-owned dealers.

EMPLOYEE SALES PROFILE

Employee Name: [   ]   Period: [   ] to [   ]

Staff Position: [   ]   Level: [   ]

Commission Rate: [   ] Service   Annual Sales Quota $ [   ] Service
                 [   ] Retail $ [   ] Retail

YTD Service Sales $ [   ]

YTD Retail Sales $ [   ]

Average Sales Ticket

	Service	Retail	Total
Daily			
Weekly			
Monthly			

Client Retention Rate

Period [ ] to [ ]	Number	%
New Clients		
Repeat Clients		

Client Referral Rate

Period [ ] to [ ]	
Total Number:	
YTD:	

Monthly Sales

	Current Target	Month Actual	Previous Target	Month Actual
Service		%		%
Retail		%		%

Month [ ] Year [ ]

Average Monthly Productivity Rate [   ] %

YTD Productivity Rate [   ] %

	YTD Target	Actual	
Service		%	
Retail		%	

Appointments

Scheduled Appointments: [   ]

Number of Cancellations: [   ]

Overall Completion Rating: [   ] %

PRINT

FIGURE 7-6 Computerized employee sales analysis.

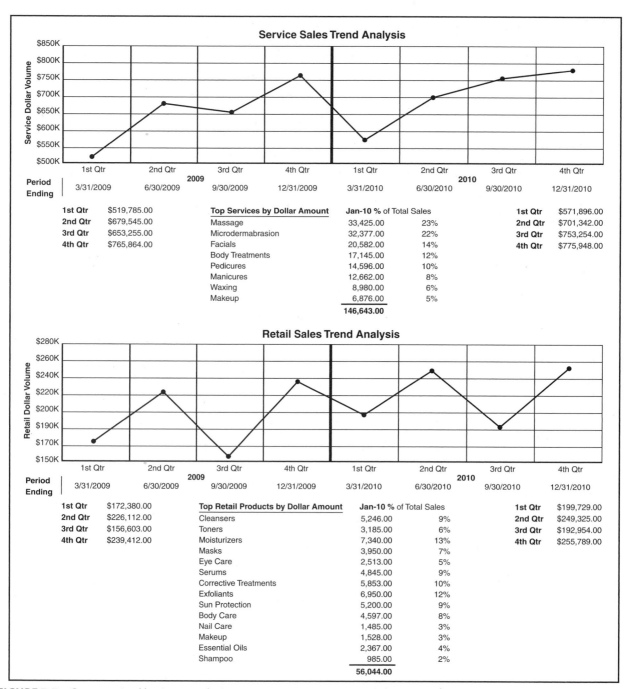

Service Sales Trend Analysis

	1st Qtr	2nd Qtr	3rd Qtr	4th Qtr	1st Qtr	2nd Qtr	3rd Qtr	4th Qtr
			2009				2010	
Period Ending	3/31/2009	6/30/2009	9/30/2009	12/31/2009	3/31/2010	6/30/2010	9/30/2010	12/31/2010

1st Qtr	$519,785.00		Top Services by Dollar Amount	Jan-10 % of Total Sales		1st Qtr	$571,896.00
2nd Qtr	$679,545.00		Massage	33,425.00	23%	2nd Qtr	$701,342.00
3rd Qtr	$653,255.00		Microdermabrasion	32,377.00	22%	3rd Qtr	$753,254.00
4th Qtr	$765,864.00		Facials	20,582.00	14%	4th Qtr	$775,948.00
			Body Treatments	17,145.00	12%		
			Pedicures	14,596.00	10%		
			Manicures	12,662.00	8%		
			Waxing	8,980.00	6%		
			Makeup	6,876.00	5%		
				146,643.00			

Retail Sales Trend Analysis

	1st Qtr	2nd Qtr	3rd Qtr	4th Qtr	1st Qtr	2nd Qtr	3rd Qtr	4th Qtr
			2009				2010	
Period Ending	3/31/2009	6/30/2009	9/30/2009	12/31/2009	3/31/2010	6/30/2010	9/30/2010	12/31/2010

1st Qtr	$172,380.00		Top Retail Products by Dollar Amount	Jan-10 % of Total Sales		1st Qtr	$199,729.00
2nd Qtr	$226,112.00		Cleansers	5,246.00	9%	2nd Qtr	$249,325.00
3rd Qtr	$156,603.00		Toners	3,185.00	6%	3rd Qtr	$192,954.00
4th Qtr	$239,412.00		Moisturizers	7,340.00	13%	4th Qtr	$255,789.00
			Masks	3,950.00	7%		
			Eye Care	2,513.00	5%		
			Serums	4,845.00	9%		
			Corrective Treatments	5,853.00	10%		
			Exfoliants	6,950.00	12%		
			Sun Protection	5,200.00	9%		
			Body Care	4,597.00	8%		
			Nail Care	1,485.00	3%		
			Makeup	1,528.00	3%		
			Essential Oils	2,367.00	4%		
			Shampoo	985.00	2%		
				56,044.00			

FIGURE 7-7   Computerized business analysis.

Be prepared to bring all of your research, questions, and concerns to the table. Good consultants will be open to your needs and wants and not push the hardware, software program, or operating system with which they are most comfortable. A consultant can also help you to select and purchase the best equipment for your money. This means products that are within your budget and are what you really need. Technology changes rapidly; so it may not be in your best interest to purchase all the bells and whistles presented to you, especially those that you are not likely to use. Most computers come with a basic package, including an operating system and word processor, spreadsheet, and database management programs. You may find these programs useful, but purchasing automatic upgrades is probably not necessary until a supplier no longer supports the program you have.

INSTALLATION

It is particularly important to seek qualified guidance on networking your computers, protecting them against dangerous viruses, and backing up your files. All of these are areas where you definitely won't want to skimp. Think about what it would cost you to replace all of your data if your computer crashes or valuable records are destroyed by a virus. Networking your computers can also present security issues, which are extremely important when dealing with confidential information such as financial data and client records.

If you intend to book appointments online, develop a Web site, or have visions of marketing and retailing your products on the World Wide Web, you will require assistance with Internet services as well. An IT consultant can help you select an Internet service provider, find a company to host your Web site, or set up a shopping cart.

Some consultants are qualified to set up all of the data communication systems you will need, including telephone, Internet, and computer connections. Others may perform specialized services but can work closely with additional service providers that can assist you. Finding the best fit for your spa is worth the time and effort when purchasing these critical business tools.

Bits and Bytes

For those lacking experience, purchasing technology can be stressful. *Bits, bytes, RAM, megahertz, hard drives, software, LANs, WANs*—the terminology alone reads like a foreign language. Familiarizing yourself with some of the more common terms used in the high-tech industry can help to alleviate some of the stress. Table 7-1 provides a quick reference guide to some of the basic terminology.

TABLE 7-1	COMMONLY USED TECHNOLOGY TERMS
ASP	Application Service Provider, a company that leases software to end users for a rental fee
Backup system	Protects against the loss of data and provides emergency retrieval; Generally refers to a system, such as a separate tape drive, remote software package, or live server that allows the user to file, back up, or restore all data for security purposes
Bit	Refers to a binary digit, or the smallest unit of data in a computer
Blog	A Web site that chronicles or logs an individual's personal thoughts and/or notes on a particular subject in much the same way that one would make entries in a journal or diary; although it should be noted that in some cases that individual may represent a larger organization
Broadband	Refers to a wideband of telecommunications frequencies that can transmit large volumes of data or carry several channels at the same time and is typically equated with high-speed Internet access that is always on. DSL and cable television are both examples of broadband connections
Bytes	Refers to units of data, or the amount of storage space available; for example, a gigabyte is equal to approximately one billion units of data.
CD-ROM	Compact Disc with Read-Only Memory
CD-ROM drive	The slot on your computer where compact discs are inserted
CD-RW	Compact Disc Rewritable, which means you can write over existing information or reuse the disc
CPU	Central Processing Unit, which is responsible for computer operations
DAP	Digital Audio Player, a portable electronic device that is capable of storing and playing a large volume of selected music or audio files; some DAPs are also equipped with video and photo features.
Desktop	The area that displays all items or programs available on your computer
DSL	Digital Subscriber Line; refers to a broadband connection that connects computers together via specialized copper telephone lines
DVD	Digital Versatile Disc, a compact optical disc capable of storing large volumes of audio, visual, or computer data
Hard disks or floppy disks	Small storage devices with a limited file capacity that are inserted into a disk drive on your computer and used to copy or back up files

TABLE 7-1	COMMONLY USED TECHNOLOGY TERMS
Hard drive and files	The storage device that houses a computer's operating system, applications,
Hardware	Refers to the physical components of your computer, such as the hard drive, monitor, mouse, keyboard, speakers, cables, and power connections
ISDN	Integrated Services Digital Network, a digital telephone line that allows simultaneous Internet access, telephone, and fax use
ISP	Internet Service Provider, a company that stores and handles Web sites and sells various Internet-related services
LAN	Local Area Network, a computer network spanning a small area that allows networked computers to share data and/or other devices, such as printers
Megahertz	Refers to the rate of speed of processing
Modem lines	A device that creates communication links between computers via telephone
Monitor	Refers to the computer screen
Network	A group of computers routed to one another to share information or devices
Operating system	Refers to the system or program manager that allows the computer's hardware and software to interact
Payment Gateway	The software that allows online shopping carts and merchant accounts, such as *PayPal* and *Verisign* to communicate
PC	Personal Computer
PDA	Personal Digital Assistant, a small handheld computer that runs simple applications to store and retrieve information
Podcast	An audio broadcast delivered in digital files over the Internet which can be downloaded or programmed for automatic delivery and listened to using computer-generated software such as *Windows Media Player* or *iTunes*; or a portable media player, such as an *MP3 player* or *iPod*
RAM	Random Access Memory, the main memory available to programs while a computer is running
Router	A device that allows two or more computers or networks to connect to the Internet

(continued)

TABLE 7-1	COMMONLY USED TECHNOLOGY TERMS (*CONTINUED*)
Server	A computer that is dedicated to providing a particular service, such as connecting other computers to each other or to the Internet
Software	The various applications or programs used to operate your computer and perform functions such as word processing, spreadsheets, and database management
Tablet PCs	Generally referred to as a wireless notebook or portable laptop with note-taking capabilities
TCP/IP	A certain set of standardized procedures or protocols, technically referred to as Transmission Control Protocol/Internet Protocol used to connect the World Wide Web
URL	Uniform Resource Locator, the unique location or address of a file on the Internet
Web 2.0	Refers to the use of the World Wide Web for the purpose of sharing information; developing people-focused connections and building communities via the Internet or social computing
Webcast	An Internet broadcast that can appear as a video and/or audio production and is capable of reaching a wide viewing audience
Webinar	A seminar or class that is broadcast over the internet using video and/or audio technology that can accommodate multiple participants; and may also include a simultaneously broadcast slideshow
WAN	Wide Area Network, or a computer network over a larger area that might connect two or more LANs
Wi-Fi	Wireless Fidelity or wireless technology that enables computers to access the Internet without a physical connection

Connecting to the Internet

The Internet is a complex communication system that consists of multiple network connections worldwide. To understand the concept of Internet connectivity, it is helpful to think in terms of multiple computers linked together. These computer connections take place through a certain set of standardized procedures or protocols, technically referred to as *TCP/IP*, or *Transmission Control Protocol/Internet Protocol*.

The *World Wide Web* is one navigational tool used to make Internet connections. The *Web*, as it is more simply referred to, is a graphics-based vehicle that uses *hypertext,* technically referred to as *Hypertext Transfer Protocol,* to link different Web sites via *browsers,* which allow users to travel from site to site. Internet Explorer and Netscape Navigator are two well-known browsers.

There are several ways to gain access to the Internet. These typically include some form of telecommunications, such as digital subscriber lines (DSL), an integrated services digital network (ISDN), T-1, or analog lines and cable television facilities. These communication lines carry information, or Internet traffic, to what is often described as the *superhighway* via a modem or router that is attached to your computer.

INTERNET SERVICE PROVIDERS

An *Internet service provider* (ISP) is a company that sells various Internet-related services, such as Internet access, domain registration, e-mail accounts, and web hosting to individuals, businesses, or organizations. To provide these services, ISPs use extremely powerful servers, or PCs that hold large volumes of information and can be accessed by literally thousands of users at a time. Many ISPs are competing for consumers' business at various rates. AOL, MSN, and Earthlink are a few, well-known examples. Many other ISPs can be accessed through local cable and telephone companies.

Before signing on with an ISP, it is wise to shop around. Many ISPs offer special package prices to businesses that include several services at a fixed rate. The cost of Internet access varies according to how you connect to the Internet. There are generally two ways to gain Internet access: either through a dedicated line which is "always on" or by connecting through a telephone or cable line. Spa businesses that use the Internet to book appointments and sell gift certificates will want the convenience of a high-speed dedicated line, which tends to cost more.

Many rating scales are available to help you compare and contrast the different ISPs. These are easily accessed online or researched through reputable high-tech and business publications. Your IT consultant can also be a valuable resource in this area.

SETTING UP A URL

The term *URL,* or *uniform resource locator,* is used to indicate the unique location or address of a file on the Internet. Web addresses are controlled by ICANN, the Internet Corporation for Assigned Names and Numbers. This international nonprofit organization created by the federal government appoints different organizations to assign and keep track of URLs and approves the creation of top-level domain names, such as .com, .net, .edu, and .org, which indicate the destination of the address. For example, .org indicates the destination for a nonprofit entity, and .edu is the destination for educational institutions.

Registering a domain, or Internet address, for a fee, is a simple process conducted through companies known as *registrars*. Internet addresses use a 32-digit numbering system translated to a set protocol for naming, which uses the prefix www, an abbreviation for the World Wide Web, followed by the name, and includes a suffix that indicates the destination. For example, *www.successfuldayspa.com* would indicate the address of a spa business at a .com or commercial destination, while *www.spauniversity.edu* would indicate a spa training facility at an .edu or educational destination.

When registering a domain, your registrar must first determine if the name you would like to use is available. Because the Internet is a worldwide network, it is not uncommon to find several businesses that use the same or a similar name, vying for the use of a single address. For example, if there is more than one spa business going by the name of Successful Day Spa, only one will be able to register its domain as *www.successfuldayspa.com*.

Domain names are registered in one-year increments, which are renewable for certain time periods. This has increased their market value. Sometimes companies will try to buy the use of a domain from another registered party. Others will find more creative ways to establish their identity, either by shortening or altering their name slightly or creating a unique association that is easily identified.

USING THE INTERNET

Businesses use the Internet to perform various tasks. The Internet is an excellent way to access general information, connect with suppliers, find out about events, participate in educational seminars, research your competitors, and advertise or promote business.

E-Commerce

E-commerce, a term used for selling products or services via the Internet, has the unique ability to reach consumers round the clock, each and every day of the year, including holidays. This incredible retailing phenomenon has quickly changed how many companies are marketing their wares and

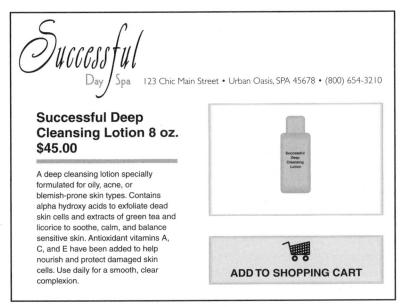

FIGURE 7-8   Internet shopping cart.

has generated literally billions of dollars for some businesses. Spas generally take advantage of e-commerce by booking appointments, selling gift certificates, and advertising special promotions online (Figure 7-8).

Scheduling appointments online has become a lot more user-friendly in recent years with most software vendors incorporating this item as a basic feature. Depending upon the software program you select your clients will be able to schedule appointments online in one of several ways: they can submit a request for an appointment that is then processed by the spa's in-house appointment administrator; they can submit a request that is confirmed instantly; or they can view the spa's appointment book and schedule their own appointment in real time, which means that an appointment is readily available at the time the client is requesting it. Whichever method is available to you, use it! Online appointment scheduling is now an acceptable method that makes it more convenient for clients to do business with you.

Real-time scheduling is a characteristic that is often critical to closing the sale; however, it may leave some spa owners feeling vulnerable. Spa owners concerned about exposing their appointment book to the world should not be overly concerned. Newer software programs are capable of limiting the amount of exposure to a spa's book, a feature that can ultimately benefit the spa owner looking to implement a yield management program, a topic that will be discussed further in Chapter 10. Other security features can be installed to prevent fraudulent activity.

Selling gift certificates online is another feature that is now commonplace and one that can be extremely lucrative for spa owners, especially during the holidays; however, not all spa software programs are equipped with technology that allows clients to produce and print their own gift certificates instantly, a feature that can be extremely valuable when it comes to harnessing last minute shoppers. Fortunately, there are third-party providers that are able to provide these services for what is generally a nominal fee.

Linking to other popular online spa resources like *Spa Finder, Spa Wish and Spa-Addicts,* businesses that sell spa gift certificates directly to the consumer have the added advantage of offering spa-goers who may be unfamiliar with your spa, or those who are seeking to purchase a gift certificate for someone in a different geographic area, quick and easy access to your spa. Spas may ultimately decide to use more than one of these types of resources; however, it is important to note that services do vary among service providers, so be sure to find out the features and benefits of each before enrolling.

Retailing spa products online is quickly becoming a popular means of generating additional revenue for some spas, however it is not for every spa owner. Creating an online shopping mart poses several business concerns for spa owners. Understanding your responsibility when it comes to protecting consumer privacy, preventing fraudulent activity, and collecting sales tax are among the most important challenges facing business owners that choose to go this route.

Whether or not you decide to sell a complete line of retail products or just gift certificates online, any spa business using the Internet to sell services or products directly to the consumer will need to take extra security precautions if they intend to accept credit card payments online (Figure 7-9). Those new to processing card payments online will want to review the Data Security Standards set by the Payment Card Industry [PCI] carefully beforehand. For more information about the PCI DSS, visit *www.pcisecuritystandards.org.* Compliance with these standards is a subject that should be covered in-depth with your IT consultant, ASP, ISP and/or ECSP e-commerce service provider. Your information security policy should always include a method for encrypting any stored data to prevent fraudulent activity.

There are other practical matters to consider in managing an online retail center, such as which shopping cart to install and what shipping methods you will use to deliver your products. There are several options for small business owners when it comes to selecting vendors for these purposes, including complete Web retailing packages that are available from

Plan for Success

The Federal Trade Commission is the primary U.S. government agency responsible for regulating e-commerce. The FTC publishes several guidebooks which can help you to understand your responsibility when it comes to marketing and advertising your products online, collecting sales tax, protecting consumer privacy, fulfilling orders, processing refunds etc. Other government agencies, including the National Telecommunications and Information Administration and the Federal Communications Commission are additional resources for spa business owners seeking more information.

Successful
Day Spa   **sophisticated beauty therapies**
(800) 654-3210

PURCHASER'S INFORMATION
(all Purchaser's information is required)

NAME:

PHONE NUMBER:
(please include area code)

ADDRESS:

CITY, STATE, ZIP CODE:

E-MAIL ADDRESS:

SHIPPING INFORMATION
(if different from purchase information)

NAME:

PHONE NUMBER:
(please include area code)

ADDRESS:

CITY, STATE, ZIP CODE:

E-MAIL ADDRESS:

PAYMENT METHOD
AMEX   MC   VISA

NAME ON CARD:

CARD NUMBER:

CARD IDENTIFICATION NUMBER:

EXPIRATION DATE:

DELIVERY INFORMATION

☐   FedEx Standard Overnight ®

☐   FedEx 2Day ®

☐   FedEx Express Saver ®

Thank you for shopping at Successful Day Spa's online boutique. All online orders are processed within 24 hours. You will receive confirmation of your order, an itemized account of all charges, and estimated shipping dates via e-mail within 48 hours. For more information on shipping rates and our return policy, click on successfulshipping&returns.

To request additional information on any of Successful's products, please contact us at info@successfuldayspa.com or call us toll free at 800.555.5555.

SHOPPING CART 🛒

🔒DATA LOCK

FIGURE 7-9   Internet purchase order form.

Plan for Success

The Internet has made booking appointments, selling gift certificates and purchasing spa products easy with online shopping carts that have the potential to generate revenue around the clock for techno-savvy spa owners. In these competitive economic times, learning to make use of this valuable online marketing tool is an option that the spa owner simply cannot afford to overlook; however, operating an online retail center poses several additional business management concerns that should be researched and planned carefully before investing in this business practice.

e-commerce application service providers like Vcommerce, Earthlink, Nexternal and Yahoo!. Your Web designer or IT consultant may also be able to set up a shopping cart for you using e-commerce templates. Shipping products within the United States is a fairly straightforward process via the U.S. Postal Service or private companies like UPS and FedEx.

Retailing your products and services online, or *e-tailing*, as it has been coined, requires another layer of administration to operate effectively. Updating product information, managing inventory, processing orders and scheduling deliveries are time consuming tasks that are likely to require extra help and training. If you are selling a successful private label line you may find that all of this is worth the investment, however not all brand name product vendors and manufacturers will be equally invested in helping you to establish an online retail store. Make this part of the information gathering process and whenever possible solicit manufacturer and vendor support to help you reach your goals.

Electronic Mail

One of the more prevalent uses of the Internet is *electronic mail*, commonly referred to as *e-mail*. Based on the concept of an ordinary mail system, the Internet allows individuals to deliver notes or messages, with attached documents, around the globe. One of the advantages of e-mail is that it can be sent to multiple parties simultaneously, which makes it ideal for sending announcements, newsletters, and sales promotions to clients. Because this is generally a cost-effective way to contact a large volume of people, e-mail has all but eliminated the use of more costly regular mail, now nicknamed "snail mail," to perform many business functions. We'll talk more about the use of electronic mail for promotional purposes in Chapters 8 and 9.

E-mail addresses can be purchased in blocks by authorized registrars, which allows a number of individuals within the same organization to be contacted directly. The standard format for an e-mail address uses the individual user name, the company's domain name, and the destination, such as *sally@successfuldayspa.com*. Companies promoting their business via a Web site typically provide a generic e-mail address, such as *info@ successfuldayspa.com*, usually located in an area identified as "Contact Us," which leads consumers to a mailbox supervised by an authorized administrator who handles correspondence.

Spa Software

Spa software programs have grown tremendously in their capabilities and are continuing to evolve as they address the increasing needs of the industry. The number of companies manufacturing software that cater to the spa business is also on the rise. To find software that is compatible with your specific business requirements, it is wise to compare and contrast several programs. Be prepared to look beyond the functional components of the program. With many companies offering similar products, other important considerations such as customer service, training, and tech support could ultimately be the deciding factor in the selection process.

FINDING THE RIGHT SOFTWARE PROGRAM FOR YOUR DAY SPA

The main question to ask when purchasing software is: What do I want technology to do for me? Today's spa software programs are multifaceted with numerous benefits and features, such as accounting, cash register, and marketing functions, to help you run your business. But keep in mind that none of these applications is of any value unless you use them. Before making a final purchasing decision, it is important to consider who will be using the software, for what purpose, and what level of expertise is required for operation.

Use the following checklist to determine which software features are most important to you in managing day-to-day business operations.

REQUEST A DEMO

Before purchasing any software program, you should have first-hand experience of how it works. The best way to do this is to request a demo, something that is usually available in CD format. Most vendors also provide online demos, but better still, have a knowledgeable customer service or sales representative walk you through it so you don't miss any of the important features. Is it user-friendly? More importantly, do you feel comfortable using it? Try a few to compare. Are you more comfortable with one program than another? Why?

A sales rep's ability to build a positive rapport with the customer is generally what makes or breaks the sale. But it is important to separate the software's benefits and features from your assessment of the salesperson. A good way to do that is to test the software on your own before making the purchase. If you have difficulty operating the program by yourself and the company provides little in the way of training or tech support, you will no doubt become frustrated and have trouble maximizing its potential.

SOFTWARE CHECKLIST

Scheduling Appointments

_____ Internet or online booking

_____ Automatic e-mail appointment reminder/confirmation

_____ Automatic procedure for scheduling multiple services or groups

_____ Automatic procedure for scheduling standing appointments

_____ Automatic reminder of client preferences

_____ Generate a waiting list

_____ Track cancellations

_____ Monitor late arrivals, no shows, and room or technician's availability

Accounting Functions (Accounts Payable and Accounts Receivable)

_____ Conduct daily bookkeeping

_____ Track invoices

_____ Pay bills

_____ Set budgets

_____ Balance checkbook

_____ Track cash flow

_____ Calculate payroll and commissions

_____ Itemize payroll deductions

_____ Track tipping for tax reporting purposes

_____ Print checks automatically

Sales Transactions

_____ Customer check-in

_____ Customer check-out

_____ Perform cash register operations

_____ Process credit card payments via the internet

_____ Scan bar codes

_____ Print receipts

_____ Track refunds

Inventory Control

_____ Establish an inventory system

_____ Sort by SKU, product, department, vendor, date, etc

_____ Generate bar codes

_____ Print price labels

_____ Determine current inventory

_____ Automatic inventory adjustment (post-sale)

_____ Download inventory control data to a PDA

_____ Automatically restock supplies

_____ Automatically restock retail products

_____ Set profit margins

_____ Track product turnover

_____ Track vendors to purchase orders

_____ Print purchase orders

Sales and Marketing

_____ Analyze product and service sales

_____ Supply graphic reports

(continued)

SOFTWARE CHECKLIST (*CONTINUED*)

_____ Generate price list(s)

_____ Track individual customer sales and service history

_____ Track discounts

_____ Analyze client demographics

_____ Develop sales profiles

_____ Evaluate product and service trends

_____ Sell gift certificates

_____ Track series and spa packages

_____ Track gift certificate and gift card sales

_____ Produce gift cards

_____ Track client retention rate

_____ Track referrals

_____ Manage customer database

_____ Create mailing labels

_____ Automatically prompt lists for promotional materials (such as referral cards, reminder notices, frequent buyer and rewards programs, and birthday, anniversary, and thank-you cards)

_____ Deliver electronic mail

Client Management

_____ Maintain client history

_____ Insert client notes and update service records

_____ Automatically generate rewards program

_____ Monitor series purchases

_____ Track client spending habits

_____ Track client referrals

Employee management

_____ Create employee schedules

_____ Provide employees with Internet or PDA access to schedules

_____ Time clock for tracking hours and absences

_____ Assess productivity

_____ Set sales goals

_____ Evaluate individual performance

_____ Calculate commission structures

_____ Automatic deductions for product usage

_____ Automatic bonus indicator

_____ Track tips

_____ Track employee purchases and discounts

_____ Store miscellaneous employee info

Business Functions

_____ Complete general ledger program

_____ Generate business reports (such as profit and loss statements and daily, monthly, and quarterly income statements)

_____ Analyze revenues

_____ Conduct comparative fiscal analysis

_____ Prompt estimated tax payments

_____ Process credit card payments

QUALIFYING A SOFTWARE VENDOR

Software vendors invested in your success will have qualified sales representatives available to conduct demos and answer any questions you may have, but this does not always translate to ongoing quality customer service or trouble-free technical support. Before putting your credit card on the table, take a closer look at the following.

SOME CONSIDERATIONS FOR SELECTING A SOFTWARE VENDOR

Reputation

- How long has the manufacturer been in business?

- What do customers have to say about the company?

Training

- Does the software vendor supply on-site training or offer conveniently located seminars? Are these free of charge?

- Does the company provide an instruction manual or other training materials? Are these easy to read and understand?

Service and Support

- What is the company's customer service policy?

- Is technical support included in the cost of the program? For how long?

- What are the hours you can access technical support day to day? Is this available online only, or does the company also provide tech support by telephone? This is important for those working beyond a Monday through Friday 9-to-5 schedule and those who prefer to speak to a live person.

- How many support personnel are there on staff? Call the tech support line before you purchase to gauge the actual processing time.

Price

- What is the base price of the software? Does this include all of the program features? Single user, multiple user, or networking privileges?

- Are automatic upgrades included in the purchase price?

- Does the company offer discounts on hardware (computers) or additional apparatus needed to run the program, such as a bar code scanner or pager system?

- Can you buy, lease, or rent the product? What are the benefits of each?

Warranty

- How long is the product warranted to be free of damage or defects?

- Is satisfaction guaranteed? Look at the fine print carefully. If you are unhappy, can you recover the full value of your initial investment?

After carefully reviewing all of these criteria with the vendor, it is wise to ask for references and conduct your own investigation. Talk to spa owners who are operating businesses that are similar in size and operation to your own. How long have they been using the program? Would they give it an A, B, or C grade? Are they using all of the features, most of them, some of them, or only a few? Why? It is important to determine if some of the features are more user-friendly or productive than others or if the spa owner simply has not attempted to use them for other reasons, such as training or personnel issues. This information can be extremely helpful, particularly if you are torn between two similar products.

FUNCTIONAL REQUIREMENTS

Before purchasing a software program, it is also important to determine the hardware requirements. For instance, certain software programs are designed to be used on either a PC or a Macintosh® computer. PCs can

generally accommodate several operating systems, whereas the Macintosh®
runs on a unique *OS*. If the software program you choose is only compatible with a specific operating system, such as Microsoft Windows® NT or
XP platform, you will need to acquire that system or choose another that is
more compatible with what you already own.

Software programs vary in terms of the amount of hard drive space
required for installation; so it is important to know how much space is
available on your computer. Processing speed, measured in megahertz, is
another significant factor that will determine how efficiently or quickly the
program will run. This is often a huge concern to those managing operations at the front desk. Note that business computers usually rely on higher
processing speeds. You will also want to be aware of the type of backup
system that can be used. Storing or recovering information in the event of
a mishap is absolutely critical to successful business operations.

Pay careful attention to any restrictions on the amount of data the
program can handle. For example, is it limited in terms of the number of
practitioners, retail items, or client files it can process? Such restrictions
can become problematic if your business suddenly takes off.

Flexibility is another issue. The ability to download information to
another program, such as Microsoft Excel or Intuit QuickBooks, can be
invaluable. For example, a program that exports financial data to Quick-
Books quickly and efficiently will make it easy for an accountant using that
application to manage bookkeeping tasks.

You will also want to be aware of any additional software that is required
to perform a specific operation, such as third-party software needed to
process credit card payments.

PRICE CONSIDERATIONS

Software prices usually vary according to the number of users, with higher
rates for multiple users or networks, and are typically restricted by licensing agreements to deter pirating.

Several programs give users the option of leasing rather than owning
or renting with the option to own, while some are only available as rentals.
In this case, the software is leased by an *application service provider* (ASP).
There are some advantages to this type of arrangement, such as automatic
upgrades and training. You will need to determine which makes the most
economic sense for you. Table 7-2 lists several spa software vendors to help
you get started in making a software selection.

TABLE 7-2	SPA SOFTWARE VENDORS*	
Clientrak!	800.397.4582	*www.clientrak.com*
Edge Salon Management Systems, Inc.	403.948.0611	*www.edgemgmt.com*
Elite Software, Inc.	800.662.3548	*www.elitesoftware.com*
Insight Salon & Spa Software	888.919.5841	*www.salon-software.com*
Innovative Computer Business Solutions	800.682.2998	*www.spasalon.com*
Mikal Salon & Spa Computers	800.448.5420	*www.mikal.com*
Milano Software	800.667.1596	*www.milanosoftware.com*
Millennium by Harms Software, Inc.	888.813.2141	*www.harms-software.com*
MPOS Management Software	706.228.4616	*www.millresources.com*
ProSolutions	800.710.3879	*www.prosolutionssoftware.com*
Priverus Software	866.488.9332	*www.priverus.com*
Resort Suite	866.477.8483	*www.enablez.com*
Salon Pro	800.830.9992	*www.salonpro.com*
Salon Styler Pro	559.266.9248	*www.salonstyler.com*
Salon Tec, Inc.	800.221.5236	*www.salontec.com*
SalonBiz Software/Spa Biz	800.632.5527	*www.salonbiz.com*
Salonware/Spaware	888.260.8181	*www.salonspaware.com*
Softbrands Hospitality Solutions	800.342.5675	*www.hospitality.softbrands.com*
SpaBoom	800.940.0458	*www.spaboom.com*
Spa Booker a division of Spa Finder	866.721.5580	*www.spa-booker.com*
Spa Soft/Spa Resort	802.253.7377	*www.springermiller.com*
Spaware	888.260.8181	*salonspaware.com*

Please note this list is not meant to be inclusive. New software programs are created all the time. Spa owners are urged to conduct their own research to obtain additional resources.

TELEPHONE SYSTEMS

In this age of computerization, the telephone still reigns as the lifeline of the spa business and one of the most important business communication tools you will purchase. Many excellent telephone systems offer numerous features, but there are only a few types of telephone systems from which to choose. These vary in complexity and include PBX, Centrex, Key, KSU-less, and Hybrid systems.

- A *PBX* or *Private Branch Exchange* is a privately owned system that is generally used in the corporate environment to accommodate 60-plus telephones or workstations. These are connected via an automated central office switch that is centrally located directly on the company's premises. Connections to the outside world are made via trunks, or telephone lines, that can carry multiple lines, such as a T-1 line capable of transmitting 24 incoming and/or outgoing calls at a time, to the public telephone network. Entry to an outside line is typically gained by dialing an access code, such as 9.

- *Centrex* systems have many of the same features as PBX, but rather than maintaining private ownership, the switching equipment is managed by the telephone company's central office. This type of system is generally used by organizations that have buildings spread across a certain geographic area, such as hospitals and college campuses, to avoid the additional expense and complications associated with wiring multiple sites.

- *Key* systems are typically used by companies that have fewer than 60 users per site. As the name implies, each button, or key, on the telephone represents a telephone line that allows the user to make or receive a call. This type of system has many of the same features and functionality of a PBX system, with the major point of difference being the connection between the central office and the key system unit (KSU). There is no need to dial an access code, and calls are quickly routed through whichever path is available, either to the key system from the central office or to the public network from the key system, rather than a central processing switch.

- *KSU-less* systems are designed to accommodate businesses with less than 10 employees. This is a much simpler proprietary telephone system with three to four lines and intercom capabilities. Because there is no central processing unit (the technology is in the telephone system), this type of system is easy to install and allows telephones to be moved from one location to another.

- *Hybrids* combine many of the features associated with PBX and Key systems, which are scaled down or adapted through the use of sophisticated software. These systems vary in the number of users they can accommodate, supplying anywhere from 30 to 200 or more workstations.

- *Computer Telephony Integration (CTI)* or *Voice Over Internet Protocol (VoIP)* is the latest in telephone system technology that allows your computer to serve as your telephone. For those small business owners looking to save money on long-distance calls or those with employees that work-off site, computer telephony can be appealing; however, there are still many issues to resolve. The inability to process a large volume of calls, poor voice quality, delayed timing, hardware and software limitations, and the problems of business coming to a standstill if your computer crashes are just a few of the concerns that have kept this out of reach for most businesses, particularly spas.

Assessing Your Telephone Needs

The size of your spa operation will determine which type of telephone system is best for your business needs. A busy spa serving a high volume of clients will need enough outside lines to schedule appointments, conduct outgoing calls, process credit cards, use a fax machine, and maintain a DSL or Internet line. If your spa employs 20 to 30 people, with two-to-four people taking and making calls, you can probably get by with four to six outside lines and 18 internal extensions, but every business is different. A qualified vendor supplied with a detailed floor plan and vital information about your business can help you to determine what is best for your spa business.

Installation

There are two basics requirements for getting your telephone system up and running—telephone wires and telephones. Most commercial spaces have existing wiring; if you can, use it. New wiring can add significantly to costs and generally is not needed unless it cannot accommodate the system you plan to install or you intend to expand operations. If you are undergoing extensive renovations or planning to build a spa from the ground up, be sure to include enough wiring to accommodate telephone jacks and data communication lines throughout the space before the walls are put up. This will ultimately save you time and money. Expect labor to be a major portion of the cost.

Equipment

Business telephones vary and can be quite costly depending on the style you choose. If you are buying telephones from an installer, they are likely to recommend a particular brand. In this case, ask for an itemized cost breakdown and check that it is a quality product manufactured by a reputable company with a long history of customer satisfaction. Many telephone system rating scales are available online and in trade publications that can provide you with cost and quality comparisons.

Selecting a Telephone Vendor

There are generally three ways to purchase and install a telephone system: (1) directly through your local or regional telephone company; (2) through a trunker, or technician who used to work for a larger corporation and now sells, installs, and services small telephone systems (usually the brand of their former employer); or (3) through a dealer-distributor that sells, installs, and services several top brands.

Many smaller day spas are inclined to go to their local telephone company first, but don't be afraid to explore the other two options. Any system you choose will require installation and programming. Look for a supplier that you are comfortable with, is conveniently located, and has an excellent reputation for customer service.

Discounts are standard when purchasing telephones, but warranties and service contracts vary. Be sure to examine these options carefully. Keep in mind that a quality system with an excellent service agreement from a reputable vendor may turn out to be more cost-effective in the long run. Unfortunately, smaller companies selling lesser-known brands frequently go out of business. If you go that route, make sure you can deal with the worst-case scenario, whether that means finding another company to support the system, replacing telephones, or installing a new system.

Many of the same qualifications used to select a software vendor apply here. Always ask for a demo of the telephone system and an itemized cost breakdown that includes all equipment, installation, labor, and service charges. Your service contract or warranty may include a certain number of service calls or a set hourly rate but exclude overtime or travel time and peripherals; so it is important to have a detailed understanding of all charges and the limitations of your warranty.

Telephone Features

The list of telephone features available to small businesses is long, with many standard items such as caller ID, hold, and call transferring included in the cost of the telephone system. Surplus features can add up; so it is important to choose extras wisely.

Spa owners should be selective when it comes to additional telephone features, particularly those that generate extra charges on a monthly, per line basis. As you run down the list of options, consider first what you absolutely need to have your business operate at maximum efficiency on a daily basis. Most small businesses do not require much more than the basics, including hold, transfer, and voice mail, to maintain the flow of business. Should your telephone vendor recommend additional cost items, make sure they will add value to your business on a regular basis. For example, an added feature such as messaging on hold, although it may not be imperative, can help to increase business by alerting clients to new treatments and special promotions. Others, like conference calling, are not vital to the success of a spa business.

Voice Mail

Voice mail is an important telephone feature that is often included in the price of a system. If it is not, you will need to find one that is compatible with the telephone system you are using (Table 7-3). Whether you decide to purchase a stand-alone system or contract a service, be aware that voice mail can be a high ticket item that has the potential to be problematic. When making a selection, remember that voice mail that is difficult to maintain, cumbersome to use, or always on, can frustrate even the most patient client and staff.

Many voice mail systems will incorporate an *automated attendant* feature that routes callers directly to a specific extension, such as a person who handles gift certificates or appointments only. The main purpose of this feature is to improve the quality of service and increase direct access to the appropriate party or information. Still, some businesses program voice mail into the direct extensions and use this feature to cut down on administrative costs, a tactic that in the personal care business spa goers may perceive as rather impersonal. Given these concerns, those interested in using more sophisticated voice mail technology, such as automated appointment reminders, should take care to personalize messages with a familiar voice and to program them with specific information that will satisfy the customer's needs. Although a small percentage may continue to be annoyed by the use of voice mail and automated attendants, when used appropriately these telephone features can be extremely beneficial to small business owners.

TABLE 7-3	COMMONLY USED TELEPHONE FEATURES
Automated Attendant	Automatically distributes calls via a programmed messaging system, for example, *Press 1 to make an appointment in the spa, Press 2 to purchase gift certificates*, etc.
Call Forwarding	Transfers incoming calls to another telephone number or extension, such as another office in the building, your cell phone, home office, or some other remote location.
Call Transfer	Allows you to transfer the caller to another extension.
Conference Calling	Allows three or more people to communicate jointly over the same line.
Hold	Places caller on hold momentarily while you complete another call.
Intercom	Allows personnel within the same office to speak to each other without picking up the telephone.
Marketing-on-Hold	Allows you to program music and general information or advertise and promote business while the client remains on hold.
Speakerphone	Allows you to hear and speak to another party without picking up the headset through a microphone built into the telephone.
Toll Restriction	Circuitry that blocks or restricts long-distance calls to specific area codes. This feature can also be password protected, which requires employees to enter a certain number or letter code to gain long-distance access.
Voice Mail	A messaging system that can be programmed with different features, such as an answering machine or automated attendant, to meet the individual needs of your spa business. Voice mail can be purchased as an individual freestanding system or included as part of a service package from a telephone company or dealer.

Marketing-on-Hold

In recent years, the *marketing-on-hold* feature has become extremely popular with busy spas and for good reason. On-hold messaging systems allow small businesses to deliver powerful marketing messages that can help promote new services, broadcast specials, or up-sell less popular menu items to what is virtually a captive audience.

The cost of such a service is typically based on the length of the recorded message or cost per minute and the frequency of editing script. Some on-hold marketing programs are incorporated in telephone system package prices, while others can be purchased as stand-alone items. If you are undecided about this feature and don't want to spend the extra money right away or wish to postpone such a service until you have an established marketing plan, this feature is generally one that can be added at a later date.

GENERAL BUSINESS EQUIPMENT

A small day spa business may have little need for more traditional and costly office equipment, such as a sophisticated copy machine that prints and collates large quantities, but it will still require the basics. These should include a fax machine, copier, printer, credit card processor, and a high-quality surge protector to safeguard all of the aforementioned technological tools, including your PC.

For many small businesses, an economical, multipurpose machine that combines several functions, such as a fax, printer, and copier is a good investment. Although prices have come down considerably for these space-saving devices, it is always a good idea to compare and contrast similar products before buying.

Printers

Printers, in particular, should be selected carefully since you will need one that is compatible with your PC and operating system. There are two basic types of printers: ink-jet and laser. Smaller day spas can probably get by with an ink-jet printer, which is typically less expensive and can print in color. Laser printers tend to be more efficient and produce a better quality image that won't smudge, a drawback to the ink-jet, but they are more costly and color models are generally altogether cost prohibitive for the small business owner.

The color printing option supplied by ink-jets is often appealing to spas and can be helpful in producing eye-catching signs, graphs, and charts; however, it is not recommended that you use a small printer to produce critical marketing pieces, or large quantities of materials, such as your brochure or business cards. If you are considering the ink-jet to accomplish these tasks, don't! Such marketing pieces should be outsourced to obtain professional quality.

Credit Card Processors

Your spa business will also need equipment to process credit card transactions, an integral part of doing business today. To obtain credit card processing equipment, you must first apply for merchant status, which is typically accomplished through a bank or, more often in the case of the small business owner, through a third-party provider. Application fees, discount rates, transaction fees, cost of leasing or owning equipment, and other miscellaneous charges vary considerably in this arena; so it is important to shop around before committing to a plan.

At the very least, the equipment needed to process credit cards will consist of a telephone line and card imprinting device (Figure 7-10). Spa businesses also have the option of processing credit cards electronically, through the use of terminals that swipe credit cards and debit cards, cash registers, and specialized software programs. This equipment can be purchased or leased, but it is generally more cost-effective to own it.

Software programs that allow transactions to be authorized online can significantly reduce the cost of processing credit cards, but be aware that these may require additional equipment, such as receipt printers. If you intend to sell products online, you will also need to make sure that the

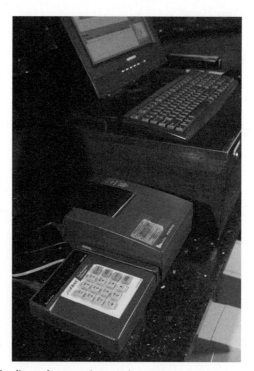

FIGURE 7-10   Credit card processing equipment.

shopping cart software you use is compatible with the payment gateway, or software program, provided by the merchant card or service provider you select. Security issues must also be addressed.

Sorting through these details can be difficult; so it is important to gather as much information as possible. Your business bank account representative is often a good resource and may be helpful in directing you to seminars and classes that will bring you up to speed on related issues, such as identity theft and credit card fraud. Take advantage of such classes whenever possible.

SPECIALIZED TECHNOLOGY

The list of specialized technology designed to aid the spa industry is growing. Two devices that are particularly beneficial to spas include pagers and digital imaging equipment. For obvious reasons, time management is extremely important to day spa owners. Clocks in treatment rooms and software programs that build turnaround time into the service schedule are useful, but to help spa managers keep service providers on schedule, many spas have adopted the use of pagers.

Pagers

Several types of pagers are available to keep guests and staff on schedule. Guest pagers given to clients that arrive early are ideal for spas located in busy shopping malls, where clients have the opportunity to run an errand while waiting. They can also be used to route clients from one service to another. Pager styles and techniques vary and can include vibrations, flashing lights, or beeps. Some are even capable of programming advertising messages, but all have the same goal—to alert the client when the service provider is ready.

Silent pagers for staff are available as numeric and alphanumeric text messaging systems. These devices are great for letting a service provider in session know that the next client has arrived without disturbing the relaxation benefit to the client. For example, a simple text message, such as "Your 10:00 am facial is here," can be sent discreetly to the service provider. Spas that take walk-ins or simply wish to optimize service can also benefit from individual treatment room units or transmitters that allow staff to alert front desk staff that a room is empty and a service provider is available. Specialized software is required to perform these tasks.

Digital Cameras

Those interested in demonstrating the effectiveness of highly specialized products or series treatments should consider the use of a digital camera. Digital photography can provide an objective assessment of skin conditions, such as wrinkles or sun damage, which can be extremely helpful to skin care specialists looking to initiate a dialogue on client goals or develop long-term targeted treatment plans. It also gives clinicians a valid way to measure client progress over time, a method that is popular in medical aesthetic spas. If your day spa works cooperatively with medical personnel this can be a useful tool that promotes better communication; however, you should be aware that archiving photographs requires strict confidentiality practices. A client's right to privacy should be taken seriously whether or not you work under medical constraints.

There are many other uses for the digital camera in the spa, including marketing and public relations efforts. Documenting an important event or showcasing a particular treatment or service with digital images that can be reproduced in brochures and Web sites, or delivered to media can be an effective part of an overall marketing strategy. We'll talk more about using salon images for marketing purposes in the next two chapters.

If you are interested in purchasing a digital camera for use in your spa, look for one that is easy to use, has flexible lighting options, offers good resolution, incorporates lenses that are suitable for close-up facial photography, and has enough megapixels to enlarge and touch up photos for publication. There are many models to choose from with all kinds of sophisticated accessories and accompanying software programs to help clinicians analyze, store and retrieve images on their computer. Some are pricier than others so be sure to shop around for the one that best fits your business needs.

Simulation Software

This type of digital imaging software is used to give the client a preview of what to expect. It is used in salons, spas, and medical aesthetic practices to discuss various options, such as hair color, make-up application, and plastic surgery techniques. Using digital photos and specialized software programs, a realistic simulation of the intended outcome is developed for the client's review. This is an excellent tool for managing the indecisive client and evaluating and establishing realistic outcomes, although it should be noted that this type of imaging equipment can be pricey and may not be warranted in all day spa environments.

Whatever imaging methods you ultimately decide to employ in your spa, make sure they are worth the return on your investment and that you are respectful of the client's right to privacy when storing, retrieving, and handling photos or exchanging information. If you intend to use any photo of a client for advertising, teaching, or promoting any treatment or service, be sure to gain the client's consent in writing.

Audiovisual Equipment

When planning your technology budget, don't forget important items such as a stereo system, television, and video equipment. A quality sound system will add to your clients' relaxation benefit and can enhance the quality of the work environment for staff; however, purchasing audiovisual equipment is no longer a simple task.

Audio systems have become extremely sophisticated with numerous options to control individual treatment rooms and areas, making it necessary to consider wiring during the construction phase. There are also choices to be made when it comes to music selection. Today, many spas are using digital music content providers, companies that offer subscriptions to preprogrammed music. This service is worth looking into to avoid copyright issues, one of the newest litigation concerns emanating from the music industry that can affect spas that play CDs in the workplace.

Those who enjoy being on the cutting edge of technology may also want to incorporate the use of *podcasts*, audio broadcasts that are delivered over the internet via digital files. While various uses for podcasts are still being explored in the spa industry, podcasts are ideal for educating clients, promoting the spa life and healthy living. Creating a unique series of meaningful podcasts is an excellent noninvasive way to stay in touch with clients in between visits. Podcasts are easily downloaded and can be listened to at the client's leisure from their personal computer or a portable media player.

Television and video equipment is usually not at the top of the list for spa owners, but don't overlook these important visual communication tools. While many spas are opposed to invading the sanctity of the spa environment with any reminder of the outside world, some are turning sleek, unobtrusive, plasma television screens into a versatile amenity that adds to the client's overall enjoyment of the spa experience. Others are incorporating cyber cafés and hosting Wi-Fi Internet connections as amenities for clients who insist on being connected at all times. Your individual spa philosophy will dictate whether or not you incorporate these items and how, but it is important to note that television and DVD equipment can serve as excellent marketing tools, helping you to introduce and sell new or specialized treatments and services. They can also be extremely useful for staff training purposes.

THINK IT OVER

Technology has revolutionized the way day spas conduct business today. This trend will no doubt continue as newer methods are developed. When considering the many ways technology can be applied in your spa, remember that in most cases technology indicates progress and can eliminate or simplify many of the more tedious and costly tasks you must accomplish to run your business; however, not all technological tools will be right for your spa. Your budget will be an important factor in the type and amount of technology you decide to incorporate. There are other important considerations, such as your ability to maintain certain operations, and how you feel about the superfluous use of technology in what many feel should be a stress-free zone for clients, that will no doubt play a role in your decision making. Perhaps the best advice you can receive in this competitive business environment is: Don't be afraid to use technology. In the end, the right technology could be what puts your spa on the map—no small feat in what is now an intricately bound World Wide Web.

MARKETING YOUR SPA

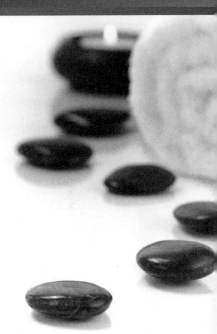

Y̶ou have all of the operational requirements in place—the right location, an impressive spa design, top-notch equipment, and efficient business technology—but without clients your business will not succeed. To attract the right clients to your spa, you need to develop and implement a good marketing plan.

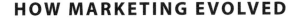

HOW MARKETING EVOLVED

In ancient times, the concept of marketing was easily understood. People went *to market* to barter or exchange goods they had for things they did not have. The key to a successful exchange was having something to offer to others that they either needed or wanted. As civilizations evolved, the concept of marketing became more complex, requiring an arbitrary value system to sustain those with limited resources. Money replaced bartering, and a definite value or price was assigned to goods and services.

This is certainly a simple explanation of the evolution of marketing, but it highlights the concept of a mutually satisfying exchange, one of the basic principles of marketing that still holds true today.

MARKETING IN MODERN TIMES

Since the industrial revolution, marketing has become a complex process that has undergone a number of significant transformations.

In the last century, the concept of marketing in the United States has progressed from a simple production model, where a scarcity of goods created its own demand, to an era where overproduction stimulated a fiercely competitive sales environment. This set the stage for a much broader *marketing concept era* that moved beyond sales toward satisfying the customer's needs and achieving organizational goals.

As we enter a new millennium, marketing has taken on a "consumer-centric" orientation that puts the customer at the core of all marketing efforts. This development has marketing managers thoroughly entrenched in managing customer relations, a concept commonly referred to as *customer relationship management* (CRM). To do this effectively, marketing teams focus on collecting and analyzing as much information as possible about their customers and competitors to create consumer value. This practice has been fueled by tremendous advances in technology that make it possible to develop consumer profiles at the push of a button, but it also relies heavily on developing a personal bond with the consumer. This is a definite boon for the spa owner, whose business naturally focuses on building a one-to-one relationship with the client.

With customer relationships at the forefront, marketing has taken yet another significant step in recent years—that of developing consumer confidence in marketing practices, building trust and establishing credibility; a situation that has elevated public relations to a leading role in present day marketing strategies.

Definition of Marketing

Although many automatically equate marketing with sales and advertising, marketing actually encompasses a much broader business strategy for how goods and services are bought and sold or exchanged.

Over the past two decades the American Marketing Association's definition of marketing has evolved from a more practical management-focused viewpoint to a much broader philosophy that currently defines marketing as "the activity, set of institutions, and processes for creating, communicating, delivering, and exchanging offerings that have value for customers, clients, partners and society at large." [AMA 2008] While the AMA's current definition of marketing continues to acknowledge core business principles, it places greater value on the education and scientific components of marketing and acknowledges its wider communal effects.

Customer Value

The current definition of marketing gives us a healthy respect for its broader reach; however, it does not deter from what is perhaps the most critical factor in marketing: customer value. All markets ultimately consist of people with specific needs and wants. To put it simply, buyers, referred to as clients in the spa industry, have certain needs and/or wants when it comes to purchasing spa services and products. As a spa owner, or seller of spa services and products, it is ultimately your job to satisfy those needs and wants. The most important thing to remember is that in the process of marketing something of value is exchanged so that ideally both the buyer and seller are each better off. As you establish goals and map out a detailed marketing plan, developing a solid understanding of what those needs and wants are should be a top priority.

NEEDS VERSUS WANTS

The debate over what consumers need versus what they want appears to be endless. What difference does it make to us in terms of marketing, and how do we differentiate between the two? *Needs* refer to basic necessities. For instance, we all need food, clothing, and shelter. *Wants* are shaped by our knowledge of a particular product, the culture in which we live, and our individual personalities. Now think about how many times you have stood in a department store trying to justify the purchase of an item based on whether you really needed it or just wanted it.

An effective marketing strategy can create or shape the needs and wants of the consumer. For example, people need clothing, but their apparel choices may be influenced by any number of factors, such as cost, color or quality of the fabric, information about the manufacturing process, and availability. If they are driven by fashion trends, their clothing choices may also be influenced by certain style magazines, a brand name label, or a celebrity endorsement. Time and convenience can also play a role in the decision-making process, making a person more apt to shop for clothes at a nearby mall, via a catalogue, or online.

WHAT DO YOUR CLIENTS VALUE?

To get consumers to buy their product, marketing managers know they must satisfy a variety of needs and wants. As the marketing manager of your spa, the big question is what do your clients need and/or want?

In Chapter 2, we learned that studying the demographics of a population is an important part of developing an effective marketing plan. Before deciding which treatments you will offer or the brand of retail products you will sell, it is important to know what your clients value. Are they looking for quality spa services at value prices, or are they willing to pay high prices for exclusive treatments and results-driven products? Are convenience and accessibility a top priority? For example, do they expect quick, efficient treatments during their lunch hour or want to be able to schedule early morning or late evening appointments? For some, customer service may be a top priority. In that case, time spent explaining procedures, home care programs and products, educational seminars, and literature or an opportunity to speak directly to you when they have a question or concern will be important to them.

All of these things should factor into your marketing program, but catering to the wants and needs of your customers does not mean you cannot influence their purchasing decisions. The right product, presented at the right time, to the right market can sway consumers' buying decisions. Who would have thought that consumers would go for breakfast in a bar, microwave meals, laser hair removal, pumpkin peels, and permanent make-up? Think about this as you develop your marketing plan.

The Marketing Mix

All marketing efforts should be based on a strategic business plan. This typically begins by establishing what are commonly known as the four Ps: Product, Price, Promotion, and Place. All of these factors, generally referred to as the *marketing mix,* form the basis of a marketing strategy. As a spa owner, keep in mind that you control these factors in an effort to market your business in the most efficient and profitable manner possible.

PRODUCT

Defining your *product* is generally the first step in developing a marketing plan. In the spa business, product refers to the complete *spa concept.* This includes all of the services you offer, the products and equipment you use to perform those services, and the retail products you sell. It also takes into account all of the nuances that make your spa unique.

To develop your product or spa concept, you will first need to identify all of the tangible and intangible characteristics associated with operating your spa business, a task you actually began in Chapter 1 when you were asked to define your ideal spa. During this phase of business development, you will need to express those objectives in more finite terms. This involves decisions about the focus of your business. For example, will you establish your spa as place to relax, remedy certain skin conditions, improve appearances, or develop overall health and wellness? What name will you use for your spa business? Will you incorporate water therapies, such as a hydrotherapy tub or a steam shower? What type of equipment will you use? Which retail items will you sell? How many people will you employ? As you develop your plan, it is in your best interest to define your spa concept in the most explicit terms possible.

PRICE

Determining a *price* or value for your products and services is a major component of the marketing mix. Your pricing should account for all of the costs associated with selling your products and services. This includes the cost of performing each service in terms of direct (labor, time, and materials) and indirect costs (rent and utilities). What the competition is charging is also a factor. How will your prices compare? Will they be competitive, discounted, value oriented, or associated with superior quality?

Another important consideration in pricing is the demand for your product or services. What can you expect in terms of volume? If there is a large population of spa-goers in your area, what percentage of the population can you expect to frequent your spa? More importantly, how much is that population willing to pay for spa services? Other factors such as economic conditions and the level of sophistication of your target market will have a direct impact on pricing as well. Of course, you are in business to do business; so be sure to calculate a reasonable profit margin into the final equation.

PROMOTION

Designing a *promotion* strategy is critical to getting your message to the consumer. Promotion involves several methods of communication: advertising, public relations, publicity, direct marketing, sales promotions, and personal selling tactics. Most businesses use a combination of these methods to enhance sales, such as simultaneously running an ad in the local newspaper and sending a direct mail piece to clients. If your spa is hosting a special event, you might seek publicity in addition to sending out invitations.

Whatever methods you decide to use, take a thoughtful approach and map your strategy out carefully for the entire calendar year. Taking a laissez-faire approach to promotions with in-spa flyers and random advertising techniques is not likely to get the sales results you are seeking.

PLACE

Place refers to the channel of distribution that is used to supply the consumer with your product or service. In marketing retail items there may be several channels of distribution with a product going from the manufacturer to a wholesaler and then to a distributor before it actually gets to the retailer and into the hands of the consumer. Products may also be available in several distribution outlets, such as in department stores, drugstores, or supermarkets.

In the spa industry, manufacturers of certain retail products, such as professional skin care items and equipment, may use a limited or exclusive number of channels or intermediaries to dispense their products. Some also sell directly to spas. As a spa owner, you are in the position to distribute your own private label products; in which case, the distribution channel is shortened.

Because the spa business is a service business, it can be hard to separate the role of place from the service provider. When looking at place from this perspective, greater emphasis is placed on the role of convenience in marketing your spa. For example, do clients view your spa as easily accessible, affordable, and customer-service oriented? As you develop your spa business, you will want to give serious thought to how clients perceive this aspect of your services (Table 8-1).

WHAT DO YOU WANT MARKETING TO DO FOR YOU?

The four Ps form the basis of a strategic design and development plan, but before you can put your plan into effect, it is important to determine what it is you want marketing to accomplish for your business. Would you like to generate a certain level of gross revenue, increase sales, double your gross income, or make it possible to give your employees an annual cost-of-living wage increase?

TABLE 8-1	MARKETING MIX FOR SUCCESSFUL DAY SPA
Product	• Successful Day Spa will offer a complete menu of superior face and body services. These services will be focused on providing clients with exclusive treatments geared toward enhancing appearance and maintaining a youthful image.
Price	• Successful Day Spa's services will range in price from moderate to high with retail products geared toward the high end. Compared to other spas in the area, Successful Day Spa's prices will be higher.
Promotion	• Successful Day Spa will use a variety of promotional strategies, including advertising, sales promotions, public relations, publicity, and direct marketing. All efforts will be geared toward attracting an upscale clientele via sophisticated media and professionally designed vehicles.
Place	• Successful Day Spa will market directly to spa-goers from a conveniently located urban facility adjacent to several other popular upscale stores in the heart of a downtown metropolis. Successful Day Spa will distribute an exclusive line of private label products under the Successful brand name.

Organizational goals will vary, but all marketing strategies require ongoing evaluation and periodic adjustments. Marketing is a dynamic process that keeps business flowing. It is unwise to think of it as something that can eventually be discontinued once you reach certain sales goals or revenue markers. It is also foolish to think you can rely on one single strategy to achieve the results you want.

Developing a Marketing Plan

In Chapter 3, we outlined the ingredients of a good marketing plan. This included: (a) understanding current economic conditions; (b) identifying your target market; (c) performing a competitive analysis; (d) establishing a unique selling position; and (e) describing the methods you will use to promote your spa business. Let's take a closer look at these important steps now.

STUDY ECONOMIC CONDITIONS

Reports that the spa industry is booming abound, but does this mean that your day spa is guaranteed to be a winner? Not necessarily. As we discussed in Chapter 2, all data should be studied carefully, especially when it comes to money. Robust economic indicators may not specify that the bulk of spa industry revenues actually come from a small group of high-end destination spas or a select group of full-service and medical spa facilities. Your goal is to find out what a spa business similar to the one you would like to open has the potential to earn in the geographic area you have selected.

Begin your search by taking the overall pulse of the nation. Is the economy strong, flat, depressed, on the upswing, or in recovery? How do these national figures compare to what is happening in the particular region and, more importantly, the community where your spa will be located? It is important to recognize that in some cases the economic viability of a community can depend on a single business, a particular industry, or even the weather if the area depends on tourism to make a living.

Examine the Spa Industry

If the economy appears healthy, you will want to examine the spa industry more closely. How many spas are currently in business across the country? What are they earning? What is the growth rate? If these preliminary findings give you confidence that the spa industry is stable, you will want to take your investigation further by studying the success rate of spas that are located in the specific geographic location in which you are interested. A downturn in the economy will require significantly more research to determine if this is the right time to set your plan in motion.

Cross-Reference Your Findings

It is important to bring the human element into your study. This means cross-referencing industry statistics with the rate of unemployment and the average household income in your community. This data is generally available through local and state government offices such as Town Hall and the Department of Labor.

How do these facts and figures stack up against your spa concept? For example, could you expect those with an average household income of $70,000 and two children to purchase your spa services? Or might they be out of their price range? What is the unemployment rate in your target area? If there is a high unemployment percentage, will spa services be the first thing clients are likely to cut from their expenditures? How will transient populations, such as those who work in the area, affect your business?

Ask around, and you may learn that a number of businesses are supported by customers who do not even live in the area. You may also discover other useful information, such as the fact that most people in the community travel outside the area to purchase an elite brand of spa services.

When all of the facts are tallied, you may decide that a good marketing strategy can prevail over certain circumstances. Many have made a fortune by taking advantage of poor economic conditions or finding creative ways to weather tough economic times, but it is always best to understand the odds.

IDENTIFY YOUR TARGET MARKET

Successful entrepreneurs understand that they cannot be all things to all people. By directing your marketing efforts toward a particular group of potential clients, or *target market,* that is more likely to want or need your services, you increase the probability of your success.

Positioning your product or services to satisfy the needs of a particular market segment is known as *target marketing.* This is an important step in the marketing process that will help your spa to become more profitable. Target marketing is used to identify the needs of those who are most likely to purchase your services. It can also help you to identify a segment of the market with unfulfilled needs. The growing interest in targeting men for spa services is a good example (Figure 8-1).

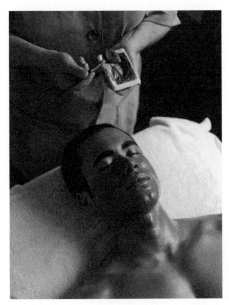

FIGURE 8-1 Men have become an increasingly sought after target market.

Your target market can be broken down in terms of age, sex, education level, economic status, and lifestyle. For example, the services in your spa may be geared toward career women ages 35–50 who have an average income of $50,000 to $60,000 per year. Or it might attempt to reach those with a certain lifestyle, such as men and women age 50 or older with a high level of disposable income who are looking for spa services to maintain a youthful vitality. You could also decide to direct your spa services specifically toward men or teens and preteens.

Most spas target a certain market to bring in the bulk of their revenue but use additional market segments to enhance their profits. For instance, a spa's clientele may consist mainly of women between the ages of 40 and 50, but a good deal of effort may be expended to attract teenage girls. A well-rounded marketing strategy will include other groups that can enhance your profitability.

As a spa owner, this means that you are likely to have somewhat of a varied clientele that will require you to use a combination of marketing strategies. Without losing sight of your primary target market, it is important to specify a plan for each additional category. Using an outline that defines *who* you will market to, *what* you will offer, *where* you will market, *when* you will market to them, and *how* you will fulfill their needs or reach them will help you to plan effective promotion strategies that satisfy all of your clients' needs and increase your profitability.

TARGET MARKETING STRATEGY FOR SUCCESSFUL DAY SPA'S "MEN'S SPA"

Who
- Men ages 25 to 45 are a secondary market for Successful Day Spa.

What
- Spa products and services for this group will be geared specifically toward meeting the personal care needs of men.

Where
- Marketing will occur in places where they spend time, such as gyms, airports, hotels, apparel shops, and sporting events as well as on the Internet.

When
- Marketing efforts will be focused on the time of the day, month, or year men are most likely to respond to ads and

> promotions, for example, at their computer during regular business hours.
>
> - As a secondary target market, we will make an effort to reach this group three times per year with targeted sales promotions.
>
> How - Successful Day Spa will segregate an area specifically for men. This will have multimedia components and masculine furnishings.
>
> - We will use media that men are most apt to respond to, such as electronic mail, direct mail postcards, print (newspaper and magazines), television, and radio advertising.

PERFORM A COMPETITIVE ANALYSIS

We discussed the importance of checking out the competition in Chapter 4 and know that an inability to recognize the competition is one of the top reasons many businesses fail, so it is critical that you take this task seriously.

An analysis of your competition should begin by calculating the number of day spas in your area; however, because there are no set standards or criteria for separating day spas from beauty or skin care salons, it can be difficult to extract this data. The board that governs spa businesses in your state, ordinarily the Board of Cosmetology, can be of assistance here. Although the board may not be able to segregate day spas, they can usually supply a list of beauty and skin care salons that might be helpful in zeroing in on those that are calling themselves day spas. If possible, ask to have the list arranged by zip code to help you distinguish the number of spas in your area, but be prepared to pay for this service. It is also a good idea to cross reference this information with state and local offices responsible for registering all businesses. This will help to fill in the gaps.

Next, you will want to compare the types of services your primary competitors are offering. Beyond the standard skin care, body treatments, and massage therapies, is there anything that makes one or the other stand out from the crowd? How so? Take time to compare all of your competitors' services to your spa menu. What crossover do you see? Are there any services that you intend to offer that are not on your competitors' menu, or are most of the services you intend to offer the same or similar?

Price is a major competitive point that should be scrutinized carefully. What are your competitors charging for their services? Here is where you must take a calculated risk. Go back to the four Ps and your original plan. Given what you have learned, does it make sense to undercut those prices, charge comparable rates, or establish your spa as one that offers premium or superior services at top dollar?

After carefully reviewing all of this data, you will want to assess whether or not the population can support another day spa in the area. But don't rely on economic conditions alone. The answer to this question also depends on your ability to establish a unique selling position.

Establish a Unique Selling Position

If you were to ask your clients the first thing that comes to mind when they think of your spa, what would you want that to be?

Establishing a unique selling position (USP) is an important phase of marketing development that describes how your business is better than or different from the competition; however, with the number of day spas growing at a rapid pace, setting your spa apart is no easy task. Too often, we see nothing more than spas mimicking one another, with the same treatments and even the same descriptions of those treatments appearing over and over again. How will you differentiate your spa services? Finding out what your competitors are offering is a good place to begin, but you will also need to look closely at the clients you wish to attract.

To create a unique selling position, you will need a solid understanding of the needs of your target market and a distinct method for satisfying those needs. Not only should this be something that clients can clearly distinguish from the competition, but also whatever you decide to offer should be something your clients clearly want and value. Think in terms of a specific experience that is reproducible time after time and one that clients come to associate with your spa. Yet unlike a signature treatment, a USP is more in line with a certain level of quality and service that clients come to expect.

Many times spa business owners looking to appeal to a wider market segment make the mistake of doing a lot of things in a mediocre way or take on more than they can handle, only to find that clients don't really associate them clearly with any one thing. If you are not quite sure of your spa's focus, take some time to develop your business skills and promote excellence. In the process, you may discover that clients actually help you to establish a unique selling position by demanding more of a particular service.

Spa business owners can also get into trouble when they confuse a unique spa design with a unique selling position. Although a fabulous ambiance can add to the client's overall enjoyment of the spa experience, it is important to note that a posh setting with lavish décor won't keep customers coming back. Without a reputation for quality, beneficial treatments, and excellent customer service, clients will soon come to see your spa as just another designer showplace.

Undoubtedly, the best USP is one that has your clients talking about how well they are treated and how great your services are. One of the more novel approaches I have seen was in a full-service day spa that employed a designated customer relations person. Along with several other public relations duties, it was that person's job to make sure that every client left the spa satisfied. To set the tone, all hair services began with a relaxing shampoo and scalp treatment. Spa treatments incorporated a hand or foot massage. At the end of their treatment, clients were asked about their experience. If a client reported anything less than a positive experience, every effort was made to understand why and correct the situation to the client's satisfaction.

As you identify your USP, remember that it can be just about anything: a proprietary product or one that is exclusively limited to a select number of spas; an exclusive treatment method; a unique philosophy; or a creative approach to delivering your services. For example, you may choose to establish your spa as ecologically conscious, using only nature-based treatment products, earth-friendly décor and cleaning products, and linens that are recyclable.

There are many other ways to establish a unique selling position. Some that have been successful include injecting elements of the local culture, topography, or climate into the spa experience, offering express treatments for those on the go, customizing treatments or products, or targeting a niche market, such as teens. Deciding what works best for your spa is ultimately a matter of answering the needs of your clientele with an economically viable marketing plan that first and foremost creates extraordinary consumer value.

Marketing Communications

In marketing, how you get your message across is just as important as what you have to say. An effective marketing communications program involves several key components that are easily clarified by addressing what, how, where, and who—that is, *what* you have to offer, *how* you present it, *where* you deliver your message, and *who* your target market is. Keep these in mind as you develop your marketing communications plan.

THE PROMOTION MIX

Without a doubt, the best form of marketing is *word of mouth*. An outstanding reputation for quality treatments and excellent customer service that has everyone singing your spa's praises is the best way to promote your business, but to get to that point, you need a carefully planned promotional strategy.

The *promotion mix* refers to the various methods that are used to communicate a company's marketing message such as advertising, public relations, publicity, sales promotion, direct marketing, and personal selling. Most businesses use a combination of these to develop an inclusive marketing program.

Advertising

Although *advertising* is used loosely to refer to any aspect of promoting business, in marketing this term refers to promotional efforts that are paid for with the direct intention of increasing business.

There are many ways to advertise your spa. More popular methods include classified, newspaper, magazine, television, and radio ads. These are appealing because they provide the advertiser with an opportunity to reach a large number of people in a relatively cost-effective manner.

Selecting the Right Media

There are literally hundreds of media vendors vying for your advertising dollar. Selecting the best vehicles to promote your spa will require the same kind of detailed demographic analysis used to evaluate other aspects of your business.

A reputable media vendor should be able to supply you with specific information about the number of people watching, listening, or reading their program or publication, as well as specific information about that population, including the average age, sex, income, and education level. Pay careful attention to this data, as it is essential that it include your target market.

Cost is another significant factor in media selection. Rates vary among print and broadcast media with more elite publications, television, and radio stations capable of demanding higher prices. All are nevertheless based on the same criteria: frequency or air time and size. *Frequency* refers to the number of times the ad is run within a certain time period and is usually based on one calendar year. *Air time* is a factor in broadcast media, where cost is measured according to the duration of the ad or amount of time, generally the number of seconds or minutes the ad will be aired. Newspapers and magazines calculate costs in terms of the *size* of the ad space, generally defined as column inches or a portion of the page, such as a full-, half-, or quarter-page ad. Because media tend to offer discounts that are intertwined with frequency, placement, and color, rates can be difficult to understand. If you find yourself puzzled, don't wait until you receive an exorbitant bill to gain clarity. Ask your vendor to break it down in language you understand beforehand.

As you sort through the countless media options, consider also which formats are most in sync with your image. If yours is a posh, high-end day spa, you are not likely to attract your target market by advertising in a suburban shopping guide that showcases best bargains. Yet limiting your advertising to one or two high-end publications is a mistake.

You need to use a variety of media resources to reach your target market. Just because you have a Web site does not mean you should skip advertising in telephone directories or avoid placing a display ad in local or regional newspapers and magazines. But don't limit your print advertising to newspapers and magazines. Consider renting a billboard at a nearby mall or placing an ad on the screen at your local theater. A good advertising program will incorporate a number of different vehicles and should be flexible enough to accommodate spontaneous opportunities, such as a display ad in a special program for a community event.

Setting Advertising Goals

The goal of any advertising plan is to increase business, but it is important that your advertising plan is consistent with your overall marketing strategy. What do you want your advertising program to achieve? Name recognition or an overall increase in sales? Do you want to prompt more visitors to your Web site? Promote a new service provider or elicit a direct response for a specific spa treatment? The answer to these questions depends on where you are at in the evolution of your business. You may be juggling multiple objectives simultaneously. To be successful, you will need to supervise your advertising program closely. (See Table 8-2). If you lack marketing experience or simply don't have enough time, it is best to hire a professional to do this for you.

Whether you intend to use a consultant or map out a strategy on your own, heed this caution: Advertising reps can be extremely convincing. Make sure account executives understand that you have targeted goals and are looking for just the right opportunities to promote them. Too many times, day spa owners are driven by an enthusiastic sales pitch from a sales representative looking to fill random time slots or space. If the media they are selling does not fit your promotional goals or budget, don't waste precious advertising dollars. This is especially true if your advertising budget is limited. Most media reps are happy to point out those issues, programs, or spots that will benefit your spa's marketing initiative; however, it is still your job to make sure that person understands the needs of your business.

TABLE 8-2	ADVERTISING CALENDAR FOR SUCCESSFUL DAY SPA						
Publication	**Ad Size**	**Cost per Ad**	**Jan**	**Feb**	**Mar**	**Apr**
Metro Newspaper	1/5 page display ad	575	✓✓	✓✓	✓✓	✓✓
Local Newspaper	1/4 page display ad	250	✓✓✓✓	✓✓✓✓	✓✓✓✓	✓✓✓✓
Metro Magazine	1/8 page display ad	1,300	✓	✓	✓	✓
Community Guide	1/2 page display ad	800 per year				
Spa Directory A	Classified	150 per year	✓	✓	✓	✓
Spa Directory B	Display Ad	395 per year	✓	✓	✓	✓
Radio Broadcast	30/60 sec. spots per week	2,000 per week	✓✓✓✓			
Cable TV	5/90 sec. infomercials per week	1,500 per week	✓		✓	
Internet	Banner	300 per month	✓			
Telephone Directory	Display Ad	3,000 per year	✓	✓	✓	✓
	Super Pages	40 per month	✓	✓	✓	✓
Miscellaneous Reserve						

Helpful Hint: Establishing a budget at the beginning of each calendar year and taking advantage of lower renewal rates will help you to get the most out of your advertising dollars.

On occasion, an account manager tuned into your marketing goals may present a last-minute media buy that has the potential to reach your target market with a great offer. Learning to distinguish a good buy that fits into your overall marketing strategy and budget will help you to spend wisely.

Look for opportunities that directly correlate to promoting your spa business, such as a special section in a newspaper that is geared toward health and wellness, beauty, weddings or holiday gift guides. Consumer guides or Web sites, such as those that list all of the businesses in an area, or help people locate spas in a specific geographic location, can also be cost-effective. Other collaborative advertising resources, such as those that target brides or a specific industry, are another viable advertising option for spa owners.

Building Name Recognition

One of the primary objectives in advertising is building name recognition. A powerful message used consistently over time in a medium that appeals specifically to your target market, such as a special section of a newspaper

May	Jun	Jul	Aug	Sept	Oct	Nov	Dec	Yr Total
✓✓	✓✓	✓✓	✓✓	✓✓	✓✓	✓✓	✓✓	13,800
✓✓✓✓	✓✓✓✓	✓✓✓✓	✓✓✓✓	✓✓✓✓	✓✓✓✓	✓✓✓✓	✓✓✓✓	13,000
✓	✓	✓	✓	✓	✓	✓	✓	15,600
								800
✓	✓	✓	✓	✓	✓	✓	✓	150
✓	✓	✓	✓	✓	✓	✓	✓	395
✓✓✓✓				✓✓✓✓				8,000
✓				✓				4,500
✓			✓			✓		1,200
✓	✓	✓	✓	✓	✓	✓	✓	3,000
✓	✓	✓	✓	✓	✓	✓	✓	480
								5,000
					Total for year with addition of directories			65,925

or magazine or a radio program you know clients read or watch, can help you to achieve this goal. But don't expect your spa's name to become a household word overnight.

Many small businesses have lost their nerve waiting for the kickback. If your ad does not bring in a ton of calls overnight, don't be too hasty to nix it. Building momentum takes time and patience. For example, several months into the program a client called to let me know that a certain magazine ad was finally pulling in customers. Many of the clients who were responding to the ad reported that they had clipped it for future reference or that they were suddenly driven to a response after seeing the ad repeatedly. If you feel the medium is definitely your target market, it is important to hang in for the long haul.

Public Relations

We hear a lot about *public relations* (PR) today. In fact, PR, as it is more commonly referred to, has replaced advertising as the top marketing communications tool. Why? Public relations is the direct result of a public that has grown leery of slick ad campaigns and broken promises and is now demanding a more ethical approach to advertising.

Most people simply equate public relations with generating free publicity. However, public relations is actually a more involved marketing process that requires careful strategic planning.

The main objective in any public relations program is to steer public opinion in a positive direction. PR accomplishes this by publicizing information about your business and backing it up with factual information to support marketing claims. In the spa business, PR is usually aimed at building credibility around a spa's products and services. The public must see the value in what you sell and do before they will buy into it. To increase your company's credibility, public relations professionals seek media coverage, plan events, and encourage businesses to do good works to get attention, rather than purchasing paid advertising. Planning and developing relationships with key people who have the authority to shape or influence public opinion is a significant part of this process.

But PR is not simply about managing the media or gaining celebrity endorsements. A good PR program will also take into account how you handle all interpersonal interactions, including customer, employee, vendor, and community relations. Think of it as a total communication plan that involves all of your business relationships.

Using a Public Relations Professional or Agency

A qualified public relations professional or agency can provide an overall communications strategy to help you promote your business. This generally includes coordinating all aspects of the promotion mix, such as public

BUILDING PUBLIC RELATIONS

A good public relations program requires:

- Effective communication and management skills

- Ethical business policies and practices

- A commitment to providing quality service

- An ability to resolve difficult situations with skill and diplomacy

- Respect for individual differences and the work others do

- Standards that foster goodwill in the community

relations, advertising, publicity, event planning, and sales promotions to create a unified and consistent message.

To present your spa business in a polished professional manner, PR professionals must conduct a great deal of preliminary work. This usually involves collecting data about your business and developing promotional materials, such as a press kit, press releases, and advertorials. Your input is a vital part of this process. Make sure they have all the facts about your business and are informed about any marketing communications efforts you are currently using. Be forthcoming about what has and what hasn't worked in the past, and be open and willing to listen to any suggestions they offer. A team effort is required to create a synchronized communications program that ties all of your media efforts together, such as your brochure, Web site, and advertising.

Some spa owners choose to contract with a PR professional to manage only certain aspects of their public relations program, such as press and media relations, rather than implement an entire strategy. If you go this route, take time to establish clear boundaries that define the role and responsibilities of each party. It is also wise to clarify fees. Some PR professionals work on a project basis, while others have a set fee schedule. Whichever you agree to, make sure you understand exactly what the terms of your contract entitles you to and that you are comfortable with how a PR professional works.

PUBLIC RELATIONS SERVICES MAY INCLUDE

- Qualifying media outlets
- Following editorial calendars
- Targeting key journalists
- Writing press releases and advertorials
- Generating publicity
- Planning events
- Providing crisis management
- Acting as a spokesperson for the company
- Positioning the client as an expert
- Conducting research that supports your philosophy, treatments, and services
- Developing relationships with key people and organizations

One of the more important services PR professionals provide is presenting your spa to the media; however, contact lists are generally not something that are handed over to clients, a point of difference that can lead to misunderstandings with those who are unfamiliar with the process. PR professionals also spend a great deal of time researching, networking, and developing relationships to achieve their goals. If you have difficulty seeing the value in these professional services, then hiring a PR person is probably not for you.

Targeting the Right Media

Media knowledge is critical to getting information about your spa in the hands of the right people. Some businesses specialize in distributing press releases to a huge volume of media outlets, but a good PR agent attuned to your needs understands that there are really only a handful of people at the local, regional, or national level, not millions, that can help you further your business.

PR professionals study the editorial position of print and broadcast media and know who to target and how to pitch stories that will pique their interest. They are also skilled at positioning the same information to a broad range of media channels, including daily and weekly newspapers, consumer magazines, trade publications, business journals, newsletters, radio and television broadcasts, and other organizations, in a way that will capture the interest of their target audience.

Small business owners on a budget are often advised to solicit such media attention directly, but it is important to understand that the media generally prefers to work with PR professionals who understand the process, know what is newsworthy, and can deliver the facts quickly.

Press Release

The press release is the standard form of communication for interfacing with the media and one that journalists, who are constantly looking for news, rely on to keep them informed. It is a succinctly written and informative news release that follows a structured format.

STANDARD FORMAT FOR SUBMITTING A PRESS RELEASE

1. State the name, address, and Web site of the spa or company that the release is being written for at the top of the page but do not include the terms *Inc.*, *LLC*, or other abbreviations unless there is a chance that the company might be confused with

some other business. Spa stationary or a logo may also be used to identify the business.

2. List the *contact information* (name, telephone number, and e-mail address) of the spa or public relations representative responsible for supplying additional information to the press.

3. Write the words "PRESS RELEASE" across the top, followed by the words "FOR IMMEDIATE RELEASE" in capital letters to let news people know the information is currently available to the public. If the information is intended as a feature story, the words "RELEASE AT WILL" may replace these words.

4. Provide a *headline* that sums up what the release is about in as few words as possible. "One-liners" are ideal, but two lines can be used if needed to form a complete thought. In some cases, a brief subheading is used to support the headline (Figure 8-2).

5. State the *dateline information* (city, state, and date) at the beginning of the first paragraph of the text to let the reader know *where* the information is being released from and *when*.

6. Use the *body of the text* to explain *why* the information is important to the target audience. The first few sentences or paragraph of your text are critical to the success of the press release and should answer *who, what, where, when, why*, and *how*. The remaining paragraphs should support this information and may include direct quotes from the spa owner, provided they are meaningful. Other legitimate resources and statistics can also be used to help validate the main points.

7. End your press release with a *closing paragraph* that gives the reader standard information about your spa and the best way to access more information about the company or topic.

8. The very *end* of a press release is indicated by the use of three consecutive pound signs "###," the number "30," or the word "END" to let the newsperson know there is no other information to follow. Note that when more than one page is used in a press release, number the pages and place the word *continued* at the bottom of the page to indicate that another page follows.

Successful Day Spa
123 Chic Main Street
Urban Oasis, SPA 45678
987.654.3210

Press Release

FOR IMMEDIATE RELEASE

CONTACT:
Janet D'Angelo
J. Angel Communications
781.545.5508
janet@jangelcommunications.com

SAMPLE HEADLINES

Successful Day Spa Launches New Product Line

Successful Day Spa Sponsors Skin Cancer Awareness Clinic

Successful Day Spa Voted Best Day Spa in Urban Oasis

Successful Day Spa Announces Appointment of New Spa Director

Spa Town, State, June 1, 2005

Body of Text

Closing Paragraph

END

FIGURE 8-2   The headline should grab the reader's attention and summarize what the press release is about in as few words as possible.

The use of a structured format lends credibility to the press release, but in order for a press release to gain media attention, it must be newsworthy. Many spa topics qualify as news, such as the announcement of a new product, technique, or service; the appointment of a new spa director; or a special event, such as a spa opening, anniversary celebration, participation in a fund-raiser, or receipt of an award.

A powerful headline that pulls journalists in and gives them an understanding of what the release is all about is critical to getting the recipient to read your press release. To increase the chance that it does, headlines are typically slanted to appeal to the editorial position of a particular media channel or news segment. For example, the opening of a new spa may emphasize the relaxation benefit to appeal to a lifestyle or health and wellness publication, while the use of new equipment and technology might be what is known as a better "hook" for a business editor. The trick is to appeal to each news medium from an angle that relates to them.

Likewise, the body of the text should place information in a context that is relevant to the readership you are targeting. For example, a press release regarding the opening of a new spa aimed at getting media coverage in an architectural digest might focus on the design and layout or the materials used, while the same news aimed at a travel guide might focus on the cultural aspects of the spa's locale. To gain the most media coverage, all possible angles should be considered.

Writing press releases is not a simple process, but if you decide to write and distribute your own, be sure to follow the standard protocol and write your release in a journalistic style. The following do's and don'ts will help you to stay on track.

Do:

- Present information in an objective format as if you were an outsider writing about your spa using the third person, for example, "Successful Day Spa Announces the Appointment of New Spa Director."

- Use good grammar that is easy to read, and always double-check for spelling or punctuation errors.

- Assign a contact person who is responsible for handling inquiries and capable of answering any questions pertaining to the release.

- Keep your format clean and easy on the eye, using 1.5 or double line spacing. If your copy is lengthy, use subheads and number the pages.

- Study the media before targeting them and slant your release to the target audience.

- Get newspeople's names right and keep your list updated.

- Confirm receipt with a follow-up call that is brief, polite, and to the point.

- Deliver your release in way that fits in with the fast-paced world of the journalist, such as e-mail or fax. Snail mail is rarely used today.

- Send a photo if it is relevant, and include identifying information along with a caption that describes the content, including names of people in the photo.

Don't:

- Use pronouns, such as "I," "we," or "us," that may be viewed as a personal account of the information.

- Overstate your point with fantastic claims that cannot be substantiated.

- Assume the reader will understand acronyms; spell all abbreviations out clearly.

- Send the press release to multiple sources at the same media outlet. It could get confusing or, even worse, irritate rivals for the same story.

- Hound the media with numerous irritating follow-up telephone calls.

- Confuse news with sales promotions. A press release is news, not a sales pitch.

Finally, remember that a press release does not assure instant media coverage, but it may result in a story down the road. As you plan your news release, consider the timing. The media generally requires information several months in advance. Be conscious of the editorial calendar, month, or season. For example, an event that includes complimentary skin care analysis to promote the awareness and prevention of skin cancer is likely to be well received for a storyline in May, National Skin Health Awareness Month, in which case the details of your event will need to be well-planned ahead of time. But don't be disappointed if your press release does not result in coverage. Some media outlets will only accept local, regional, or national news.

Self-Promotion

While many are choosing to use public relations professionals, spa owners can still generate media attention on their own. At the top of the list is developing a reputation as a person with exemplary business practices. The public must see you as someone with integrity. How do you achieve that?

- **BE A LEADER:** Establish yourself as the industry resource in your area.

- **BE AN EDUCATOR:** Take the time to write articles, publish your own newsletter, or contribute to someone else's.

- **BE OUT THERE:** Speak at engagements, participate in community events, and distribute your business card wherever you go.

- **BE CHARITABLE:** Volunteer to help others, and participate in worthy causes.

- **BE CONSCIOUS OF THE BROADER SCHEME OF THINGS:** It's not just about treatments and services; address how your business contributes to the betterment of society in general.

- **BE APPROPRIATELY PROVOCATIVE:** Take a stand on controversial issues, incorporating research and data that support your beliefs.

- **BE A SPA AMBASSADOR:** Learn to think collectively and maintain individual standards that promote the industry.

Finally, remember that as a spa owner you represent not only yourself, but also the entire profession. Think before you act. Everything you do makes a statement about the spa business.

Develop a Press Kit

To present your business in the best possible light, you will need what is known in the trade as a *press kit* or *media kit*. At the very minimum, this should include your brochure or menu of services and photos of your spa. You might also include a biography and photo of yourself. This is a good place to let people know how your expertise can be used; for example, you might list your availability to speak at public engagements or write articles. Any press releases, awards, or articles that place your name in the news should be included.

A fact sheet that highlights important information about your spa can also be helpful to journalists looking for more detailed information about your business, or specific items that can be developed into a story. Include such information as the number of treatment rooms and specific hydrotherapy or other equipment used in your spa; the type of products you sell; your staff's qualifications; your target market; the location of your spa if that is noteworthy; and any unusual amenities or special treatments your spa offers. Make a point of highlighting what you are doing that no one else is doing. Address all of these points in a concise bulleted format that is easy to read.

Responding to Media Inquiries

Public relations is first and foremost about good communications. If you are fortunate enough to receive a direct call from the media, be sure to answer it promptly; most journalists are on tight deadlines and require a quick response. If you are not available immediately, return the message as soon as possible, but don't hound them. If they are interested, they will call you back. If someone else acts as the spokesperson for your business, provide his or her name and telephone number and alert that person immediately.

If the press has requested a personal interview for an article, make sure that you are familiar with all the information provided in your press kit, and be prepared to talk about your services in an enthusiastic and confident way. If you have the luxury of knowing the story line in advance, ask what the author is looking for and do your homework on the subject matter. Don't be afraid to take a stand on controversial issues, but make certain you can back up your opinions with hard facts. If possible, give the author several references that will enhance his or her understanding of what you do and your position. Confirmation by a reputable third party will increase the validity.

Unless the story is a human interest feature that allows you free rein to talk about yourself, keep the focus on what they want. Don't try to lead the story or get journalists interested in something else you are doing. A reporter interested in your signature treatment does not want to hear about your new laser hair removal equipment.

Occasionally, a journalist may accept an invitation to receive a treatment to develop a story line or to glean a better understanding of your services; however, keep in mind that journalists have an obligation to maintain a neutral position. While you would always want to put your best foot forward, it is unethical to offer free services or bribes to elicit a favorable story. When you open your doors to the media, expect an honest unbiased appraisal of your spa and its benefit to the public. Good, bad, or indifferent, you must be willing to accept the risk.

Measuring the Effects of PR

It can take months to see tangible results from a public relations campaign. PR is a cumulative communications process, not an exact science, and can often take years to develop. Look at the most-noted authorities in the spa industry. It is unlikely that they will tell you they developed recognition overnight or that it was the result of a single initiative.

If you are working with a PR professional, that person can help you to develop a consistent message and become clear about your goals. For example, do you want to achieve national recognition for your spa or position yourself as an expert in the field? Be wary of anyone who guarantees results. A successful public relations campaign is measured by steady progress and increased consumer recognition. The best advice anyone can give you is to keep track of your efforts and work on your business.

PUBLICITY

Publicity refers to those methods of bringing attention to your spa without paying for it. This free form of advertising can be stimulated by a number of carefully focused public relations efforts such as a press release, public speaking engagement, or special event.

There are countless ways to generate publicity. For instance, your spa could sponsor a fund-raiser or provide a worthwhile community service. Most spa owners are quick to take advantage of announcing important milestones in the evolution of their business, such as grand openings and special anniversaries, but even something as simple as a dynamic window display can be newsworthy.

The key to getting free publicity is pitching the right story to the right person. Many spas are beginning to use professional publicists to get their name in the news. Professional publicists, like public relations agents, study the various media outlets, understand what they are looking for, and know the best way to pitch a story. Although hiring a professional involves some costs and may seem counterproductive to efforts focused on acquiring "free" press coverage, the result is often worth the increased mileage a spa gets out of it. A story generated on its own merit often has a much greater impact than one that the public obviously construes as paid advertising.

When it comes to generating free publicity, don't be shy. Do whatever you can to attract attention to your achievements. If you receive a special award or participate in a valuable continuing education or community service project, be sure to let everyone know.

Handling Negative Publicity

Of course, publicity can also have a negative connotation. While no spa purposely looks for bad publicity, an unfortunate situation can affect the best of businesses. A spa may suddenly find itself in the position of being associated with a product or treatment that has been shown to be harmful or of no recognized value. In a worst-case scenario, it could be held responsible for a highly publicized malpractice incident.

If your spa is the target of negative publicity, be certain to counteract it as quickly as possible. A good public relations agent can be extremely beneficial when it comes to damage control, responding to a crisis with immediate honest, concise, and diplomatic answers that satisfy the consumer's need for facts and keep the press from spinning out of control.

If you decide to act as your own spokesperson, supply the facts in a brief, straightforward manner, and above all, don't lie! Untruthful remarks are likely to come back to haunt you. Whenever possible, include data that will support your position. For example, if laser equipment used in your spa receives negative attention but in reality such equipment has been proven to be used successfully 99.9 percent of the time, you would want to share this information with your clients. You would also want to inform clients of the measures you have taken to ensure that the equipment is used safely in your spa, perhaps highlighting the training and competency of your staff or the direct supervision employed.

Sales Promotions

Sales promotions are an extremely important part of the promotion mix aimed at stimulating sales. Most spa owners would agree that sales promotions also give them an opportunity to be creative and reward valued customers at the same time.

Sales promotions are an excellent way to generate excitement and get people talking about your spa. But to be effective, clients must perceive that the sales promotions have some added value. This usually takes the shape of a special offer or discount available for a limited time period.

Establish Targeted Sales Objectives

In the spa business, sales promotions are designed to stimulate growth by targeting one of the following key areas:

1. Create an ongoing interest in standard offerings.
2. Encourage repeat business.
3. Fill in slow periods.
4. Promote new services and products.
5. Increase retail sales.

This can be accomplished by incorporating any number of routine sales promotions, such as referral cards, reward programs, series discounts, and point-of-sale coupons, to name a few. You can also use themes to target specific business goals on a monthly or seasonal basis. Body scrubs, facials, and pedicure treatments that incorporate specific lotions or creams fall naturally into "flavor of the month" and seasonal categories.

There are many other ways to create excitement around sales. The key to success is to be original—the more creative, the more memorable. Throw a party to introduce a new product; delight clients with a handsomely packaged free gift or coupon; or introduce a new service by giving clients an opportunity to sample the treatment on a smaller scale. Entire books are devoted to the subject of sales promotions. The important thing is to keep them coming. The goal of all sales promotions is to add value and increase customer satisfaction 7 days a week, 52 weeks a year, a topic we will discuss further in Chapter 10.

Direct Marketing

Direct marketing refers to any attempt to reach the consumer directly with an offer, such as a sales letter, note card, postcard, coupon, e-mail, newsletter, telephone call or text message.

In recent years, direct marketing has become an extremely popular promotional technique—for good reason. Targeting potential or existing customers directly is one of the best ways to build business. It is also an excellent way to develop a one-to-one relationship with the consumer, a concept that fits well with the present consumer-concentric marketing orientation; however, the real key to its success depends on two critical factors: the offer and the target audience. First, the offer must be one that has value, and second, the offer must be aimed at the right group of people.

Many times business owners make the mistake of thinking the creative aspect of the promotion pulls customers in, and while direct marketing guru Robert Bly points out a well-designed piece can get people to read something they might otherwise put aside, in direct marketing, the "40-40-20 rule" generally applies; that is: 40 percent depends on the offer, 40 percent depends on the list, and only 20 percent actually depends on the creative aspect. Therefore, spa owners are wise to spend more time figuring out what to offer and who to offer it to, rather than developing the perfect creative piece.

Call to Action

All direct marketing is geared toward soliciting a direct response from the consumer, but once again, your goals are an important consideration. Think about the action you hope to achieve. Do you want to attract new clients; promote a new treatment or product; enroll potential or existing clients in a seminar or event; increase your share of a particular market segment such as men or teens; or reward your regular clients?

In creating the offer, be aware of your motives, but remember the bottom line is to increase business. Clients must want what you're offering. The trick to creating a win-win situation is finding a way to add value. This doesn't always mean a discount. Learn to question consumer value. An appealing offer gives the client some incentive to act. It is also straight forward and truthful. As a general rule, do not make promises you cannot deliver or incorporate too many disclaimers in fine print. Honest value is the key to the success of any direct offer.

Direct Mail

Certain direct marketing techniques, such as telemarketing and spam, have forced marketers to find more user-friendly and less invasive ways to bring their message to clients. Direct mail pieces such as postcards, flyers and sales letters sent via regular mail are ideal for presenting your offer to a specific group of people without the risk of invading their privacy.

To create an effective direct mail program, you will need a targeted mailing list. Most day spa owners are comfortable with the idea of using their own database, but they may be concerned that targeting a larger population will be cost prohibitive. There are many ways to expand your database without spending a lot of money. Inviting prospective clients to subscribe to your newsletter, participating in community events that give you an opportunity to interface directly with the consumer, or having contests that invite new customers to provide their home or business address are several low-cost solutions to increasing your mailing list.

Renting mailing lists once or twice per year is another convenient and affordable option for many spa owners. If you go this route, it can be helpful to tap into industry organizations beforehand to establish a list of criteria of those that are likely to go to a spa. Some professional and nonprofit organizations and community groups may also be willing to share lists for a small fee or donation. Coupon vendors, local mail houses and printers are other resources for generating customized mailing lists.

Direct mail provides the added bonus of updating your database. This is a great way to correct address changes and remove clients who have moved away or no longer do business with you.

The key to a successful direct mail piece is to make it appealing enough to get the recipient to read it. Unusual pieces, boxes, and those with small gift items such as pens and magnets tend to get opened first, but direct mail does not have to break the bank. A simple postcard on colorful stock can be just as effective as an expensive mailer. We'll talk more about designing eye-catching direct mail pieces in Chapter 9.

Track Your Efforts

Direct mail can be a cost-effective way to market your spa, but it is important to determine if you are getting enough return on your investment. Several methods can be used to measure the success of direct mail. Special codes and telephone numbers are easy to apply to mailings, but perhaps the best way to track your efforts is to ask the recipient to bring in the mailer or attach a tear-off sheet to redeem the offer. This should give you a fairly accurate accounting (See Figure 8-3).

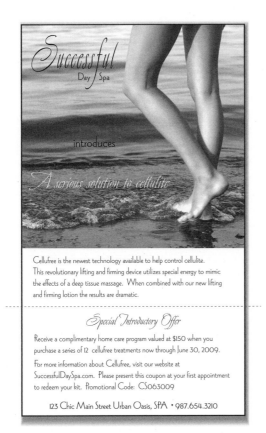

FIGURE 8-3 Perhaps the best way to track your direct mail efforts is to ask the recipient to bring in the mailer or attach a tear-off sheet to redeem the offer.

If you find that your response is too low or you have not managed to cover your costs, take time to explore all the variables. Did you target the right group, or was there too little value in your offer? Look critically at all possible reasons before you decide to discontinue this method. A word of caution is in order here: When sending a large volume of direct mail pieces, such as 5,000 postcards, it is not uncommon to receive a 2-to-3 percent return; so don't be alarmed if you do not receive a huge number of responses.

It may take a few trials to work out the kinks, but in the end, a good direct mail campaign should actually pay for itself and stimulate business. You know you have a winning series when clients call to make sure they haven't missed one of them.

The Internet

The Internet has become a commonplace direct marketing tool that is typically used to supply clients with important information about your spa. Most spas accomplish this goal by creating a Web site. There are several things you can do to increase the value of your Web site as a direct marketing tool. For example, incorporating a simple request on your Web site that gives visitors the opportunity to be added to your mailing list, receive a brochure, or subscribe to your newsletter can help to increase the volume of your business. We'll talk more about how to make your Web site a more effective marketing tool in Chapter 9.

Electronic mail is another extremely powerful direct mail approach that is being used successfully by many spa owners. In fact, this can be one of the most cost-effective and convenient ways to reach clients directly. Unfortunately, spam, or unsolicited e-mail, is generating the same response that has caused the public to dread telemarketers. If you decide to use this method, be sure to filter your lists and clearly identify yourself as well as the purpose of your correspondence. Send e-mail only to clients or potential clients who have requested information about spa services and limit the frequency of your e-mails. Otherwise, you are likely to be perceived as a nuisance.

As a general rule, if you are running both monthly and seasonal promotions, delivering one e-mail message per month along with a quarterly newsletter that includes seasonal specials is appropriate. You may also want to consider an occasional bonus offer to give business a boost, but it is important not to let this tactic get out of hand. Anything more than two e-mails per month could have clients asking to be removed from your list. Hopefully your messages will be well-received, but it is important to provide an easy vehicle for clients to opt out or be removed from your list.

Web 2.0

There are many other creative uses of the Internet in development today. "Web 2.0," or the advanced use of Internet technology for the purpose of sharing information, developing people focused connections, and building communities via the Internet, a practice commonly referred to as *social computing* or *networking,* is a growing phenomenon that is rapidly gaining the attention of many business owners as a viable form of marketing.

The terms *social marketing* and *social media* are often used interchangeably and generally refer to the use of *blogs, podcasts* and *viral marketing* techniques that are used to spread the message about a particular product or service across the internet. The use of this technique for advertising and promotional purposes has gained considerable interest in the last few years for several good reasons. Studies reveal that social forums like Friendster, Facebook, and LinkedIn are being used by all ages in record numbers. This combined with the knowledge that consumers generally have a lot more confidence in the opinion of their peers, has many businesses turning to this new media outlet for marketing purposes.

Blogs

A blog is a Web site that chronicles an individual's personal thoughts and or notes on a particular topic; however, in some instances that individual may also represent a larger organization. Blogs typically have an interactive component that allows readers to share their own views on the subject matter, and may also supply links to other Web sites that support their opinions, or provide additional information on the topic.

As blogs become more popular a number of spa industry leaders and organizations are using them to invite discussion among peers and colleagues that might not otherwise have a forum. Others are simply using blogs as an advertising vehicle to promote goods and services. Blogs can be very useful to companies seeking new and more cost-effective methods for reaching their clients. However, given the dynamics of this new technology, one of the problems that exists is that it can be hard to separate personal interests from business interests, or to determine if the host is actually being compensated to represent the interests of another party. This has raised a number of ethical questions for business owners, marketers, and consumers that have yet to be clearly defined. Still one thing is certain, the use of the Internet for the purpose of social media has many relevant marketing applications and can ultimately be an excellent vehicle for spa owners and managers to better understand and respond to customers needs.

Podcasts

A podcast is an audio broadcast that is delivered in digital files via the internet. It can be listened to on your computer with the aid of music playing software, such as Windows Media Player or iTunes, or downloaded and played back on a portable media player such as an MP3 or iPod at the listener's leisure.

The use of podcasts has only begun to be explored in spas; however, there are a number of cost-effective applications for its use. Podcasts can be used to increase the relaxation benefit of certain services, educate clients on the benefits of spa treatments and products, promote new products and services, or deliver important messages about healthy living and

Plan for Success

The use of viral and stealth marketing techniques poses several unique challenges for any business owner interested in using these methods of marketing. Of primary concern is the question of "truth in advertising." While to date the federal government has not mandated specific laws with regard to viral marketing, the FTC, in compliance with the Federal Trade Commission Act, does prohibit the use of deceptive advertising. If you decide to use viral marketing in any shape or form, study the FTC's guidelines carefully, and be cautious.

Although viral marketing can be used in a creative and cost-effective manner, if the recipient is unaware that the messenger is being compensated the issue of nondisclosure can be problematic. To make the most of social media spa business owners are urged to follow ethical marketing practices as outlined by the FTC and other reputable agencies such as the American Marketing Association, the American Advertising Federation, the American Association of Advertising Agencies and the Better Business Bureau.

TIPS FOR SUCCESSFUL E-MAIL MARKETING

- Stick to your own database and people who have requested information from you.
- Do not send more than two promotions per month.
- Always give clients the option to be removed from your list.
- Clearly identify yourself and the purpose of your e-mail.
- Use a service to distribute your electronic mail.

maintaining the spa lifestyle at home. If you decide to develop your own podcasts and would like to incorporate music there are several royalty-free music outlets available to avoid infringing upon copyrights.

Viral Marketing

Viral marketing generally refers to the spread of marketing messages across the Internet via a social network. This is typically accomplished through the use of electronic mail messages which are sent from one person to another, although viral marketing may also involve word-of-mouth techniques.

Similar to traditional rewards based marketing programs, for example, client referral programs, viral e-mail messages may offer the sender some type of incentive to forward the message to another individual, for example, a coupon reward, free gift, or some other offer. In some instances, stealth marketing techniques are used to promote the spread of viral messages, a topic that is currently the subject of much discussion among business owners, marketing professionals, and organizations.

PERSONAL SELLING

This method of promotion involves a one-to-one exchange with the customer that typically takes the form of a sales dialogue. Given the tremendous opportunity for face-to-face interaction with clients, spas clearly have an advantage when it comes to personal selling. Nonetheless, this form of promotion requires all spa personnel to hone their interpersonal communication skills.

As a spa owner, it is your responsibility to train your staff to communicate effectively. Teach staff to be thoughtful in terms of how they listen and how they present themselves to clients. It is not enough to simply supply the client with a list of recommended products at the end of a treatment session and expect them to buy everything on the list. To be effective, spa service providers need to take extra care to build rapport and take an interest in the needs of clients. Built-in consultation and designated call-in times are a good way to open the lines of communication, but to be truly effective you will need an inclusive program that encompasses every level of client interaction. From your front desk manager to your massage therapists, everyone should be able to communicate your spa message clearly. We will talk more about personal selling in Chapter 10, but it is important to note that when used appropriately and as part of a complete customer service program, the personal dialogue is an extremely beneficial form of promotion.

WORD-OF-MOUTH ADVERTISING

When it comes to purchasing products and services research indicates that most people have more faith in the recommendation of friends and family. Today social computing has expanded that vote of confidence to include online reviews by other people who have used the product or service who an individual may not know personally but whose opinion they are likely to consider. This has further cemented word-of-mouth as the best form of advertising, however, the new "buzz," as it is often referred to, may also involve face to face stealth or guerilla marketing techniques.

Stealth advertising refers to the use of covert marketing technique(s) whereby the individual being solicited does not necessarily associate the individual promoting the product with the company. For example, some companies plant people in public places or at events with the goal of engaging others in a dialogue about a particular product or service. Unlike personal selling, where the connection between the buyer and the seller is directly understood, or a genuine referral between two friends or acquaintances, the goal in stealth marketing is to initiate conversation in a way that appears spontaneous or natural rather than a sales pitch. The catch is that the person responsible for spreading the word is usually receiving some sort of compensation, although the consumer may be completely unaware of this. As you might imagine, these marketing techniques raise a great deal of legal and ethical issues which have yet to be fully resolved in terms of government regulation.

GUERILLA MARKETING

Guerilla marketing is a phrase coined by Jay Conrad Levinson whose book on the subject, *Guerilla Marketing,* was first published in 1984. Since then a number of small businesses have been drawn to this alternative marketing strategy which promotes the use of creative and cost-effective techniques to spread the message about a product, service, or brand. Guerilla marketing often combines the use of several methods, such as viral marketing word of mouth, publicity, referrals, etc, and is designed to appeal primarily to the entrepreneur who is encouraged to target both personal and professional contacts to reach his or her goals. Guerilla marketing tactics typically employ low- or no-cost efforts which may include staging an unusual event or activity to generate free publicity. Today guerilla marketing is often used as a generic term for viral, buzz marketing and other unconventional marketing methods.

Determining a Marketing Budget

When it comes to marketing, every spa business owner has the same question: How much money should I spend? Although there are many theories and a wide range of calculated formulas, there really is no magic number. Several guidelines can help spa owners to set limits. To begin the process, ask yourself three important questions:

1. Where am I in the evolution of my business?
2. Where would I like to be?
3. What can I afford to spend?

Historically, marketing budgets have been based on a certain percentage of gross, or projected gross sales figures, depending on where you were in the life cycle of your business. For example, a business just starting out might spend 10 percent or more of its projected gross sales on marketing, whereas an established business might level its marketing expenditures to 3 percent of gross sales after several years. While this method satisfies those looking for a precise formula, it also implies that there is a direct correlation between sales and marketing that can be measured exactly. For example, it suggests that 10 percent of gross revenues of $500,000 can be actualized by spending $50,000 or that 3 percent of gross revenues or

$15,000 could generate the same $500,000. This is where I think many get into trouble. The goal of marketing is to increase sales, but marketing is not an exact science that can produce precise correlations.

It makes more sense to plan your marketing budget in terms of goals and objectives, employing those strategies you think will help you to achieve your goals and track the effectiveness of each initiative. If the strategies you are using do not bring the results you want, it makes sense to adjust your plan accordingly. It does not necessarily mean that how much or how little you are spending is the problem.

Whatever marketing strategies you employ they should be based on sound professional judgment, the amount you can afford to spend, and a complete understanding of what it will cost you to implement those strategies over a set period of time. There are many cost-effective marketing techniques. The key is to tailor those that meet your particular needs.

DEVELOP REALISTIC EXPECTATIONS

Smaller day spa owners often tell me they cannot afford to spend much on marketing or advertising and would rather focus on getting their name in the news through free publicity. Remember the old adage that there is no such thing as a free lunch? It may be a cliché, but it's also true. Any marketing plan should be considered a long-term investment that provides enough flexibility to adjust to the needs of your business at any given point in time.

If you are just starting out, it is likely that you will need to spend a bit more on marketing, adding the initial cost of developing basic collateral materials such as a brochure, business card, or a Web site to the budget. Once your business is off the ground, you are likely to reach a point where it plateaus or suddenly spirals downward for some reason and needs that extra shot of marketing adrenalin. This is where I see many day spa owners make a serious mistake by assuming they cannot afford to spend money on marketing when business is slow. In reality, the opposite is true. A creative marketing plan can help small business owners survive critical downtimes and weather adverse economic conditions.

However, even if a spa business is making steady gains, those who have been in business for several years will attest to the fact that they are in no position to be complacent. The need to continually provide value to your clients, attract new clients, and protect your business from the competition is reason enough to maintain a long-term effective marketing strategy.

Measuring Your Success

If you are going to direct a good deal of energy into marketing, you will also want to take time to measure its effectiveness. One of the easiest ways to find out what is working is to ask. A conversation with any new client should always begin with "How did you hear about us?" Make it part of your intake form as well. Then be sure to enter the data in a reliable format. This is easily done by incorporating a field in your database that categorizes all of your marketing efforts by code. For example, if your marketing plan includes a radio ad, several print advertisements, and a Web site, you will want to make sure these are listed by name, such as *WABC, Daily News, Metro Magazine,* and *Successful Web Site,* in a pop-up list. Don't forget a category for the most important form of advertising—word-of-mouth referrals. Computerization of this information makes it easy to call up the different categories at the end of the week, month, or year.

You will also need to pay attention to sales numbers on a weekly, monthly, and yearly basis. Are sales higher during certain sales promotions or at certain times of the year, such as the holidays? Note the correlation between ads, promotions, and sales. If you are not paying attention to these numbers, you are throwing your marketing dollars out the window.

However, even under the best circumstances, it can be difficult to measure exactly which efforts are producing results or how well your strategy is working compared to your competition. If a certain ad or other promotional strategy does not produce immediate results or the results you want within a specific time frame, does it mean that the strategy does not have any real marketing value or that you should discontinue the program? The answer to this question is complex.

Studies have shown that a potential customer needs several exposures to a brand before buying. Just like the client who reported her ad was finally pulling customers in, expect the number and type of exposures your clients need to vary. You should also consider that clients may not necessarily remember how they heard about you. If your telephone suddenly starts to ring after you have employed several strategies, it may be the overall combination of your efforts rather than one single initiative that turns the tide.

Ethical Issues in Marketing

It is no secret that marketing tries to influence what we buy; however, this often sounds more self-serving than it actually is. In the end, all the products and services your spa sells must provide the consumer with an honest value.

Ideally, marketing should make it easy for buyers to act as educated consumers. A good marketing program creates awareness, informs, and in many instances attempts to educate the consumer about your product, service, or idea. This is an extremely valuable service. Unfortunately, the use of deceptive promotional practices by some businesses has caused the public to be wary of advertising and marketing. To build confidence in your spa's marketing message, it is important to develop good business ethics. Ethics are standards designed to uphold moral behavior. The following guidelines will help you to maintain consumer confidence in your marketing program.

- Develop policies and procedures you can uphold.
- Be honest and truthful in all your endeavors.
- Be able to substantiate all claims, written and verbal.
- Be knowledgeable about your products and services, and make sure you can stand behind them.
- Avoid "stretching the truth."
- Stand behind any guarantee or warranty you assign to products and services.
- Avoid making false or misleading statements about your competitors.
- Use good judgment when advertising and be conscious of using materials or language that might be offensive to the general public.
- Avoid deceptive techniques, such as bait and switch advertising, or advertising at a lower price to get consumers through the door and then trying to sell them a higher-priced item.
- Think carefully about the people and organizations with whom you choose to associate or conduct business.

CONSUMER PROTECTION

Today, businesses are being held accountable for misleading advertising practices and products that have the potential to cause harm. Laws to protect consumers against fraud and unsafe products have been adopted at both the state and federal levels. As a spa owner, it is important for you to be familiar with how these laws govern your spa's marketing efforts.

Three important federal government agencies exert influence over marketing practices: the Federal Trade Commission (FTC), Food and

Drug Administration (FDA), and Consumer Product Safety Commission (CPSC).

1. The FTC is responsible for regulating all business conduct.
2. The FDA has authority over packaging and labeling of food, drugs, and cosmetics.
3. The CPSC files suit over unsafe or defective products.

State and federal government offices, such as the attorney general, have the authority to protect public interests against fraudulent promotional practices. In addition, the Council of Better Business Bureaus and other private agencies help to set standards for advertising and promotion. News media also have considerable clout and can be quite powerful in their efforts to bring public attention to deceptive or misleading practices or defective and unsafe products.

As a spa owner, it is important for you to become familiar with FTC, FDA, and CPSC regulations, as well as those set forth by state and local agencies. Remember that if you get called on any claim, you will need to supply evidence to back it up. The FTC supplies a list of frequently asked advertising questions on their Web site to help the small business owner understand their responsibility. Get in the habit of checking your advertising message against these and other reliable standards such as those guidelines set by the Better Business Bureau, American Marketing Association, American Advertising Federation, and American Association of Advertising Agencies.

There are also numerous legal channels, books, articles, and reference guides available to those who wish to become more familiar with the legalities of advertising. When in doubt, use them or bring your questions to an attorney who specializes in advertising law.

THINK IT OVER

Because marketing attempts to influence the buyers' purchasing decisions, developing a marketing program that stimulates business and provides a real benefit to consumers requires careful planning and implementation. Consumers are naturally wary of what they perceive as clever ad campaigns to get them to part with their hard-earned dollars. And why shouldn't they be? How many times have you been disappointed by the fine print in an ad? Shouldn't we question the value of the products and services we buy? Absolutely!

As you develop your marketing program, take time to evaluate how your marketing plan will benefit your business and how it affects consumers. Do your products and services provide a solid value to the consumer? Is your message perfectly clear? Does your approach make it easy for customers to readily accept your offer? For marketing to work, in the end it must always be a win-win situation.

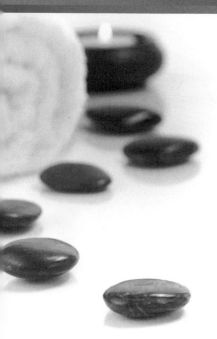

PRESENTATION IS EVERYTHING

The quality of your treatments, customer service, cleanliness, and ambiance of your spa are all important factors in presenting a polished professional image. But before clients even step foot into your spa, they will most likely be basing their opinions and, more importantly, their expectations on your marketing materials. What can you do to ensure that their first impression is a good one?

In this chapter, we will discuss what goes into putting your best media presentation forward. Whether a client's introduction to your spa is a business card, brochure, or a Web site, you will want your marketing materials to send the right message.

BRAND RECOGNITION

Brand recognition is an important part of developing a positive image and should be viewed as an integral part of an inclusive marketing strategy. For example, a good public relations program and the right amount of publicity are key factors in spreading the message about your spa business. But to make it simple for consumers to positively identify a business, companies typically use a brand name or symbol that is easily recognizable.

A brand name is a basic marketing tool that is used to distinguish a business from its competitors. This can include a name, phrase, or slogan, a certain design or symbol, or a combination of these, which people come to associate with your company. Typically a *brand name* refers to the spoken word that is used to identify your company's product or service. For example, Nike is a brand name that most consumers instantly associate with running shoes or sports gear; most can easily identify the symbol, or logo, that is also connected with the product.

As a spa owner, you may want to register or trademark your brand name, or *trade name,* the commercial or legal name under which a company conducts business, along with the logo, tagline, or slogan associated with your spa. This protects your business from others who might want to infringe upon its use. Trade names are registered through the U.S. Patent and Trademark office and are commonly identified by the symbol ™ and ® which are placed at the end of a registered trade name. (For a quick review of trademarks and service marks, see Chapter 4.)

WORKING WITH CREATIVE AGENCIES, DESIGNERS, AND COPYWRITERS

Readily available software programs that offer desktop publishing have tempted many small business owners to create their own marketing materials, including logos, brochures, business cards, and flyers. If you are among those who feel you can develop sufficient materials on your home or office PC, or feel this task is easily delegated to an administrative assistant with good computer skills, resist the temptation. When it comes to developing marketing materials, it is important to hire professionals. Poorly written copy and amateur designs send the wrong message about your business and will forever brand your spa as lacking a professional image.

This does not mean that your ideas, likes, and dislikes do not matter. Spa owners generally have an idea of the look they would like to achieve; they may even wish to incorporate certain language, a particular piece of artwork, or a symbol they feel is important in representing their spa business. This can be helpful. In fact, a good design team or freelancer will welcome your input and work with you to bring your vision to life in a way that is both unique and marketable.

Marketing professionals work hard to please their clients, but it is important for spa owners to understand the process. The design of a logo and other marketing materials typically begins with developing a general business profile. Gaining an understanding of the client's goals, target market, and the image the spa owner wishes to project is critical to success. This typically requires a team approach and may include a number of professionals, for example, a marketing consultant, art director, copywriter, graphic designer, and production or project manager who will work with you to shape materials that reflect your vision.

Once the team has a good understanding of your business and the information that should be included in your materials, they will be able to present several design ideas for your review. Be prepared to offer explicit feedback, defining what it is you like or don't like about the design. This is a significant part of the process that helps the team to refine the design accordingly but it is important to be open to constructive criticism that will help you to better market your business.

Most design teams will work with you until you are satisfied but expect limitations. Restricting the number of design choices or copy revisions is not uncommon. These guidelines vary among designers. Prices will also differ, which raises an important concern about fees. Some agencies establish set prices for creating a logo, developing an ad, or writing and designing a spa brochure. Others work on a commission basis or a combination of fee plus commission-based structures. Independent consultants and freelance designers may charge an hourly rate. Fees may take into account the timeline for completing the project, number of revisions, and/or number of meetings involved. If you go beyond the set limit, you will most likely be subject to additional fees. Before entering into any agreement, always ask for an itemized proposal that specifies the terms in language you can understand. A contract or proposal should also discuss any additional charges, such as the cost of photography, printing, or paper that are necessary to complete the project. If you are still unclear about any of the items listed, ask. It is best to have a clear understanding of all possible charges before you begin. This will help you to work within your budget.

KEY ELEMENTS IN DEVELOPING MARKETING MATERIALS

The development of marketing materials begins with several basics: the design of a logo and the selection of typography, colors, paper, and photos that are woven into the fabric of all your marketing materials.

Logo Design

A logo is a graphic design that is used to identify a business. This typically takes the shape of text and/or a symbol and is usually some adaptation of the name of the company (Figure 9-1).

Creating a logo is an integral part of establishing your spa's identity and is critical to developing brand recognition. It is best done by a professional graphic designer. Graphic designers are artists who specialize

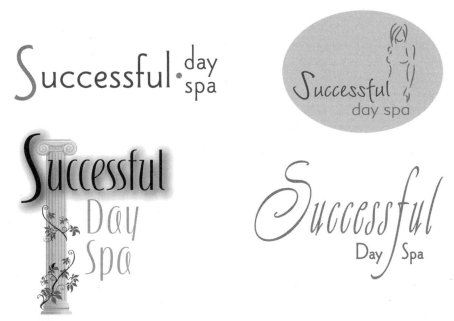

FIGURE 9-1   Designers typically offer several logo design choices to clients.

in developing visual communication tools for electronic or print media, such as logos, brochures, business cards, ads, newsletters, and Web sites.

Sometimes small business owners are confused by what a logo is, thinking that it must incorporate some form of artwork or symbolism. A logo can be designed using simple typography, a symbol, or both. A good example of a typographic logo design is the one used for Coca-Cola, the trade name of the Coca-Cola Company. Although there are many cola beverages, you can easily identify the Coca-Cola brand by its distinguishable typeface. Other companies combine symbolism and typography. An excellent example of this is the "golden arches," a logo that the entire world has come to associate with McDonald's fast food chain. Study logos in the spa industry. How many can you find that use a combination of typography and symbols? Are they effective? Why? Compare these to several text-only designs. Which do you prefer?

A logo is generally something that stays with a business for a long time. It also forms the basis for all other visual communication tools. Think carefully about what you want it to communicate. A good logo should reflect the overall image and philosophy of your business, but it is just as important to consider how others receive it. Many times, small business owners rely on employees, friends, and relatives to help them evaluate logo designs. Although they may offer valuable suggestions, to get a good idea of how your logo will be received, seek the opinion of your target market. It is also wise to look at the logos of your competitors and others in the industry, such as product vendors. In fact, many find it helpful to begin the process by creating a checklist of what they like and don't like about particular designs.

A professional designer can walk you through all facets of the design process, pointing out critical factors that should be considered before committing to a final design. For example, how easily can the elements of your logo be separated and incorporated into letterhead, business cards, promotional items, shopping bags, buttons, and T-shirts? How will it look in black and white, a factor that is important when it comes to advertising? You can take some creative license with a logo design as long as it does not cause embarrassment or misinterpretation and fits in with the strategic development of your spa. However, too often clients get caught up in the semantics of language, insisting on prefacing their spa's name with an article, such as "The Successful Day Spa," which can ruin an otherwise good design. This is just one example of why it is crucial to let marketing and design professionals guide you.

Tag Line or Slogan

Chances are you would have no problem identifying the companies associated with the simple phrases "Just do it," "You deserve a break today," and "Because I'm worth it." Such taglines or slogans are instantly recognizable, which was the goal of the marketing professionals who created them for Nike, McDonald's, and L'Oreal.

Along with being a catchy and memorable phrase, a tagline should embody the company mission. A clever tagline or slogan can sum up the purpose of your business in just a few words and has a good chance of surviving for generations. Unfortunately, many business owners become impatient and look to experiment before their tagline is recognizable. If you like the idea of using a tagline, hang in there. In most cases, it takes at least one year for consumers to recognize it, so it is important to give it time to take hold. In fact, changing your tagline midstream can destroy precious momentum. Once your tagline has taken hold, stick with it. The time to change is when you decide to take an entirely new approach to your spa business.

Coming up with clever phrases is the work of marketing professionals, but if you decide to create your own tagline or slogan, keep it simple and pertinent to what you do. You should also check that it is not in use through the U.S. Patent and Trademark Office and take the proper action to copyright it.

Typography

Typography is an integral part of the design of all marketing materials and refers to the way the printed word appears on a page. There are literally thousands of typefaces, or *fonts,* as they are commonly called. These are generally broken down into two main categories, those with *serifs,* or hooks at the tops and bottoms of each letter, and those without hooks, known as *sans serifs.* Fonts with serifs are easier to read and are commonly used in lengthier text, while sans serif fonts tend to be more legible, which makes them great for short copy or headlines that need to stand out. Typefaces are also classified according to the style of the design, such as a *script* or *decorative* style.

The fonts that you select for your print materials will set the overall mood or tone of the piece and should be chosen not only for their legibility and reading ease, but also for the ambiance you wish to suggest. For example, if your spa specializes in ancient healing techniques, you may choose to use a font that is reminiscent of hieroglyphics or early letter symbols, while an Old World style font might be a good fit for a spa with a European-based philosophy.

Fonts are further categorized in *families,* which include several variations of the basic design. These will differ in weight and stroke, such as Arial Narrow, Arial Black, or Arial Rounded MT Bold (Figure 9-2). Using font families is a good way to give typographic unity to a piece yet allows enough difference to create interest. Although many times designers will vary the font styles in a piece to create a unique or interesting look. The blending of various font styles is an art that is best left to graphic designers who are trained in this area. But whether you prefer a significant contrast or subtle variations, it is best to limit the number of fonts used in any one piece to two or three that are easily identified with your business.

Other Typographic Features

When working with designers, it is helpful to become familiar with the technical terminology used for typographic features, such as point size, bold, and italics. *Point size* refers to the height of letters, which ranges from 8 to 72. Varying the point size often adds an artistic dimension that makes a piece more appealing and is commonly used to emphasize titles or bring attention to more important language in the copy. The *bold* feature is used to make text stand out. *Italicized* text gives a font a slanted appearance, which again brings attention to the word or phrase and may also be used to indicate the title of a publication, pronoun, or name brand. Bolded and italicized words are generally used for emphasis, but both should be used sparingly as they are otherwise difficult to read. This defeats the attention-getting purpose.

Serif Family

Times

Successful Day Spa offers an exclusive selection of sophisticated spa services in Times 14 point.

Times Bold

Successful Day Spa offers an exclusive selection of sophisticated spa services in Times Bold 14 point.

Times Extra Bold

Successful Day Spa offers an exclusive selection of sophisticated spa services in Times Extra Bold 14 point.

San Serif Family

Arial

Successful Day Spa offers an exclusive selection of sophisticated spa services in Helvetica 14 point.

Arial Black

Successful Day Spa offers an exclusive selection of sophisticated spa services in Helvetica Bold 14 point.

Arial Rounded MT Bold

Successful Day Spa offers an exclusive selection of sophisticated spa services in Helvetica Italic 14 point.

FIGURE 9-2   Examples of a font family.

Script Family

Snell Roundhand

Successful Day Spa offers an exclusive selection of sophisticated spa services in Snell Roundhand 14 point.

Snell Roundhand Bold

Successful Day Spa offers an exclusive selection of sophisticated spa services in Snell Roundhand Bold 14 point.

Snell Roundhand Black

Successful Day Spa offers an exclusive selection of sophisticated spa services in Snell Roundhand Black 14 point.

FIGURE 9-2 Examples of a font family. (*continued*)

Changing the *case* or *formatting* of words is another way to draw attention, such as integrating lower and upper case lettering; however, it is important to note that the use of all capital letters can be difficult to read. Dropping the capital letter at the beginning of a paragraph and rotating or positioning words on the page in a curved or angled fashion are other ways to create diversity in a piece (Figure 9-3).

Loosening or tightening the tracking, or space between the letters in a word or in between lines, is another typographical feature that can be adjusted to give text either an open, light feeling or a heavy, dense look (Figure 9-4). The technical terms for tracking are kerning and leading. *Kerning* refers to the amount of space between two letters, while *leading* indicates the space between lines.

Alignment is another important factor that affects the ease with which copy is read. Copy can be aligned in four ways: right, left, center, and justified (Figure 9-5). Ordinarily text is aligned from left to right, with jagged edges to the right of the page; however, marketing materials such as brochures and newsletters that contain concentrated blurbs of text may be *justified,* or set in even lines or columns across a page to make them more attractive and readable. In certain instances, text is aligned to the right with jagged edges facing left to create interest or to wrap text around a

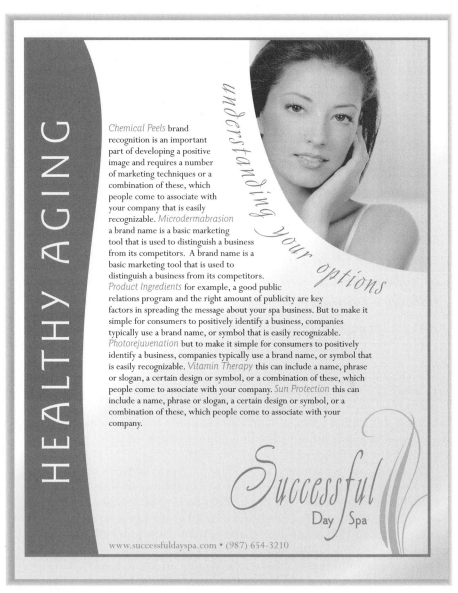

FIGURE 9-3   Formatting can change the look of a piece entirely.

supporting graphic. However, this technique is rarely used as it is difficult for the reader to follow. Centered text is generally used to bring attention to words, such as when highlighting the title of a piece or creating a tiered effect for an announcement or invitation.

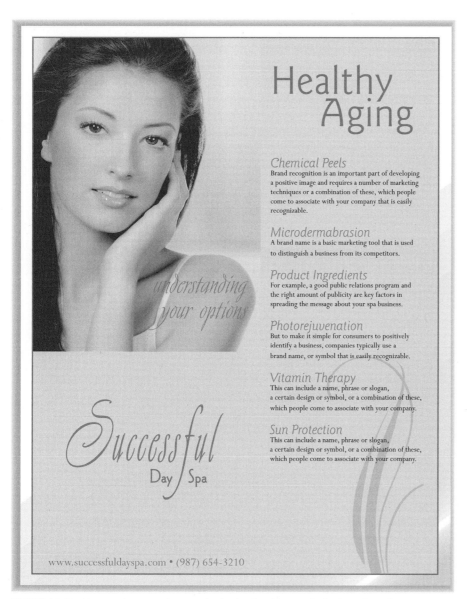

FIGURE 9-3 Formatting can change the look of a piece entirely. (*continued*)

You can experiment with all these typographical features by using the menu or tool bar and formatting tools on your computer's word processing or desktop publishing software.

Kerning	
Normal	
Successful Day Spa	
Loose	
Successful Day Spa	
Tight	
Successful Day Spa	

Leading	
10/10	
Successful Day Spa offers an exclusive selection of sophisticated spa treatments to promote healthy aging and wellness. All of our services are delivered in an elegant and relaxed atmosphere that protects the privacy of our spa guests.	
10/12	
Successful Day Spa offers an exclusive selection of sophisticated spa treatments to promote healthy aging and wellness. All of our services are delivered in an elegant and relaxed atmosphere that protects the privacy of our spa guests.	
10/14	
Successful Day Spa offers an exclusive selection of sophisticated spa treatments to promote healthy aging and wellness. All of our services are delivered in an elegant and relaxed atmosphere that protects the privacy of our spa guests.	

FIGURE 9-4   Variations in kerning and leading.

Colors

The colors used in your marketing materials send a strong message about your business and should work harmoniously with the décor and ambiance of your spa.

Left	Center	Right	Justified
Successful Day Spa offers an exclusive selection of sophisticated spa treatments to promote healthy aging and wellness. All of our services are delivered in an elegant and relaxed atmosphere that protects the privacy of our guests.	Successful Day Spa offers an exclusive selection of sophisticated spa treatments to promote healthy aging and wellness. All of our services are delivered in an elegant and relaxed atmosphere that protects the privacy of our guests.	Successful Day Spa offers an exclusive selection of sophisticated spa treatments to promote healthy aging and wellness. All of our services are delivered in an elegant and relaxed atmosphere that protects the privacy of our guests.	Successful Day Spa offers an exclusive selection of sophisticated spa treatments to promote healthy aging and wellness. All of our services are delivered in an elegant and relaxed atmosphere that protects the privacy of our guests.

FIGURE 9-5 Text alignment.

Remember that light soft colors and pastels tend to be calming and soothing and create a more subdued image, while bold bright colors tend to be stimulating or energizing and create a more dramatic presentation. Either can be appropriate for marketing materials depending on the ambiance and philosophy of your spa. For example, dramatic color schemes may be perfect for a spa focused on results-oriented treatments, while soft, restful colors that blend in with the environment might be better suited to an ecologically conscious spa based on wellness.

A good designer is instrumental in the color selection process. Designers are skilled at tying marketing materials together with colors that will complement a spa's décor. They can also suggest different shades and hues that work well with your main collateral pieces for use in other key pieces, such as postcards and flyers where the need to grab the consumer's attention is critical. Designers also look at color in terms of market trends where the creative use of color can make a big statement about how innovative your spa appears to potential customers.

As we learned in Chapter 5, color also has a psychological effect and is often tied to particular cultural or personal beliefs that can have different meanings for different people. When making color selections, it is always a good idea to get the opinion of your target market before making any final decisions. As a business owner, you are likely to have your own biases. Listen to your inner voice.

Color can also have gender connotations. Think back to your childhood days when pink was a symbol for girls and blue was the color for boys.

Unless you are trying to make a point about the gender focus of your spa, or involved in a breast cancer awareness campaign where pink is symbolic, you probably won't go to such extremes, but it is true that certain colors can help to create a more feminine or masculine mood. Tones of black, brown, tan, and navy have a stronger masculine feel, while softer shades of lavender, pink, green, and yellow are likely to appeal more to women.

Variations in Color

Everyone sees color differently, which makes it difficult to determine color exactly. This is complicated by the fact that color appears differently in different mediums. The use of color charts that show various shades or hues and group various combinations together can be helpful if you have a hard time distinguishing variations in color or wish to explore the use of complementary colors. These are available through printers, designers, and art supply stores.

A color wheel can also be useful in understanding the primary, secondary, and tertiary colors associated with basic color theory. Primary colors—red, yellow, and blue—are the basic "building blocks" of all color. Secondary colors are those located halfway between each of the primary colors, and tertiary colors are a mixture of primary and secondary colors. Complementary colors are located directly across from each other on the color wheel.

Printers and designers often talk about the hue, value, and saturation level of color. The word *hue* is synonymous with the word *color* and stands for each of the colors on the color wheel. *Value* explains the lightness or darkness of color in comparison to black or white, while *saturation* refers to the intensity, brightness, or dullness of a color, or how pure it is. Variations of color are achieved by creating tints (lighter) or shades (darker) of color. This is accomplished by adding white or black to a hue. Color can also be muted or toned down by adding its complement, black, or gray. Color also has *temperature* and can be perceived as warm or cool. Which would you use to describe your spa?

As you process the colors that will be used in your marketing materials, consider all of these factors and make sure you are looking at true color— that is, how it will appear in the medium being presented. Note that the same color may appear slightly different from one computer screen to another and the same ink used on the same paper can vary slightly from printing to printing.

Cost may ultimately be the deciding factor in your color decisions. Color paper and one-print color is the most economical way to go, while printing materials in full color is the most expensive. Using two colors or spot color is often a cost effective solution that can add to the diversity and appeal of a piece.

Paper

There are literally thousands of exciting choices when it comes to paper. In fact, there are often too many from which to choose. Look to your graphic designer and printer to help you select those that are best for your particular design needs.

Texture and Weight

There are three important considerations when it comes to paper: color, texture, and weight. Paper is available in numerous shades of white, and just about every color imaginable, but if you don't find one that meets your needs, remember that the color of your choice can be applied directly on the paper during the printing process. Paper is also available in a variety of interesting designs that may include stripes, specks, and splashes to give it a marbleized look.

The *texture* of paper adds another dimension that can make an ordinary piece look extraordinary. Texture can be rough, smooth, or ridged with a variety of finishes, such as linen, sheer, vellum, opaque, cotton, silk, and metallic. Paper can be coated or uncoated. The right texture and finish can give your marketing piece a simple, sophisticated, elegant, or dramatic look. It can also make a big statement about your philosophy. For example, a "green" spa may decide to use only recycled paper in its marketing materials.

Paper is measured in several standard grades, such as writing, bond, text, cover, and card stock. These come in varying weights and sizes. For example, writing paper is generally 24 lb.; text can be 60 lb., 70 lb., or 80 lb.; and cover stock ranges from 100 to 130 lb. Paper is usually delivered in large sheets and then trimmed to obtain the size needed for the project, such as brochures or business cards. Some papers come with standard-sized matching envelopes; others need to be custom ordered, which costs more.

Not all papers print easily in mass quantities, and some papers are better suited to certain production methods, such as a four-color process or offset or digital printing. A designer can help you to narrow your choices to several that are compatible with the theme of your spa and the purpose of the piece, pointing out text, cover, and card stocks that will work well with the piece and the production methods to be used.

Photos

Quality photos add a great deal to the appeal of marketing materials (Figure 9-6). They are also important in presenting your spa to the media. It is a good idea to have several digital photos of your spa on hand that are readily available for electronic transmission should an opportunity to obtain free publicity arise.

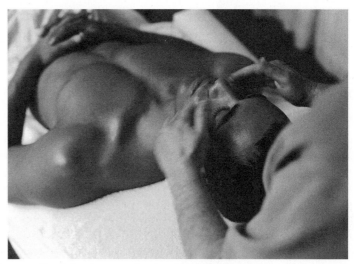

FIGURE 9-6   The right photos will enhance the quality of your marketing materials.

Any photos you use should represent your spa's image and philosophy. They should also have a broad appeal to your target market. Use faces that represent the culture of your clientele and do not discriminate based on age, sex, or race.

Professional photos of professional models are ideal, but it is certainly more cost effective to shoot your own, provided you are good at it. If you are, invite clients, not employees, to act as models, and be sure to have them sign a release that gives you permission to use their photo for advertising purposes. If you are not a good photographer, seek out a professional photographer in your area. Some photographers are willing to trade services or take photos for you in exchange for media credit, such as a mention in your brochure, which can save you money.

Conducting a photo shoot in your spa can be fun. It is also a great deal of work that requires careful planning and organization. Engage the staff in readying the spa and be prepared with a list of photo options, models, and all the props you will need to ensure things go smoothly.

Your list of marketing photos should include shots of the spa with and without people. Include pictures of the interior and exterior of the building, service providers performing the different treatments you offer, and several human resource poses such as the front desk manager with a client. Give special attention to the more aesthetic areas of the spa, such as a boutique, outdoor gardens, or a pretty sitting room. Anything related to your unique selling position is significant. Take photos of specialized apparatus, services, and products that make your spa unique. And remember that photos of happy, satisfied customers are invaluable when it comes to demonstrating dramatic before and after results derived from your treatments.

If a photo session seems like too much work, you can always purchase or rent stock photos from a broker or agency. Stock photos range in price and are available in different resolutions. Newspapers are generally able to work with a lower resolution of 150 dpi, whereas a glossy magazine usually requires 300 dpi. A quality photo purchased at 300 dpi is typically your best bet since it can be adapted to a variety of mediums.

When using stock photos, it is important to understand the limitations of their use. Some photos are subject to a one-time use, while others are royalty free and may be used more flexibly, although these too generally have certain restrictions. If you are working with an agency or graphic artist that has purchased a set of stock photos on CD-ROM, this can give you access to a wider portfolio of images. Posters and other stock photos may also be available through product vendors and equipment manufacturers. Many will allow you to use these photos in ads, brochures, or on your Web site. However, they may also insist that you mention their product.

Nonphotographic art such as charts, graphs, illustrations, and diagrams can add to the readability of your marketing collateral. In fact, studies have shown a good percentage of people enter reading material via a photo or design, and captions have seven times the readership of copy, which is why it is so important to have photos ready for the media.

Plan for Success

Most photos can be sent electronically, but when sending prints to the media, be sure to supply the name, address, telephone number, and Web address of your spa on the back. Include a brief caption of what is going on and a list of all the people in the photo. Don't write directly on the photo; use a label to avoid damaging the print.

PRIMARY MARKETING MATERIALS

The primary purpose of marketing materials is to inform consumers and increase business. Several key pieces will help you to accomplish this goal, and no spa should be without them. These include a brochure, price list, business card, and gift certificates.

Brochure or Menu of Services

The marketing of your spa business begins with an appealing brochure that describes all of the treatments and services your spa has to offer, presented in an honest and appealing fashion. Your brochure is the most important marketing piece you will develop and one that represents the core of your entire business. It should be put together thoughtfully with the utmost attention to detail.

Many brochure styles can be used to present your spa services, but a brochure's effectiveness depends on how it is received by your target market. Is the material well written and easy to understand? Will potential clients find it interesting or amusing? A brochure can be straightforward, whimsical, or highly descriptive. Avoid overly technical explanations and detailed descriptions of services, which can be overwhelming to clients and may end up leaving them with more questions than answers.

In addition to informing clients about the services you offer, your brochure should give customers a good idea of what to expect when they arrive at your door. It should reflect the type of business you operate. For example, if your day spa operation consists of two or three treatment rooms with a limited number of services and a single shower, don't lead people on with an elaborate piece that gives them the idea they will be entering a destination-style retreat. This does not mean a limited number of choices will automatically translate to a boring brochure. There are many ways to present your services creatively. What is ultimately most important is that you provide enough information for clients to book services in a way that meets their expectations.

Some spa owners decide to focus their menu of services around a particular product brand. Think twice before stating the brand name of a product in your brochure. Unless you are dedicated to representing a particular product line and receive some benefit or have an exclusive agreement with the company, it is wise to be cautious. If one of your competitors starts to use the same brand, the product suddenly becomes unavailable, or the company goes out of business, you have lost your unique selling position.

Layout and Design

Design is an integral part of an appealing brochure and should reflect the ambiance and philosophy of your spa. It does not matter whether you provide 10 or 35 treatments. What matters is that the information is presented in an alluring way that is easy to follow and characterizes the mood of your spa.

Numerous techniques can be used to create a visually pleasing brochure, but a great deal depends on the style of your spa. Is it trendy, funky, sleek, natural, clinical, sophisticated, or elegant? A good designer will work with you to communicate the style of your spa on paper by integrating typography, color schemes, and photos that reflect the true nature of your spa business. Your logo will be a major component in the design and should be placed on the front cover of your brochure to develop brand recognition. It can also serve as a springboard, integrating elements that are carried throughout the entire layout.

The organization of your brochure plays an important role in making it easy to follow and pleasant to read. The use of subheadings can be extremely helpful in creating an easy flow. If you have numerous treatments use categories, such as face, body, waxing, massage therapies, body work, hair, nail, makeup, and teens' or men's services, etc., to make it easier for clients to select the appropriate service. In contrast, a simple menu with a limited number of choices is often better served by categorizing treatments in terms of skin types and conditions, such as basic, deep cleansing, hydrating, and problem skin types, or by function, such as cleansing, exfoliating, hydrating, and nourishing treatments.

Brochure designs range in size and shape from simple inexpensive gatefolds or panels to more complex booklets, die cuts, and pocket styles with inserts or slots to hold business cards and price lists (Figure 9-7). If you are concerned about costs, use a simple layout and streamline the copy as much as you can without compromising the integrity of your business. Odd sizes and shapes and lengthier brochures will cost more money to print and to mail, especially if you will be inserting them into a custom made envelope. To defray some of the cost, you can turn your brochure into a self-mailer; however, this is not recommended for an upscale spa.

During the initial phase of developing a brochure many spa owners express concern about menu changes and the cost involved. Cost concerns are valid, but keep in mind that investing in quality materials will benefit your marketing strategy for years to come. No matter what type of design you choose, initially you can expect the cost of design fees to drive the price of producing a brochure higher. Still, it is possible to produce a beautiful piece cost-effectively. If you are just starting out and not sure how clients will receive particular treatments or plan on adding more services down the road, it makes sense to use an adjustable format, such as a folder with inserts. This is also a good technique for incorporating regular seasonal treatments. To maintain the consistency of your design, any additional materials should use the same size and format of your spa menu.

Main Components of the Spa Brochure

Brochures come in many shapes and styles, but several key elements make it easy for clients to understand how your spa operates. These include a philosophy or mission statement, a description of your treatments, business policies, spa etiquette, hours of service, location, and a detailed price list.

1. The *mission* or *philosophy statement* is a significant component of your spa business and should provide customers with the basic ideology to which you adhere. Keep it relevant to the way you conduct business and the underlying theory of your treatments and be sure that your entire staff has the same understanding of what it means.

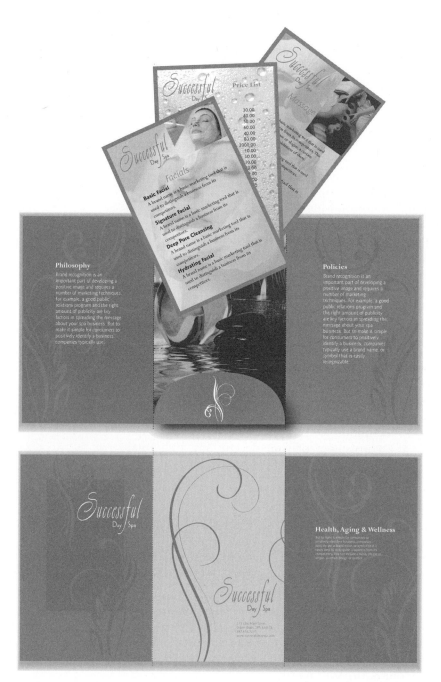

FIGURE 9-7   Various brochure styles.

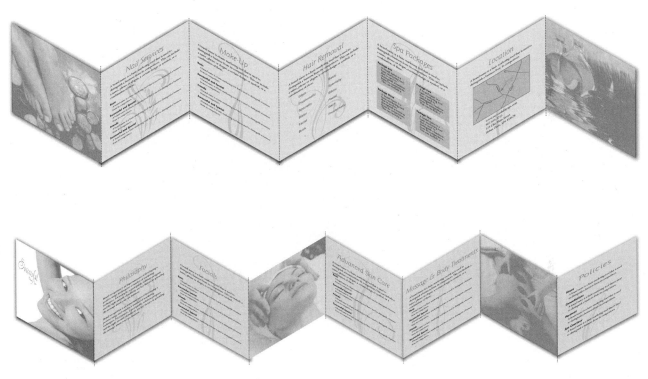

FIGURE 9-7 Various brochure styles. (*continued*)

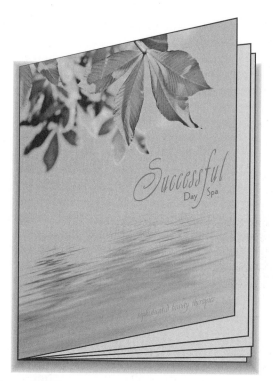

FIGURE 9-7 Various brochure styles. (*continued*)

2. The *description of your services* should help clients to make informed purchasing decisions. Use language that is easily understood, yet enticing, and create an order that is easy to follow. The format should be consistent throughout. For example, if you decide to use catchy names to describe your treatments, give all of your facials and body treatments interesting names. While you can take some "poetic license" in describing treatments, the content of your brochure should be truthful, grammatically correct, and double-checked for spelling and word usage. It is also important for copy to be legible. As a general rule, if you have to strain your eyes to read it, the print is too small.

3. Your *business policies* tell people the standards by which you operate your business. Spell these out clearly and concisely, including important information such as what forms of payment are accepted and how the spa handles gratuities, cancellations, and late arrivals. Any fees associated with cancellations should be explicit.

4. *Spa etiquette* sets the standard of behavior expected in your spa. Let clients know you are concerned with their comfort and safety in a way that puts their best interests at the forefront. Include information about what to wear or bring, personal storage facilities, limitations on the handling of valuables, the use of cell phones, and so forth.

5. The *hours of operation* are vital to the continued flow of business. List the days of the week and daily hours of operation that the spa is open, specifying at what hour you take the last appointment. If you have special hours for groups, parties, and special events or require reservations for these or all appointments, spell this out clearly. Spas that take walk-ins should include this information.

6. *Directions* to your spa make it easy for clients to find you. Don't rely on computerized maps to do the job for you; test them before putting them in your brochure. Provide graphics and text for those who require a visual, and list several landmarks that will let people know they are headed in the right direction, particularly if you are in a remote location.

7. The *telephone number, address,* and *Web site* of your spa are basic information that should be printed on all marketing materials.

8. If you have a simple layout that is easy to reprint and you will not be making changes more than once per year, it is okay to list *prices* directly in your brochure. Otherwise, include a separate insert that lists the cost of every service you provide.

As a spa owner, you may choose to incorporate a number of other individual items that are important to you. Two of the most frequently asked questions I receive from spa owners are: (1) Should I include a biography of myself? and (2) Should I include a photo of my staff in my brochure?

The answer to these questions brings up a couple of issues. First, a spa operation is often a team effort, not an individual providing services; therefore, I do not recommend including a bio of yourself in your spa brochure unless you are a one-person operation. Save this for your press kit; however, if you feel you would like to add a personal touch, consider writing your mission statement or philosophy in a letter format and include a personal signature.

A staff photo can be appropriate in some cases, and may work well for medical spas, but it depends on the image you are trying to project. Your staff turnover rate will also factor into the equation. If you are looking to present a warm, friendly, casual atmosphere that provides personal service and you have had the same loyal staff for five years, include the staff photo.

But if you are just starting out, it is wise not to take the chance. More than one spa owner has been disappointed by an employee who left within a couple of weeks or, even worse, never started after a good deal of money was invested in developing personalized marketing materials.

Updating your Brochure

Your brochure is a major presentation piece that requires a huge investment of time and money. It should be reviewed on a regular basis. Keep a running tab of corrections and edits, and note those services that are not popular. It is also a good idea to have one person responsible for maintaining inventory and reordering; otherwise, you may suddenly find yourself running short.

Finally, if you are thinking about bypassing a brochure and replacing it with a Web site to save costs—don't! A brochure is a necessary and personal statement about your business that should be included with gift certificates, gift baskets, your press kit, charitable donations, and community welcome packages. Make it the most beautiful presentation piece your budget allows.

Price List

You would not go to any store and select merchandise without knowing what the price of that product is, would you?

Clients have a right to know the charge for each service before they buy, but a lot of spa owners, concerned about changing prices and the high cost of printing new brochures, are often hesitant to publish their prices in large quantities. This worry is easily eliminated by using a separate price list that can be inserted into your brochure (Figure 9-8). There are several ways to do this cost effectively. You can add a simple fold at the end of a gatefold, or panel-style brochure, where you can insert a matching card; place your price list in the center of a booklet as a separate booklet; or insert a matching text and weight flyer, carefully folded to the design's specifications. There are many other creative possibilities that make it easy to reprint price lists as needed.

Business Card

A business card is your "ticket" to the world of commerce and provides important contact information. As the owner of your spa, it is likely that you will use it as a calling card to introduce yourself and your business in various situations. Although it is a much simpler and straightforward marketing piece, it should be given the same attention as a brochure.

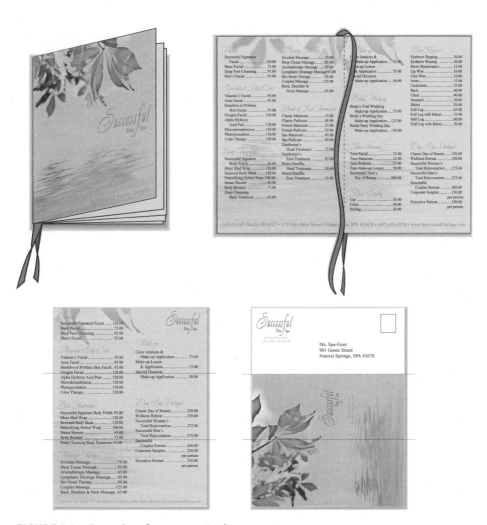

FIGURE 9-8 Examples of separate price lists.

Your business card should incorporate your spa logo and coordinate with all of your other marketing materials to create a "family" look (Figure 9-9). This is particularly important if it will be inserted in *slots* or *cutouts* in your brochure. Business cards are printed on card stock that is generally available in most paper collections and typically coordinated with the paper and ink colors used in your brochure; however, your business card can be a different color provided it works with the general theme. Business cards, like brochures, can be printed using either a two-color or four-color process. The use of more than one color will add dimension, but it will also increase the

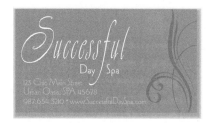
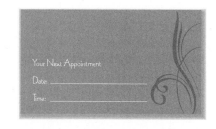
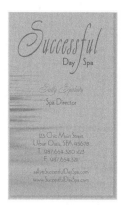
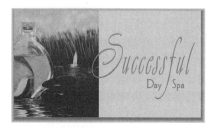
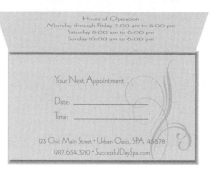

FIGURE 9-9   Examples of business card layouts.

cost. This is not always clear until you receive a quote; so be sure to ask the designer about color options up front.

There are many styles of business cards that include elaborate designs such as die cuts, folds, tiny envelopes, and odd sizes. These can make a big statement, but they can also be pricey. If you are on a budget, steer clear of these more expensive designs. A standard size card that fits neatly into a wallet or card case is generally a more practical and economical option.

What is most important is that you include all of the basic information about your business, such as the name, street address, telephone number, e-mail address, Web site, and, if necessary, the title of an individual employee. But don't turn your business card into a mini-brochure. Too much information condensed on a small card can make it difficult to read. It can also make it look messy. To avoid a cluttered look, highlight the name of your spa and keep information organized in a way that makes sense. For example, group the name of the cardholder along with his or her credentials in one area and keep the telephone number, street, and Web address together.

Several types of business cards can be used in the spa, including individual, generic, and appointment cards. What you use will depend on your business needs and your budget. Do you want or need to have a separate business card for each employee, or can you get by with generic business and appointment cards? Perhaps you can combine the two. Smaller day spas that allow clients to request individual service providers may choose to provide all of their employees with a personalized business card that has a place to write appointment information on the back. In most cases, however, a generic appointment card that gives the option to list the service provider will suffice. Note that in some cases listing the name of a specific service provider can become problematic should scheduling conflicts arise.

Gift Certificates

Plastic gift cards have become increasingly popular and are available in almost every business enterprise from supermarkets to coffee shops, boutiques, and retail stores. They are particularly popular with younger people and can be a good way to go with series and membership programs. You simply apply the dollar amount to the card and subtract it at the point of sale or assign a certain value, such as $25, to each card. Plastic gift cards are a great convenience, but they can't beat the presentation value of a paper gift certificate.

Paper gift certificates have tremendous gift appeal. When wrapped up in ribbons and bows or an attractive gift box, they make a glamorous presentation. They are also one of the easiest ways to drive sales during the holidays. No spa should be without them for special occasions, such as birthdays, anniversaries, graduations, and last-minute gifts.

Many attractive pre-designed paper gift certificates are available through stationers, but it makes a lot more sense in terms of marketing and brand recognition to have one designed specifically with your spa logo. The style of your gift certificate can be as varied as the style you choose for a brochure (Figure 9-10). In fact, the more you think outside of the box, the more likely it is that your gift certificate will be remembered. A beautifully designed gift certificate is an excellent advertising tool that lends credibility to your business.

From a business perspective, several important items should be applied to all gift certificates, including a place to write the names of both the giver and the receiver; date; dollar amount; an authorized signature to verify receipt of payment; and expiration date, if appropriate. It is particularly important to incorporate security features such as an embossed logo, special paper, numbers, or codes to identify each certificate. All gift certificates sales should be tracked through a financial software program and dated for escheatment purposes, a subject we will discuss further in Chapter 11.

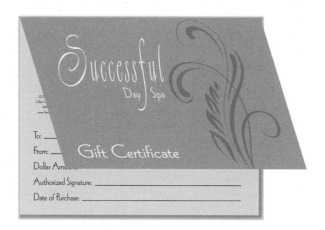
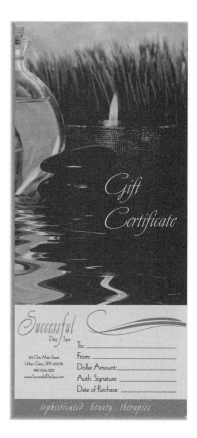

FIGURE 9-10   Examples of gift certificates.

Spa Stationery

Beautiful stationery is a great way to polish your presentation. A few simple pieces, such as letterhead, note cards, and matching envelopes, can improve the quality of your spa's image tremendously (Figure 9-11). In addition to these standard writing materials, several straightforward items can help you to further your marketing efforts with a minimum of effort. These include thank you, referral, birthday, and reminder cards (Figure 9-12).

A thank-you note to first-time customers is a nice way to let them know you appreciate their business and would like to see them again. Handwritten thank-you notes are always in vogue, but if you are operating a large day spa, you may not have time to handwrite notes to all of your spa guests. A standard phrase with a personal signature from the spa owner or service provider can add a nice touch.

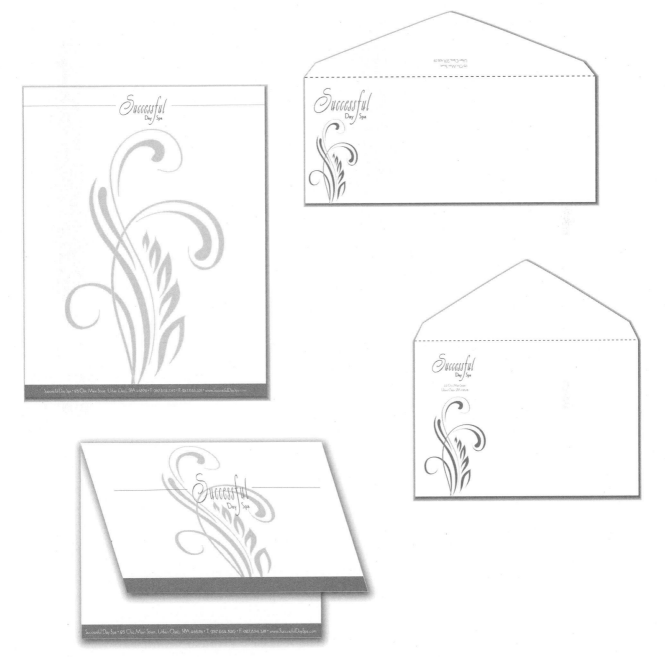

FIGURE 9-11 Stationery helps establish a spa's image.

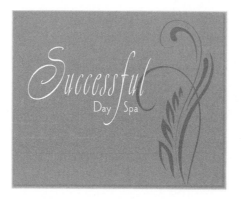
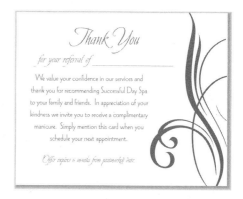
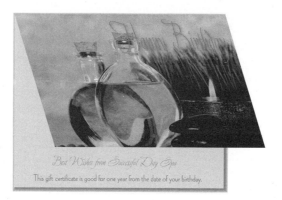
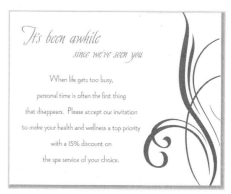

FIGURE 9-12   Referral, birthday, and reminder cards are an ideal way to develop positive client relations.

A good marketing program rewards regular customers for referring friends and relatives. In this case, a simple "Thank you for your referral!" with a special offer or discount on their next service will let customers know you appreciate their confidence in your services. A birthday card that includes a "special gift" is another way to let regular clients know their business is appreciated without any strings attached. For those you haven't seen in a while but wish you would, a "friendly reminder" with some incentive to return is always appropriate. All of these simple marketing pieces can be produced and reproduced cost-effectively. They also go a long way in developing good public relations. If you are concerned about the cost of delivery or the impact on the environment these items are easily transformed for electronic delivery.

Special Announcements

On occasion, you may need additional pieces, such as invitations, an announcement for a new staff member, an open house, or a notice that you are expanding or relocating your spa. All of these can be developed using a simple format based on your "family" look. When developing these materials, work from your standard layouts and always incorporate your logo to make the piece instantly recognizable.

Series, spa club, and corporate membership cards are other pieces that are easy to create from the same layout used for your business cards.

Don't Forget the Frills

There are a wide range of choices when it comes to wrapping it all up (Figure 9-13). Shop around for the best price on bags, ribbons, bows, tissue, and boxes. Have your logo and name printed on gift bags, or use a seal if you are trying to cut costs.

Sheer-colored mesh bags in sparkly tones are ideal for small samples and make a great presentation when enclosed with your business card. Samples can also be attached to postcards with sticky gum and inserted in gift bags at the point of sale.

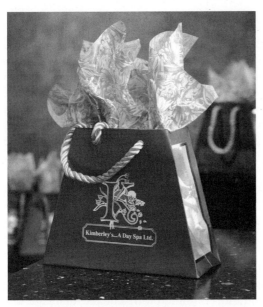

FIGURE 9-13 Handsomely packaged gift bags will enhance your spa's image.

ADDITIONAL MARKETING MATERIALS

Postcard

The postcard is a simple, yet effective, direct marketing tool that is well received and inexpensive to produce. Postcards come in various sizes and styles, such as single cards and double cards with perforated tear-offs (Figure 9-14). Tear-offs are great for surveys and client feedback as well as measuring the return on your investment. The most popular postcard sizes are the 4×6 inch, or standard size postcard, and the 5×7 inch, or jumbo size. If you are concerned about rates, consider that the U.S. Postal Service reserves postcard rate for standard and smaller-sized cards, while the cost of the jumbo is the same as that of mailing a first class letter, although it is often worth the extra money in terms of impact. For more information about postcard mailers and current rates, visit the official Web site of the U.S. Postal Service.

The postcard is the perfect venue for delivering a powerful marketing message using relatively few words in an eye-catching format. But remember the "40-40-20 rule": The key to customer response is more about your offer and your list and less about the creative. That said, you needn't go further than your own mailbox to understand that your postcard still has to stand out.

An effective postcard is one that captures recipients' attention and immediately lets them know why they should take advantage of your offer. It also provides customers with all the information they need to follow through. Keep it simple and straightforward, and provide a big incentive to act quickly. Let clients know exactly what they will receive, when it is available, and when the offer expires. If the offer cannot be combined with any other promotion or if there is a limited supply, let them know in language that is easy to understand, such as "not to be combined with any other offer" or "while supplies last." The important thing is not to mislead clients with a promise you cannot deliver.

While the design does not need to be elaborate, it should fit in with the image of your spa and the objective you are trying to achieve. For example, a generic postcard designed to help you build a clientele should embrace the ambiance of your spa and let potential customers know the types of services you provide. When using this format, it is wise to provide an incentive for trying your spa, such as a complimentary skin analysis or discount on a particular treatment for first-time guests.

An enticing headline combined with a beautiful image will help to pull the recipient in, but you don't need to use expensive stock photos or fancy

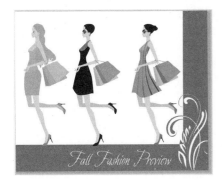

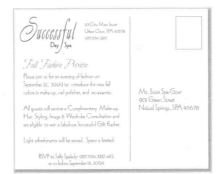

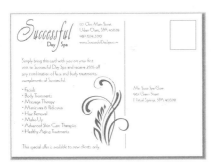

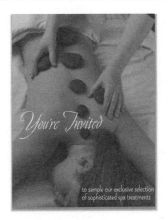

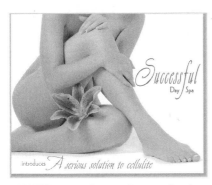

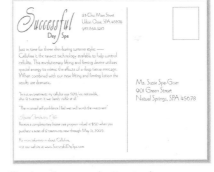

FIGURE 9-14 Postcards are a simple, cost-effective direct marketing tool.

artwork to get people to read your mailer. A brightly colored postcard with an attractive font printed in one or two colors on plain card stock can be just as powerful as a four-color piece on glossy card stock. A plain white card with a clever message and simple illustration can also be quite effective. A lot depends on the ambiance of your spa, the aura you wish to create, and the amount you want to spend on design and production.

To make an impression, use themes, colors, and styles that are easily identified with your spa and that you know will be attractive to your target market. For example, a clever caricature or a series that promotes head-to-toe body treatments can be fun and is a good way to keep customers interested as long as it complements the image of your spa. Remember to incorporate your logo and include the name, address, telephone number, and Web address of your spa on the postcard. When space is at a minimum, consider using your logo as part of the return address.

Postcards are a fun and creative way to promote business and are easy to track, but if you find you are getting little return on your investment, take time to figure out why. Is it simply that you have forgotten to ask the recipient to return the postcard to redeem the offer, or is there no real value in your offer? What about the creative: Does it demonstrate good taste and bring attention to the offer? Look at all the information with an open mind before discontinuing what is typically a very effective direct mail piece.

Newsletter

Newsletters are an excellent way to build client and business relations; however, publishing a newsletter is an ambitious project that often takes more time than busy spa owners have (Figure 9-15). If writing a newsletter appeals to you, limit the number of issues until you gain some experience. For many, following a seasonal schedule with a winter, spring, summer, and fall newsletter makes sense. Others may find two or three newsletters per year sufficient.

The key to managing a successful newsletter is organization. Look to newsletters from professional associations and news publications for ideas, and then develop categories with which you are comfortable. Devoting a column to new products and treatments and seasonal promotions is a natural. Depending on the focus of your spa, you may also wish to include a section for spa recipes and health and wellness information or show off your staff's expertise with a "Professional Spotlight." Brainstorm ideas for columns with your employees and involve your clients. What are the most frequently asked questions your staff receives? What topics would interest clients? Would your employees be willing to contribute a feature article? Consider a "Q&A," assigning topics to staff based on their expertise or

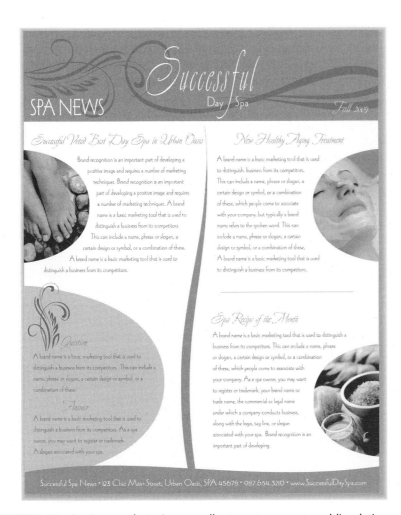

FIGURE 9-15 A print newsletter is an excellent way to promote public relations and can be adjusted easily to fit the format of your Web site.

inviting other professionals that offer complementary services to write a column for your newsletter. Vendors may also allow you to use materials from their literature.

Some professional organizations and trade publications supply reusable newsletter formats. You can also use software to develop a template on your own; however, your newsletter is likely to look more professional if you hire a graphic designer to develop a masthead that includes your logo and a format that is in sync with your "family" image. Keep your newsletter format

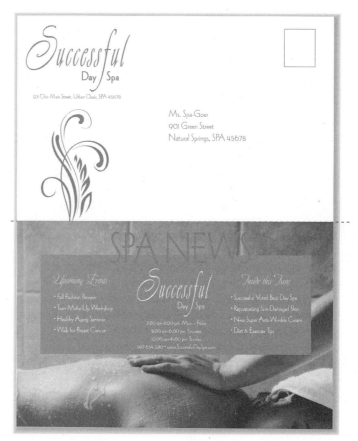

FIGURE 9-15   A print newsletter is an excellent way to promote public relations and can be adjusted easily to fit the format of your Web site. (*continued*)

simple, and limit the number of words that can be used in each column. A spa newsletter need not be lengthy to be informative. A template and concise format will also make it easy to plug in new text on a regular basis.

Your newsletter will require well-written feature stories. If you do not have a qualified writer on your staff, consider hiring a professional copywriter to write material for you. This can save time and money in the long run and will give your newsletter a unified and professional tone. If you are concerned about authenticity, supply the writer with reference materials that uphold your philosophies and/or summarize the information you would like to include. Interviews conducted with you and your staff for articles and material will help to maintain the true voice of your spa. You can also take a more active role by contributing a personal note from the spa owner in each issue.

It is a good idea to have several hard copies of your newsletter available in the spa, but the most economical way to distribute your newsletter is via the Internet. There are a number of Internet mail services which provide distribution lists that can help increase circulation, but it is best to "invite" people to subscribe to avoid "spamming." This is easily accomplished by providing an option on your Web site to subscribe or by asking existing clients if they would like to receive your newsletter electronically. If you decide to purchase lists or solicit subscribers on the Internet, be sure to qualify your leads as people who have given their permission to be contacted and provide them with an offer that invites them to receive your newsletter. Always provide the reader with an option to unsubscribe.

Once your newsletter is available to customers online, you will want to take full advantage of its potential to increase your customer base. Link it to your Web site and special promotions and provide options to multiply your database by supplying customers with an option to e-mail your newsletter to a friend. A coupon or special offer can help to increase the popularity of your newsletter.

Newsletters provide a great opportunity to promote public relations and are a good way to build trust in your professional services. They also require a good deal of time and energy; so it is important to look closely at the return on your investment. If you distribute your newsletter via the Internet, there are tools available that allow you to measure how many people actually open your newsletter, read it, or forward it. Your Webmaster or IT consultant should be able to supply you with more information on Web analytics.

Flyer

A flyer is a standard 8.5 × 11 letter size sheet of paper that can be used for multiple purposes: to create awareness, present information, or promote new services, products, and equipment. This simple and inexpensive method of advertising does not need to be boring. Jazz it up with a splash of bright color, photos, or artwork, or use glossy paper for a more sophisticated and polished look.

Flyers are a great way to announce events or introduce new products. They can also be used to highlight your name in the news or bring attention to current ads (Figure 9-16). For example, most publications will supply you with 8.5 × 11 reprints of a news article in which your spa appears. If not, ask for permission to reprint the article and hire your own typesetter to create a flyer for you. This is great material for a press kit. You might also consider

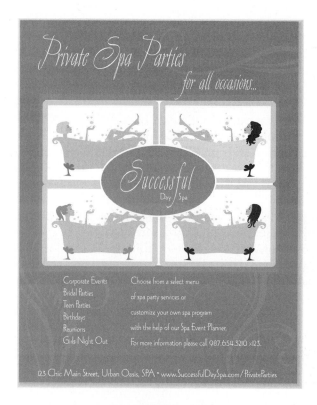

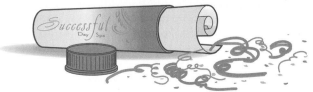

FIGURE 9-16   Flyers are an easy way to attract attention to special promotions.

turning a popular ad into a flyer. This technique works well for larger display ads, such as those that appear in kiosks at the mall or on screen at the cinema, and can help to reinforce the connection. Use your imagination. Create reprints of other existing marketing materials, such as the home page of your Web site, or blow up an article from your newsletter.

Vendors are another great resource for marketing materials and often have flyers pertaining to new products and equipment. Many will include a supply with the purchase of a product; others may charge a fee. Insert them in gift bags at the point of sale or place them near retail displays to promote products.

Sales Letter

Sales letters are not all that popular in the spa industry, but they are a great way to build client relations. Addressing business topics in a letter format involves the customer at a personal level. For example, if you are introducing a new technique or piece of equipment, a conversation about why you are in favor of this method or why you chose this particular piece of equipment, and how you anticipate your clients will benefit from it will leave clients feeling they are an important part of the decision-making process.

The main purpose of a sales letter is to promote business, but it can also be used to further public relations. Consider a trend-setting New Year's letter that thanks valued clients for their patronage, talks about spa trends or your spa goals for the year, and includes a special value, such as a spa club membership for the coming year.

Writing an effective sales letter is not easy. Provide enough information for the consumer to make an informed purchasing decision without making it too long. Highlight the benefits and features of your product or promotion, and provide a response form or tear sheet that allows the client to redeem the offer. Again, this has the added benefit of measuring the response rate.

A masterfully written sales letter is a great marketing tool. Unfortunately, many impersonal looking letters end up in the recycle bin. To make sure yours is not one of them, try handwriting the envelope or put something inside that people will be compelled to open, such as a product sample or a pen. You can also print a message, such as "valuable offer inside," on the outside of the envelope to let customers know your mail piece is worth opening. Mailing your letter in an unusual package, such as a translucent envelope, tube, or box will increase the chances of it being opened as well; however, this can raise the cost.

PRODUCTION

A great deal of time, energy, and money are spent creating quality marketing materials, but the job is not done until you have a neat supply of printed materials available for use.

Production is an important part of the process that is often overlooked until it is time to go to print. In this age of computer wizardry, many do not realize that producing quality marketing materials is not an overnight job and must be planned well in advance of the actual printing. This is particularly important when dealing with intricately designed pieces, such as brochures that are die cut. Allow at least three weeks from a final design to a finished product, but depending on how involved the piece is, production could take longer.

The amount of time it takes to go from proofs to print varies according to the scope of the project and is subject to the length of time it takes to order paper, incorporate artwork, review preliminary designs, develop mock-ups, print bluelines and color proofs, and produce the film used to make printing plates. After materials are printed, they need to be cut, folded, and delivered.

Most printed materials are first presented as *mock-ups,* which are generated by the designer from their personal computer to give the client a general idea of what the piece will look like. The mock-up is then edited to the client's liking and followed by bluelines or preliminary proofs that demonstrate exactly how the piece will look when it is printed. Bluelines are so-called because they are produced on special paper that uses blue ink. In those instances where color is a concern, a color proof may also be ordered. Color proofs cost extra but are usually well worth it if there is a concern about the exactness of the color(s).

The production of your brochure, business cards, ads, and other marketing material is best left to professionals, who are aware of the restrictions and limitations of any given piece and know how to interface with printers and production staff. Still, you should expect to be an active participant in each stage of the production process (Figure 9-17). When reviewing mock-ups and proofs, look for overall balance, proportion, and the use of white space; as tedious as it may be, you will also need to proofread the copy of each proof presented to you.

Everyone wants to keep production costs down. If you are on a budget, the best advice is don't choose an elaborate design and insist on three quotes. But never base your decision on price alone. Agencies and designers use a number of printers and have a good feel for those who can do the job best. Listen to their advice.

PRINT ADVERTISING

The Internet has taken the world by storm, and public relations is the new media darling. But neither has completely stopped people from reading newspaper and magazine ads. Print ads are still one of the most powerful and popular methods of advertising.

Print ads are used for a variety of purposes: to generate awareness of what your business has to offer; announce an event or a sale; introduce a new product, service, or staff member; or simply to build an image. They also appear in a wide range of print mediums, such as newspapers, magazines, newsletters, event programs, telephone directories, bulletins, and billboards. Despite the wide range of purpose and mediums, all ads share the same common goal: to attract, inform, and call the consumer to action.

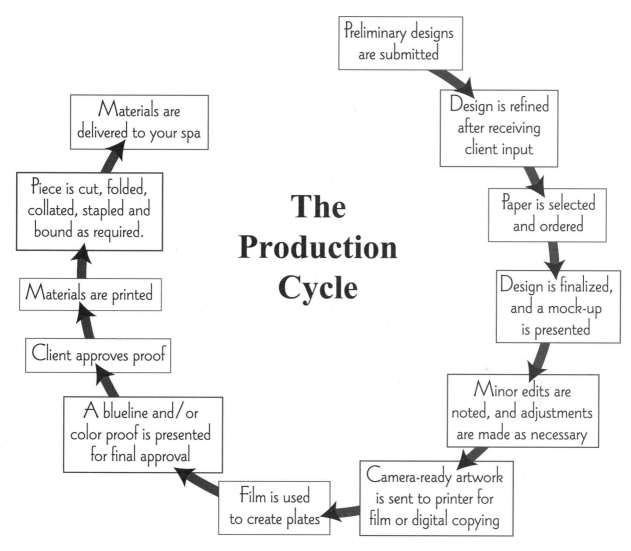

The Production Cycle

Preliminary designs are submitted

Design is refined after receiving client input

Paper is selected and ordered

Design is finalized, and a mock-up is presented

Minor edits are noted, and adjustments are made as necessary

Camera-ready artwork is sent to printer for film or digital copying

Film is used to create plates

A blueline and/or color proof is presented for final approval

Client approves proof

Materials are printed

Piece is cut, folded, collated, stapled and bound as required.

Materials are delivered to your spa

FIGURE 9-17   The Production Cycle.

Key Elements of a Good Ad

Print advertising is one of the most expensive media buys, a fact that is often a deterrent for small day spa owners on limited budgets. But don't let this stop you from using this powerful form of advertising. A single ad has the capability of reaching millions of potential spa-goers. To get the most for your advertising dollar, you will need a polished and professional-looking ad. If you are not in the position to hire an advertising agency, use a professional copywriter and graphic designer or marketing consultant to create an ad for you. A good ad does not necessarily require a lot of copy or expensive artwork, but it does require a professional presentation.

Some newspaper publications will produce your ad for free; others have set rates and editing fees. Because graphic artists who work for newspapers and magazines usually have access to a huge portfolio of artwork, this can be a viable option for the smaller day spa that cannot afford to hire a professional, but it is important to note that most in-house graphic artists simply do not have the time to develop a good understanding of your business. If you decide to work with staff designers, it is often helpful to supply examples of ad styles that you like and provide as much input as possible about your business goals and the look you are trying to achieve. The production of your ad may or may not include copywriting services, in which case you will need to provide copy as well.

COMPONENTS OF A SUCCESSFUL AD

- A logo that immediately identifies your spa
- A great headline that captures the reader's attention
- Copy that reads well and lets people know why they should do business with you
- Artwork that represents the image you wish to project
- A memorable tagline
- All the information needed to reach you
- An incentive to pick up the phone and call you or book an appointment online

Transforming the components of an ad to one that jumps off the page is not easy. How can you make your ad stand out? A great ad is limited only by imagination, but to get started, you will need to establish certain criteria. What is the purpose of your ad? Where will it appear? Who will it target? What information needs to be included to get your message across?

What restrictions may limit size and color? The answer to these preliminary questions forms the basis of your ad.

Ad Copy

Modern advertising methods have in many instances reduced the ad to an art form. This philosophy has led many advertising professionals to use bold images and relatively few words to make a big statement. Depending on your goal, this strategy may work in your favor; however, words still hold tremendous value within the context of an ad, particularly when it comes to making an offer.

An attention-getting headline is critical to pulling the reader in and defining the purpose of your ad. It should immediately let consumers know how they will benefit from your product or service or deliver some important news. For example, the headline "Beautiful Healthy Skin" sends a strong message of what they can expect to gain by taking advantage of the offer, whereas the headline "Grand Opening" supplies important information or news about an upcoming event.

Headlines are supported with subheadings, bulleted information, and/or text that describe the benefits and features associated with it. Many think this text should be kept to a minimum in print ads, but don't be afraid to use lengthier copy if it serves your purpose and you have the space. An interesting narrative can put a unique spin on what are often rote bullets and simple phrases used to describe spa fare. Testimonials from satisfied clients can also add flavor to an otherwise ordinary spa ad. This is a great technique for spas that cater to corporate events and bridal parties. The important thing is to use language that flows well and is easily understood. If space is at a premium, a good tagline that sums up the essence of your spa in just a few words can be a great approach.

An attractive design can only enhance your copy, but again don't lose sight of the offer. You can spend a lot of money on design, but it is ultimately your offer that brings in clients. Spell this out as clearly as possible in unambiguous language.

Layout and Design

The content of your ad is shaped by three important design elements: typography, artwork, and placement. There are millions of ways to use these and many opinions about what constitutes a great ad, but the size of your ad space will have a great deal to do with how these elements are used (Figure 9-18). Ad size is often deceiving, particularly when the design

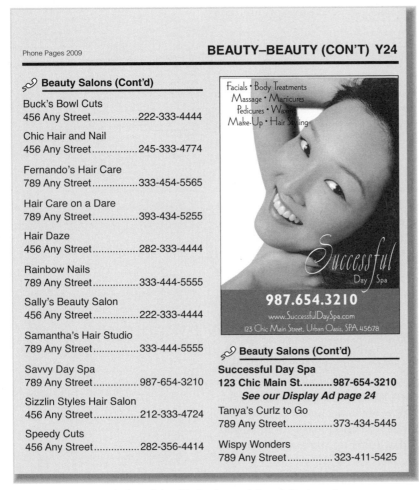

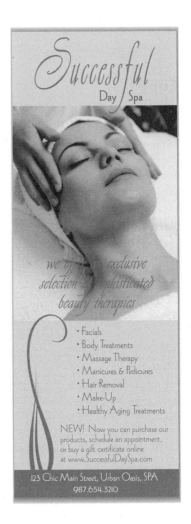

FIGURE 9-18   Examples of classified, advertorial, and display ads.

is presented out of context, such as in an isolated e-mail or by fax. Before looking at ad proofs, take a look at the layout of the publication in which your ad will appear.

Most newspaper and magazine publications sell ad space by the column inch. This is often a difficult concept for the lay person to understand and is complicated further by varying dimensions and formatting. Advertising representatives are generally pretty helpful when it comes to purchasing ad space and will typically supply you with a graphic display of all of the ad sizes that are available along with specifications and

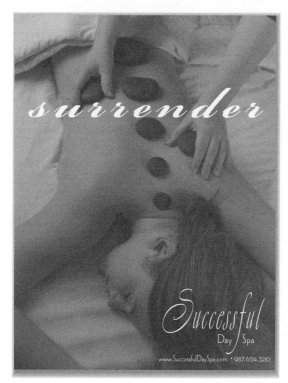

FIGURE 9-18 Examples of classified, advertorial, and display ads. (*continued*)

guidelines for setting up and delivering your ad, but it is important to have the different ad sizes pointed out to you in the actual print medium. This will give you a much better visual understanding of how your ad will present.

Typography can greatly enhance your message and helps to distinguish your ad from the competition. Placing your logo in an ad supports brand name recognition and connects the reader to typography that is automatically associated with your spa. It should be complemented with typefaces that are compatible and extremely legible. The point size will also have an impact and should bring attention to headlines, subheadings, and other important information, such as your telephone number. If the reader needs magnifying lenses to read the fine print in your offer, your advertising dollars have been wasted. The use of other typographic features, such as upper and lowercase lettering, italicized print, and boldface can also bring attention to your ad.

Research shows that consumers respond better to ads that include photos. Choose these carefully. Whenever possible, use your own photos or illustrations that are in sync with the image you wish to project. The use of various other artistic elements, such as symbols, lines, borders, shading, splashes of color and so on, can add to the quality of the design. They can also take away from it. Be careful with techniques, such as reverse type, which can "chop up" an ad if used inappropriately, and shading, which can make an ad look "dirty" or "muddy" in certain mediums, such as newsprint.

Color ads are generally more appealing, but keep in mind that they appear better in glossy magazines than in newsprint, where spending the extra money for color may not be worth it. Four-color ads are expensive, but if you get a bargain, take advantage of it. If you can't afford to run a four-color ad, you might try spot color as an accent, but this too can have an adverse effect and in some cases creates an ethereal quality where none is desired. The result can be less appealing than a black-and-white ad, which costs less.

The placement of your logo, artwork, and copy is ultimately what ties all of the elements together. Be aware of how the eye is pulled into an ad by a photo, typography, or artwork. The use of spacing and white space is an important part of the overall flow of an ad and helps to focus the reader's eye, moving it in the direction needed to take action. All elements should work together to steer the reader toward your offer and then toward your spa's telephone number.

There are many ways to have fun with placement. Circles and swirls of print, sidebars, text that wraps around photos or images, layers, and borders can turn an ordinary ad into an extraordinary one, but don't underestimate the value of a simple layout. An ad with an attention-grabbing headline, supported by a simple phrase or tagline, combined with a great offer and your logo, can make your phone ring when it is placed in the right publication.

Studies have shown that the position of your ad on the page rarely makes a big difference in terms of readership; however, certain sections of the newspaper have a higher readership of men versus women and can make a difference in terms of your target market. Think about this when attempting to reach a particular audience. At times you may want to advertise in the sports section to reach the male market, or place an ad in a section of the newspaper with a high female readership to reach women.

Cooperative Advertising

On occasion, you may wish to join forces with a product vendor. This can be a good way to feature a new product or promotion and can save you lots of money, provided you are an exclusive distributor of the product in your area; however, if the spa down the street is selling the same product, remember that you are advertising for them, too.

When engaging in joint advertising, make sure your spa name is prominently featured and check with the product manufacturer for any special requirements before placing their brand name in your marketing materials. Some companies will insist that you identify their brand name in a certain way, incorporate their trademark or copyright symbols, or use their logo to identify the product. To prevent any miscommunication, you should always supply a proof of the ad before printing.

Classified Ads

Most people are familiar with the classified section of the newspaper, where you will find ads for real estate, employment, garage sales, and business services in a condensed line-by-line format. As a spa owner, it is likely that you will have a need to place an ad in the "help wanted" section of your newspaper at some point. There are many other valuable classified ad venues.

Classified ads provide a useful service listing the most essential information about your business, such as its name, address, telephone number, and Web address. The most common use of a classified ad is the telephone directory but you can also find classified ads in magazines, newspapers, and various other print and Web-based directories. Because rates are based on a per-line or per-word basis and space is typically at a premium, this is often a good place to use a tagline or slogan that sums up the ideology of your business. If space allows, incorporate your logo as well.

TRUTH IN ADVERTISING

In Chapter 8, we discussed ethical issues in marketing. All the same guidelines apply to print advertising, in addition to the following:

- Your ad must be truthful and factual with no intent to purposely mislead or dupe the consumer.

- Use simple, easy-to-read language to avoid misinterpretation.

- Choose your words carefully when offering specials and discounts, inserting language that is clearly understood, such as "not to be combined with any other offer, special, or discount."

- Be conscious of FDA standards for cosmetic versus drug claims.

- If you claim an offer provides substantial savings to the consumer, make sure you can prove it.

- Don't copy text verbatim from someone else's ad. You can use a similar format or borrow ideas, but use your own photos, images, and language.

- Obtain permission for the use of any photos placed in your ads.

- Avoid advertising extremes. Lots of advertising today is focused on image building rather than a call to action. The ad as an art form has its place, but it is important to balance this technique with ads that supply useful information.

- Declare any kind of public recognition, such as an award for "Best Spa," in an honest, straightforward manner.

- Never use false testimonials from clients or any other person or organization.

- Weigh your advertising against standards set by the American Advertising Federation and American Association of Advertising Agencies.

Radio and Television Ads

Higher priced radio and television advertising is often out of the question for smaller day spas; however, there are some affordable deals available through cable television, smaller broadcasting companies, and public

Successful

Day / Spa

Figure 9-1a

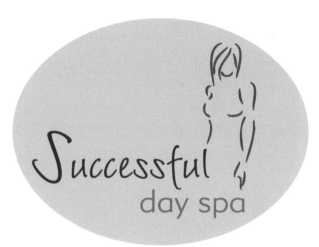

Successful
day spa

Figure 9-1b

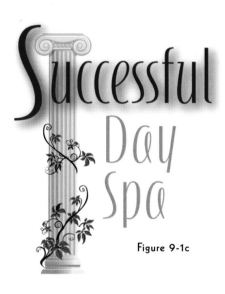

Successful
Day
Spa

Figure 9-1c

Successful·day
spa

Figure 9-1d

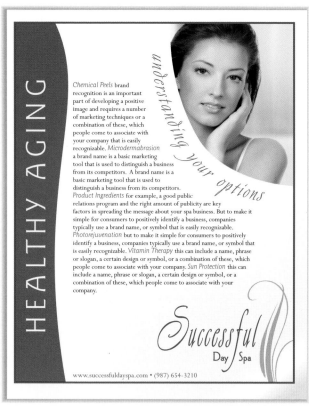

Figure 9-3A

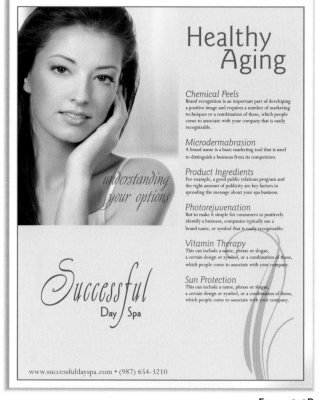

Figure 9-3B

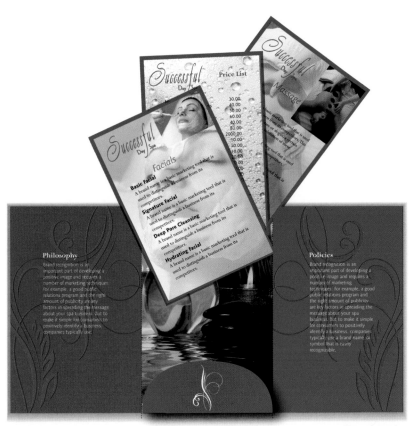

Figure 9-7A

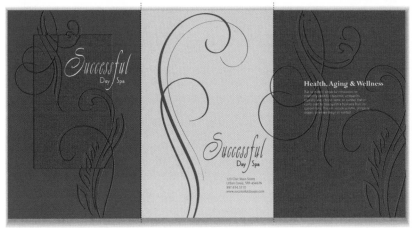

Figure 9-7b

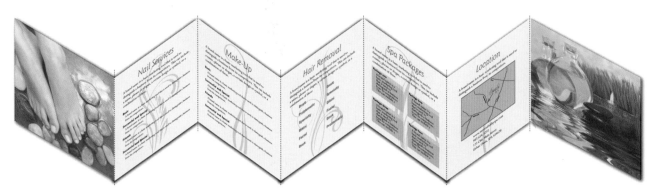

Figure 9-7c

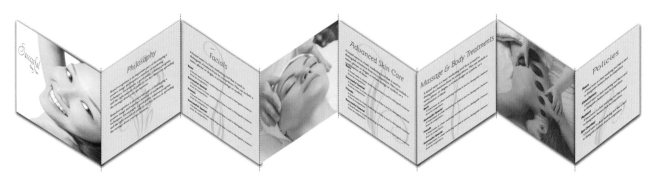

Figure 9-7d

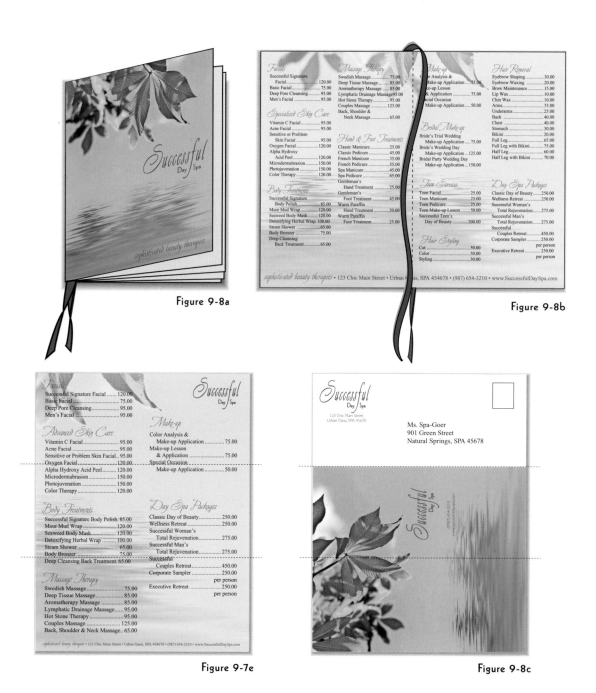

Figure 9-8a

Figure 9-8b

Figure 9-7e

Figure 9-8c

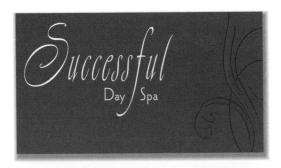

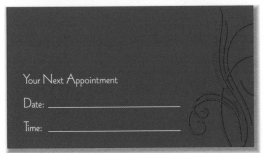

Your Next Appointment

Date: _____

Time: _____

Figure 9-9a and 9-9b

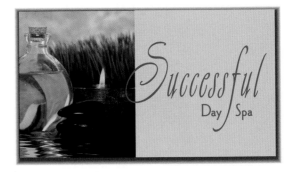

Hours of Operation
Monday through Friday 7:00 am to 8:00 pm
Saturday 8:00 am to 6:00 pm
Sunday 10:00 am to 6:00 pm

Your Next Appointment

Date: _____

Time: _____

123 Chic Main Street • Urban Oasis, SPA 45678
987.654.3210 • SuccessfulDaySpa.com

Figure 9-9D, Front + Inside

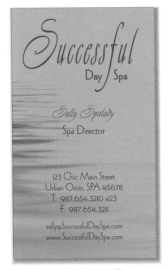

Figure 9-9c

I-6　　Business Cards

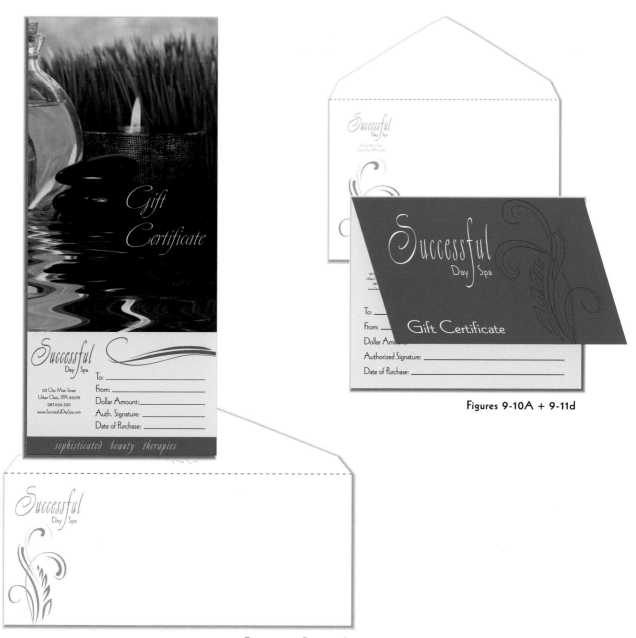

Figures 9-10A + 9-11d

Figures 9-10B + 9-11b

Figure 9-11a

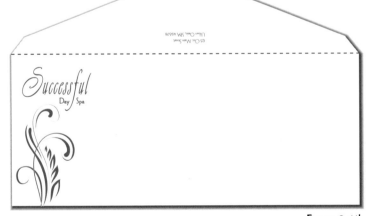

Figure 9-11b

I-8   Spa Stationery Letterhead and Envelope Example

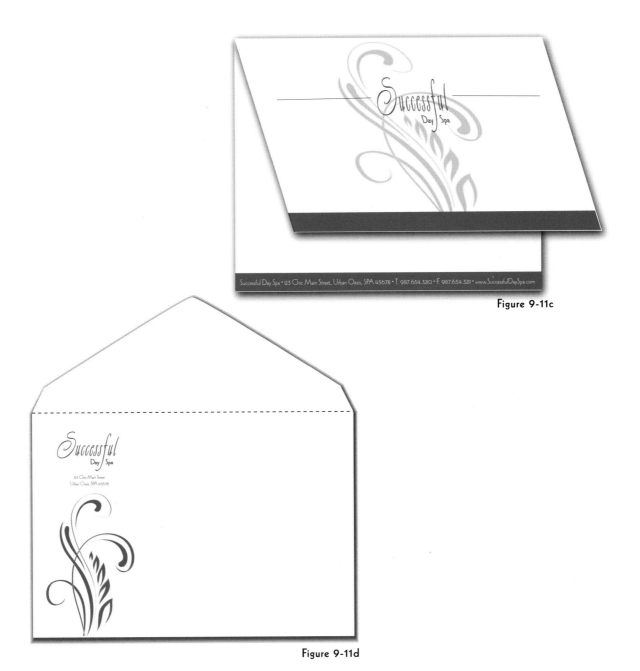

Figure 9-11c

Figure 9-11d

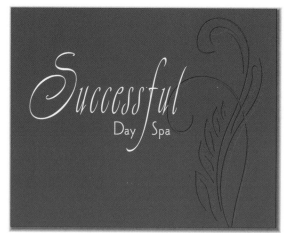

Figure 9-12A

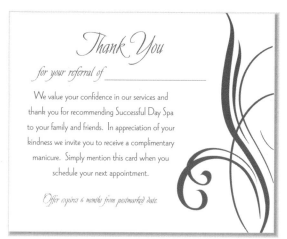

Thank You

for your referral of _____

We value your confidence in our services and
thank you for recommending Successful Day Spa
to your family and friends. In appreciation of your
kindness we invite you to receive a complimentary
manicure. Simply mention this card when you
schedule your next appointment.

Offer expires 6 months from postmarked date.

Figure 9-12B

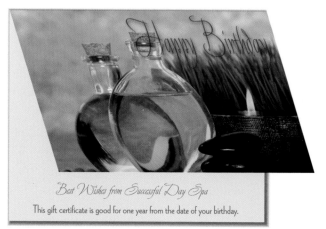

Happy Birthday

Best Wishes from Successful Day Spa

This gift certificate is good for one year from the date of your birthday.

Figure 9-12c

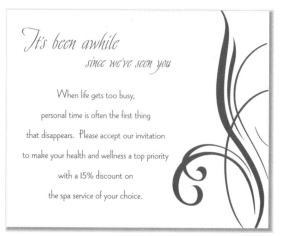

It's been awhile

since we've seen you

When life gets too busy,
personal time is often the first thing
that disappears. Please accept our invitation
to make your health and wellness a top priority
with a 15% discount on
the spa service of your choice.

Figure 9-12d

I-10   Referral, Reminder, and Birthday Cards

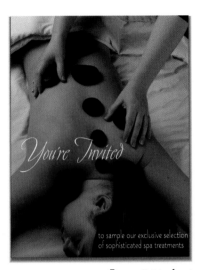

Figure 9-14a front

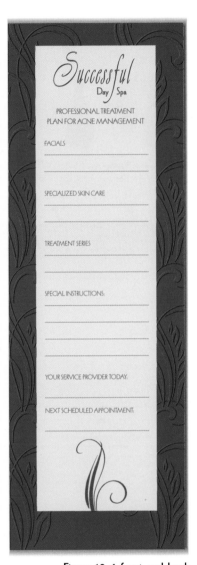

Figure 10-6 front and back

Figure 9-14a back

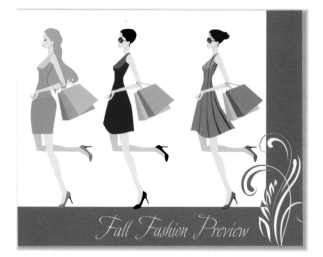

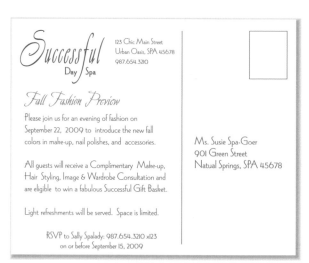

Fall Fashion Preview

Please join us for an evening of fashion on September 22, 2009 to introduce the new fall colors in make-up, nail polishes, and accessories.

All guests will receive a Complimentary Make-up, Hair Styling, Image & Wardrobe Consultation and are eligible to win a fabulous Successful Gift Basket.

Light refreshments will be served. Space is limited.

RSVP to Sally Spalady: 987.654.3210 x123 on or before September 15, 2009

Figure 9-14c

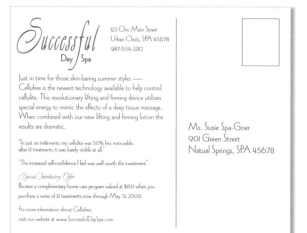

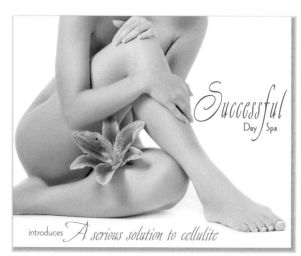

Figure 9-14D

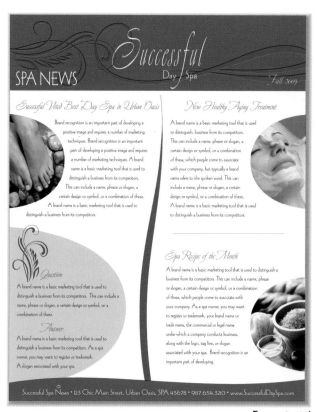

Figure 9-15A

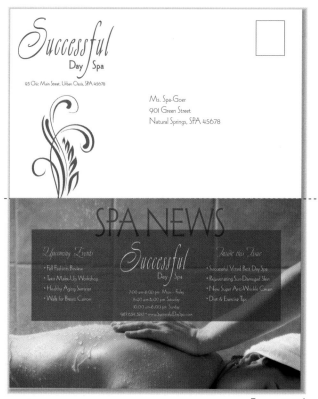

Figure 9-15b

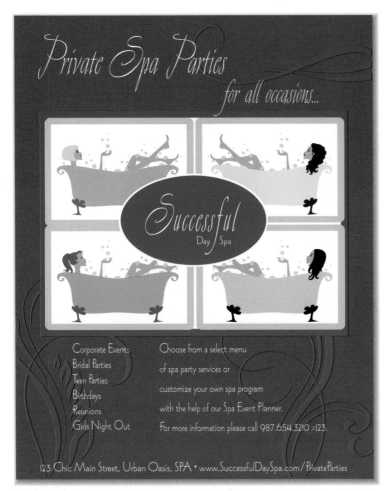

Figure 9-16A

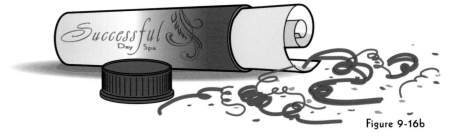

Figure 9-16b

I-14   Flyer and Mailer

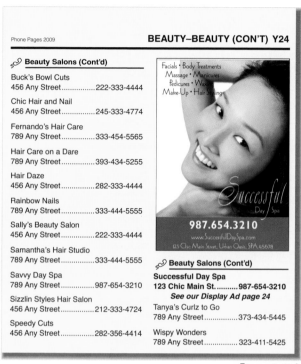

Figure 9-18A

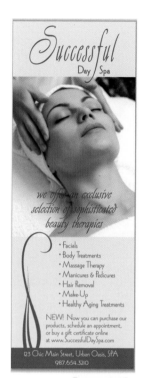

Figure 9-18b

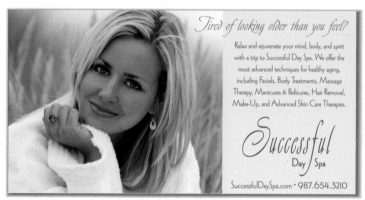

Figure 9-18c

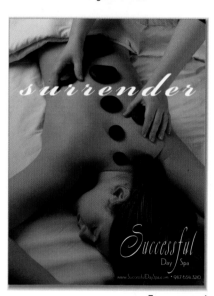

Figure 9-18d

Spa Advertisements   I-15

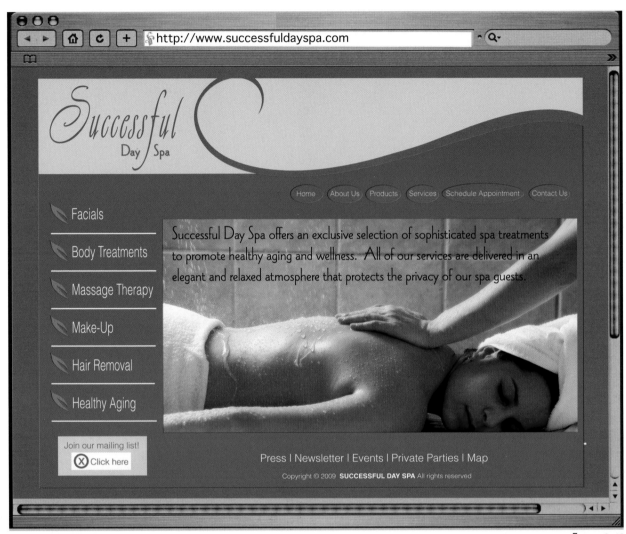

Figure 9-19

broadcasting stations. If you have the opportunity to advertise on radio or television, let broadcast professionals guide you but look at the demographics and ratings carefully before you buy. Money spent on costlier broadcast advertising can often be put to better use in other mediums.

Radio and television *commercials,* as ads are termed in broadcasting, have the same objective as print advertising, but they use additional audio and visual components. Radio is an audio message that relies on the listener accepting your offer in a short time frame, generally within 60 seconds or less. This means your message must be communicated clearly in a voice and tone that calls people to action in an enthusiastic and memorable, yet brief, manner. It is an excellent opportunity to use a tagline or slogan. Radio stations generally use professionals to write the text for a commercial and typically supply an announcer to perform the *voice-over.* If you have an excellent speaking voice and your identity is closely tied to your business—for example, you are the owner of Annabella's Day Spa and a well-known persona—using your own voice-over can add personal appeal. Background music and sound effects also play an important role in delivering a message that reflects the mood of your spa. Rely on broadcast professionals to help you sort through the millions of musical compositions that are available. If you bring in your own music, be aware of copyright issues.

Television has the added advantage of a visual component. This is where presentation is critical. If you include images of your spa in an ad, pay close attention to every detail and be conscious of the effects of harsh lighting. Clean, polish, and "dress up" all areas of your spa with fresh flowers, candles, fluffy robes, and towels. Professional models are recommended. If you decide to include staff, supervise makeup and dictate the dress code to perfect your image. Many small business owners choose to represent their company in television ads, but not all achieve the same measure of success. If you choose to be involved in the production of your own spa commercial, follow the advice of professionals and do not insist on doing it your way. The production of television commercials is an art that is best left to professionals.

Many radio stations include production in the cost of advertising, but this is not always true in television. Before signing a contract, ask about production fees. If production is not included, shop around for a vendor. There are many small independently owned production companies with professionally trained staff. Ask for references and video and audio demos.

If you find that radio and television commercials are cost prohibitive, be creative. Produce a video or podcast of the latest spa therapy technique with the help of your marketing team, and hand it over to a publicist or public relations agent for promotion, or use your website as a vehicle to present your own *infomercials*. If you are lucky enough to get a spot on the local news or a television program, capitalize on it by sending an e-mail broadcast to all of your clients.

DESIGNING A WEB SITE

For many, the first introduction to your spa will be your Web site. This is one of the most powerful and cost-effective direct marketing tools you will develop and one that virtually markets itself since the viewer typically elects to search for your business.

In Chapter 7, we discussed the technical aspects of Web development, and in Chapter 8, we noted the versatility of a Web site as a direct marketing tool. Here, we will focus on what goes into making a positive visual presentation.

Design and Development

The World Wide Web has its own language and what often seems like a great deal of technological wizardry associated with it. But building a Web site is really not a terribly difficult project; so first of all, don't be intimidated.

The standard format for creating Web pages is HTML, or *hypertext markup language protocol,* a program that allows Web pages or sections to be linked to each other. Writing in HTML requires a certain knowledge base, which can be cumbersome if you want to create your own Web site.

Fortunately, several reasonably priced, easy-to-use software programs are available for building Web sites, such as Adobe Dreamweaver, Microsoft FrontPage, and Adobe GoLive! If you are familiar with graphics-based programs such as Adobe PageMaker and QuarkXpress, you will be able to work with these programs as well. In fact, it is a good idea to go this route even if you hire a professional to create your Web site, since most Web designers work in these programs. Should you decide to change your Web designer at some point or choose to edit your Web pages on your own, using one of these types of programs will give you the flexibility to do so.

Many inexpensive templates are available through private companies and communications vendors, and a number of free templates are available online. The question is: Do you really want to look like everyone else? Consider also that unless you are a graphic artist, it is unlikely that you will be able to manipulate one of these programs to the artistic level needed to create a high quality Web site. But most importantly, do you have the time to do it yourself?

Various Web development firms, small marketing and advertising agencies, freelance graphic artists, and copywriters create Web sites; however, not all provide the same services. For example, some Web designers do not write copy. Before signing a contract, ask for references and a complete breakdown of all of the services that will be provided. In general, the best option for the small business owner is to hire a professional marketing agency or graphic designer and copywriter who can create a Web site using one of the more versatile Web development tools.

If possible, it is wise to use the same design team or individual(s) who developed your print materials. This has several advantages, mainly that the team is already familiar with your overall business and marketing plan and has a good handle on your brand, competition, and the target market your spa business is trying to reach. In addition, the same design team is completely knowledgeable when it comes to the color scheme and style of your marketing materials, which makes integrating the elements of the design that much easier.

Web Harmony

An effective Web design is enticing and functional, critical factors in maintaining the viewer's relatively short attention span, which is quickly diverted with the click of mouse. A visually appealing design can be simple, but it must be in harmony with the overall image of your spa and congruent with the look of your other marketing materials.

Although a good Web design can be created cost-effectively, this is definitely not a place to skimp. Unlike print ads and direct mail, the Web is available to millions of viewers who will base their opinion on the image you present online. If your marketing materials are not cohesive, you lose brand recognition. Pay attention to the colors, type, and images that are incorporated, and use icons and navigation tools to build brand recognition.

Basic Components of a Good Web Site

Organization is the key to a user-friendly Web site; before tackling yours, it is often helpful to browse other sites, particularly those in the spa industry. Note ones that you find exciting, well organized, and easy to navigate.

Web site architecture is a fancy name for the outline or structure of your Web site. As you develop an outline, think in terms of the most important and interesting information you want people to have about your spa business. If you do it yourself you will need to map out the number of pages, sections, and links you will include, but keep in mind that too many layers and links can become confusing.

The amount of information you include will determine the length and number of pages. This should be organized in a consistent and logical way that flows easily from one page to another without the need to backtrack through a confusing maze of links to get what you need. Each page should have an option to return to the home page. It is also important that your Web site does not take too long to download. Fancy multimedia flash technology may be on the cutting edge of Web design, but if it takes too long to download, visitors are likely to become frustrated. Be conscious of the number and size of the images, how many colors are contained in those images, and the length of the copy that you incorporate as well. Cramming too much information onto one page will extend download time.

For most, several Web pages that include a home page, an overall description of your spa philosophy and staff, services and products, special promotions, and a way to contact you for more information will suffice. If you have a newsletter, it is a good idea to include that as well. Many spas are now incorporating additional options to purchase gift certificates and products or book appointments online. These can be pluses if you are equipped to manage them. The same goes for social media components. Soliciting client feedback through the use of forums and surveys or pointing clients to your spa's blog can deepen your understanding of customer value, but it does take time.

Visual Organization

A Web site is a graphically-based program that relies heavily on visual organization (Figure 9-19). The navigation links on your Web site are critical to the overall design and should be consistent on each page. This is the list of categories that appears on the top or side of your screen, which directs users to the various Web pages. Navigation elements, such as icons, buttons, bars, borders, pop-up lists, typography, and color coding, help to maximize efficiency. Because the Web is an interactive media, the combination of categories and icons should be logical and user-friendly.

It is important to realize that what viewers see on their computer screen often varies depending on the size of the monitor and the browser (usually Internet Explorer or Netscape) they are using. This makes it difficult for Web designers to have complete control over the design. Designers work around this by sticking to a standard Web color palette and using fonts that are readily available on most computers, such as Times New Roman and Arial, and by limiting the length of text on each page to avoid excessive

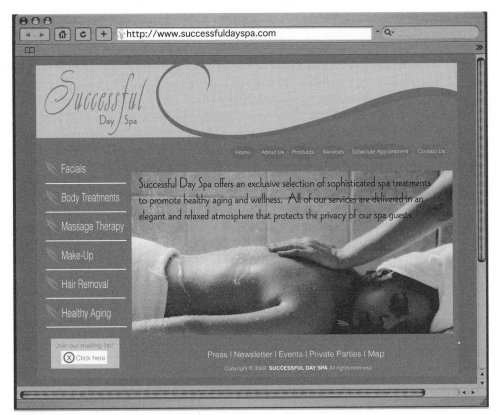

FIGURE 9-19 Visual organization is critical to a user-friendly Web site.

scrolling. A good designer will also take time to cross-reference the appearance of the design in various browsers and make adjustments to achieve a uniform look.

The home page is the first page the viewer sees and the link to all other Web pages. It is critical that it makes a good impression and does not take forever to download. If you would like to incorporate a visual tour of your spa or a musical introduction with flash media technology, give the viewer the option of skipping it.

Photos are an excellent visual tool. Use them to demonstrate the ambiance of your spa or the before and after results of specific treatments, but make sure they are relevant to your marketing purposes and can be displayed promptly. Photos are contained in various formats with differing download times. The use of smaller thumbnail images with an option to enlarge can help to decrease download time, but it is still a good idea to give viewers the option not to view images to avoid losing the impatient ones.

Web Text

The content of your Web site is vital to marketing your spa and should supply the basic information needed to take the next step to make an appointment. Don't forget to include your address, telephone number, hours of operation, and directions to your spa. Many small business owners think a Web site should duplicate their brochure or menu of services, but it is a mistake to simply paste your brochure on a Web site. The goal of a Web site is to entice viewers to take some action, so do not turn yours into what is known as *brochureware,* which amounts to using the same material that appears in a company's print brochure on a Web site.

It is okay to let people know what your spa offers, but the ultimate goal is to get viewers to take some immediate action. This can mean calling to make an appointment, purchasing a gift certificate, joining a membership club, or signing up to receive your newsletter or special promotions. Your Web site is an important communication tool that puts you directly in front of the consumer. Optimize that time by supplying additional information that will help consumers to make more informed decisions, such as a tutorial on chemical peels, answering frequently asked questions about a treatment, or how to make the most of their spa visit. This will help you to establish credibility and build consumer trust.

When soliciting a call to action, use simple terminology such as "Click here to get directions to the spa" or "Purchase a gift certificate" to make it easy for viewers to respond. It is also important to give potential customers a way to contact you for more information, but don't incorporate too many restrictions. Data entry forms that are user-friendly will help you to achieve your goal, which is to get viewers to identify themselves.

Publishing prices on the Web depends on how you are using your Web site. If you are using it to sell products and book appointments, it is important to let people know the cost of those items and services. You may choose to make your price list available "by request only," in which case it is a good idea to use a PDF format. To avoid confusion about any of the services or products your spa offers, let viewers know the last time your Web site was updated and place the date that prices are effective on your price list.

Using Your Web Site for E-Commerce

In Chapter 7, we noted that many spas are now using electronic booking and selling products and gift certificates online. Give serious thought to the main purpose of your Web site before traveling down this road. Do you want to conduct e-commerce or provide information? If you are interested in e-commerce, talk to your Web host provider and IT consultant regarding all of the mechanical and security requirements first.

Allowing spa guests to schedule their own appointments or purchase gift certificates online can be a marvelous hook, but if you are not ready to deal with the additional software programming or to set up a shopping cart, consider online purchase order forms that can be downloaded, mailed, or faxed in a PDF format, or use a dedicated toll-free number for Web purchases. If you use these methods, respond promptly, generally within 24 to 48 hours.

Improving the Visibility of Your Web Site

There are many ways to improve the visibility of your Web site. Look for opportunities to link your site to other Web sites that can help you, such as national and local directories or complementary business networks. Some links may involve fees, but it is often worth the cost to be linked to a major resource. Links increase your visibility, but you should keep in mind that they can frustrate the viewer if they are not relevant to your business or do not function properly. Before linking to another site ask yourself, how will this Web site complement my spa business?

Surveys and contests are another great way to attract visitors to your Web site on a regular basis, but again take extra precautions and seek qualified legal and technology advice before soliciting personal information for this purpose.

Search engines, such as Yahoo! and Google, are critical to helping prospective customers find your Web site. These search tools rely on key words to call up information about your business and should be located in the content of your Web site. This is one of the reasons it is so important to pay attention to copy. When developing your Web site, make a list of key words that define your spa business and test the validity of those words by conducting your own search on the Web beforehand. Your Web host provider and/or IT consultant can be a great resource in helping you to maximize your visibility and can assist you in using any analytical tools that might be available. You can also contract with companies that register and track your Web site listing on the different search engines.

For those who would like to learn more about marketing online and e-commerce, there are entire books devoted to the subject. As a spa owner, it is important for you to understand that developing a Web site is a lengthy project that requires excellent organizational skills. An attractive design is important, but do not become so consumed with design that you forget about the content. The information you provide on your Web site is a significant part of its success and should be updated regularly.

PROOFREADING TIPS

It is ultimately your message and your reputation; so don't be surprised when you are asked to review the content of all of your marketing materials. It is the agency or freelancer's job to provide you with well-written copy based on the information you provide about your business. It is your job to

PROOFREADING TIPS

- Use spell-check, but don't rely on it. Conduct your own spell-check. Many words have double meanings and should always be checked within the context.

- Focus on problematic grammar. Watch out for plurals, noun-verb agreement, and use of possessives.

- Check all punctuation and be on the lookout for periods, apostrophes, quotation marks, and commas.

- Review all headings. Cutting, clipping, and pasting text into layout can accidentally eliminate a heading or change the emphasis, such as bolding and italics.

- Note repeated letters, words, and paragraphs, which often go unnoticed.

- Hyphenated words are easily misspelled, and conjunctions and contractions are generally best spelled out.

- Aside from those listed in your price list, spell out numbers within the body of text, for example, "a series of six treatments."

- Avoid hyphenating words at the end of the sentence, whenever possible.

- Watch out for widows and orphans (those words left dangling at the top or bottom of a column or paragraph) and never leave one word on a line.

- Scrutinize your price list carefully, following line-by-line items with a ruler.

- Always double-check the accuracy of your business name, address, phone, fax, and Web address.

make sure that it is accurate. And as hard as everyone works to create the perfect piece, there is always room for human and/or technological error. As you proofread your marketing materials, review each piece: (1) once for content, (2) once for grammar and spelling, and (3) once for formatting issues (bold, paragraph alignment, etc.)

THINK IT OVER

Presentation is everything when it comes to marketing materials. Whether you are developing a brochure, ad, or Web site, your marketing collateral sends a strong message about your spa business. Materials should be well written, attractive, and professional. Think carefully about what you want to say and do not rush the creative process.

Initially, it is important to have all of the basics at your disposal, including a brochure, business card, price list, an effective ad, gift certificate and Web site, but don't stop there. Design beautiful stationary, send personal letters, offer membership cards, write newsletters, and create eye-catching postcard promotions that have people begging to be placed on your mailing list.

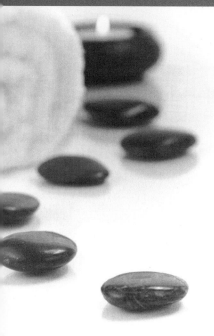

SALES AND SERVICE

SIXTEEN SIMPLE RULES FOR A SUCCESSFUL SALES AND CUSTOMER SERVICE PROGRAM

A good marketing program will get your phone to ring, but once the client walks through the door, the rest is up to you and your staff. The goal of marketing is to drive sales, but the best marketing plan in the world is ineffective without one important ingredient—*customers*.

Successful spa owners understand that every client is important and treat each client as if he or she is the most important one they have. They know that managing the customer relationship is the key to increasing sales and view customer service as an integral part of their overall marketing strategy and a genuine business skill, welcoming clients into their spa as honored guests. They know that when clients are honored, appreciated, and respected they develop trust, and when clients trust you, they believe and follow your recommendations. This is the core of every good sales and customer service program and one that all spa personnel must buy into to achieve success.

Making the Connection between Sales and Service

The spa business is a service business that thrives on providing clients with a pleasurable experience. This represents different things to different

RULE #1

Customers are the most valuable asset in any business.

SIXTEEN SIMPLE RULES FOR A SUCCESSFUL SALES AND CUSTOMER SERVICE PROGRAM

1. Customers are the most valuable asset in any business.

2. Selling products and treatments is a professional responsibility that adds value to the client's overall experience.

3. You must be confident in your role as a spa professional.

4. You can't sell something that you don't believe in.

5. Credibility is the key to having clients feel confident in your recommendations.

6. A strong interpersonal relationship with your clients will enhance sales.

7. Give your employees a strong incentive for meeting sales goals.

8. Attractive user-friendly retail displays invite clients to explore and buy.

9. A carefully mapped-out strategy for sales promotion will increase sales.

10. Enlist others to support you in your efforts.

11. Give clients what they want.

12. Earning the client's trust is critical in the spa business.

13. Listen, listen, listen!

14. Education is at the core of every successful client relationship and sales program.

15. If you want clients to remain loyal, you must be dedicated to giving them a superior level of quality care and excellent customer service time after time.

16. Long-term relationships require tender loving care.

people, but for the small spa business owner looking to increase profits in an extremely competitive environment, it means they must go beyond the client's expectations to create an experience that absolutely wows guests and leaves them wanting more.

Encouraging repeat business is a top priority for spa owners and involves two of the biggest challenges in the industry: (1) getting staff to sell and (2) maintaining a superior level of customer service. Recognizing that the two go hand in hand is the key to building a profitable spa business.

Selling in the Spa

There are generally two ways to increase revenue in the spa business: You can either increase the number of clients you serve or increase the amount you sell to the same number of clients. In the spa business, increasing revenue involves "selling" services and retail products. But the big question on every spa owner's mind is, "How do I get my staff to sell?"

We've heard it over and over again: spa service providers loathe selling. I would agree that the majority of service providers such as estheticians, massage therapists, and nail technicians did not choose a career in the personal care industry to become salespeople. However, that does not mean that the current influx of spa professionals are anti-sales. Spa professionals normally understand the value of repeat treatments and enthusiastically encourage clients to take advantage of series or book their next appointment before they leave the spa. They also know that retail products add value to the services they provide; in fact, some become licensed with the sole purpose of becoming better spa managers or product vendors.

Successful spa professionals understand that selling products and treatments is a professional responsibility that adds value to the client's overall experience. They know that a single treatment performed in isolation is not likely to generate significant change in the client's health and well-being. To enhance the benefit of the treatments they provide, they must empower clients with products that add real value to their services.

The problem is often that most spa therapists see their role as "healers" and do not make the connection between healing and selling products. This is compounded by the false belief that selling is somehow rooted in duplicity. Getting past this disconnect is usually the first step in getting your staff to sell. Encourage your staff by reinforcing that everyone sells—businesses, medical professionals, educational institutions, and organizations. When portrayed in a different light—educating, advising, and recommending, selling generally has an entirely different and positive connotation.

Confidence is Key

It seems as though some people are born with a sales gene or have a naturally personable disposition that makes it easy to get people to buy things from them. Others are eager to learn the skills needed to sell; however,

---

RULE #2

Selling products and treatments is a professional responsibility that adds value to the client's overall experience.

RULE #3

You must be confident in your role as a spa professional.

when it comes to sales, I often hear that many spa employees would prefer to get by with doing the bare minimum to meet their job requirement. In fact, some managers say you are simply wasting your time on staff with average sales techniques and no inclination to be more. That's going a bit too far when it comes to the spa business. In taking a closer look at "sales phobia" in the spa industry, I believe the real reason service providers do not like to sell has more to do with the fact that they feel ill-equipped to answer all of the many questions sales talk raises.

To sell products, you must be confident in your role as a spa professional. This means you must be knowledgeable and believe in the value of your expertise as well as the efficacy of the products you sell. In many instances, fear prevents service providers from selling: fear of their own inadequacy, fear that the product or service will somehow fall short of the client's expectations, or fear of being rejected. Your job as a spa owner or manager is to help your staff dispel those fears. The strategic value assessment in Chapter 3 can be useful in helping service providers to understand the value of the services they provide.

Another piece to the sales riddle is information overload. Many spas are now integrating multiple product lines and high-powered technology. With so many products, treatment protocols, sophisticated ingredients, and apparatus, limited knowledge and training are often at the core of a technician's feelings of inadequacy. If you find that your staff is overwhelmed by the sheer volume of products and services your spa provides and you cannot supply adequate training, you are doing your business a great disservice. It is best to limit the number of products and services that you provide until your staff is comfortable managing more, or hire professional retail sales personnel specifically for this purpose.

RETAIL SALES

It's no secret that retail sales increase a spa's revenue stream; however, to drive sales, all staff must understand that retail products are a significant part of the overall treatment plan. This involves recommending or selling retail products for home care (Figure 10-1).

The right retail products enhance the work you perform in the spa and increase your credibility as a professional; however, as we learned in Chapter 6, the key to running a successful retail program lies in selecting products that are in sync with your spa concept and your target market. Sales success also depends on your staff's endorsement of the retail products you promote.

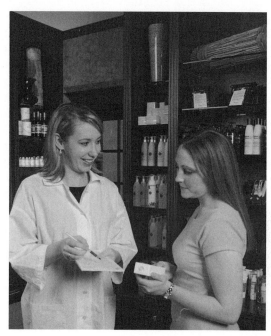

FIGURE 10-1 Recommending products to clients for home care is a professional responsibility in the spa business.

Passion

The key to selling retail products is passion. This requires the wholehearted and enthusiastic support of your staff. Their passion is what will drive sales. Because spa therapists are more apt to see themselves as healers, they need to feel that the products they sell provide a real value to their clients. If they would not use certain products themselves or recommend them to family and friends, spa therapists will do a mediocre job selling to clients. Adding to this dilemma, clients seem to have built-in radar that lets them know if your staff is genuinely convinced about a product's effectiveness or just trying to make a commission. If you cannot get your staff to feel passionate about the products they are being asked to recommend, don't expect them to sell them. It's as simple as that.

Connect Retail Products to your Spa's Services

Clients too have concerns about the usefulness of products. "Why do I need it?" they want to know. To sell retail products, it is important to attach significance to their value.

The retail products you sell in your spa should enhance the benefit of the treatments you provide. Sometimes this means remedying a certain skin condition. Other times, it means bringing the spa experience home with them. Your job is to train staff to recommend or suggest products that will enhance the treatment they have just provided. If it is a cleansing treatment for problem skin, then your staff should be recommending products that will keep the skin clean and blemish free. If it is a relaxing massage or body exfoliation, then it might be a moisturizing lotion or scrub. It could also be something that helps clients to create the spa experience at home, such as an aromatherapy candle, robe, slippers, or essential oils.

If your staff has trouble identifying products for home care, conduct workshops to educate them on the various products that are available for the different skin types and conditions. Supply charts and manuals that will aid them and create sales promotions that tie specialized products to treatments to reinforce the connection for clients.

Consider a Private Label Line

The products you promote should set you apart from the competition. If the market area is saturated with the brands you find appealing, consider adding a private label line. Quality private label products send a strong message to clients that you are selective about the merchandise you sell and can help to establish you as a noted authority in the field. Because the cost tends to be lower, they can also be an excellent source of revenue. To be successful selling your own brand name products, you must first determine what will motivate clients to buy your brand. Find out how loyal they are to their current products. Are they completely satisfied with the products they are using? Is there anything their current brand does not offer that they want? Would they welcome a lower-priced product that does not compromise quality?

The key to successfully selling your own brand is figuring out what is already selling well and what is missing from your shelves. Consider targeting certain skin conditions or selling products that fill a void, yet complement your other brands. Developing a specific item such as a signature body scrub, massage oil or body lotion that extends the spa experience can be a good way to get started and has the added value of enhancing your unique selling position (USP).

Whatever you put your name on, make sure the packaging is great and your advertising is superb. A lot of spa owners see private label products as a way to make more money but don't want to go to the trouble or the expense to market them in a way that will enhance their image. To get the best value from a private label line, you need to market it with a professional label that has your brand name on it and promote it as you would any other product on your shelf. Develop a sales dialogue. Let customers know why you have developed your own product line and how they will benefit from it.

Sell with Integrity

How many times a week do you hear media reports that caution buyers to beware? Whether it is a product, service, or unethical practice, we are exposed to negative consumerism every day. Sensationalized accounts of unscrupulous practices by physicians, police officers, and other professionals often leave us feeling vulnerable to those we trust most. Combined with reports that a previously benign substance or product ingredient is suddenly cause for alarm, such incidents naturally have consumers wary.

Because spa professionals provide personal care, they are particularly susceptible to backlash stemming from unethical behavior. One allegation of inappropriate conduct can lead to condemnation of the entire profession. And after years of consumers feeling duped by what they perceive as slick advertising tactics, spas that focus on improving appearances must also be prepared to substantiate every product and technique that claims to change the way clients look and feel about themselves.

You can hardly blame consumers for their skepticism, but you can be proactive in how you deal with the backlash. Credibility is the key to having clients feel confident in your recommendations. Before you can expect clients to buy anything from you, they must feel confident that you are invested in their well-being. Have you conducted a thorough analysis of their skin conditions and goals? Does the client need the products that are being recommended? Stick to the client's agenda. Can you actually put into words how they will benefit from using a product?

If you want clients to have faith in your recommendations, be honest and sell only those products you can stand behind. Manipulative tactics are inappropriate in the therapeutic relationship and will ultimately hurt your business. Clients want to know that the products you are promoting have been thoroughly researched and that they have been used by others with positive results. They also want to know that the selling techniques of your staff are genuine—that staff members recommend the product because it will benefit clients.

Because they know high-pressure sales tactics can backfire in a spa environment, some spa owners are now marketing their spas as "stress-free sanctuaries" and selling retail products with the same attitude. This type of sales program works in some spas. But whether you endorse a product by simply placing it on your shelf or go out of your way to advise and

RULE #5

Credibility is the key to having clients feel confident in your recommendations.

recommend, remember that in today's marketplace, truth sells. When a product or treatment is truly beneficial to clients, your staff will feel comfortable suggesting it, and clients purchasing it will feel cared for. This creates a win-win situation for both parties.

PERSONAL SELLING

Personal selling is where spa professionals have the advantage. Spa therapists are in the enviable position of being able to interact with clients on a one-to-one basis every day. This provides them with an excellent opportunity to find out directly from the client what she or he wants and expects from spa services. It is also an ideal situation for building a trusting partnership.

A strong interpersonal relationship sets the stage for a positive sales dialogue; however, in many cases, personnel lack the communication skills necessary for making the most of the situation. This is where your leadership and management skills are instrumental in creating the right sales climate.

Numerous power-selling books, audio and video tapes, and sales seminars are available to help you reinforce sales skills. Many offer specific dialogues for interfacing with customers. Researching several may help you to define your own strategy. The most important thing to remember is that they are all based on good communication skills.

Many of the important components of communication are referred to as *soft skills*. In reality, soft skills are the crux of good business communication and take into account tone of voice, rate of speech, vocabulary, the way we make eye contact, our facial expressions, hand gestures, and body language. Essentially, these things amount to *personal presentation,* a critical factor in how we come across to clients and how well we represent the products and services we are recommending. If your staff falls short of your desired expectations, remember that personal presentation skills can be learned.

Interpersonal Skills

In the spa business, excellent communication and interpersonal skills are based on several important characteristics: empathy, respect, authenticity, responsiveness, and appropriate boundaries. Empathy is the quality that allows you to simply be with a person and embrace his or her feelings. When we respect a person, we can show positive regard without passing judgment. This makes it easier to be empathic. Unfortunately,

RULE #6

A strong interpersonal relationship with your clients will enhance sales.

BASICS OF POSITIVE COMMUNICATION

Effective communication is based on strong interpersonal skills. These include six important character traits:

1. *Empathy:* the ability to truly be with the other person

2. *Respect:* the ability to show positive regard without passing judgment

3. *Authenticity:* the ability to be genuine and truthful

4. *Attentive listening:* the ability to stay focused and give the person your undivided attention

5. *Responsiveness:* the ability to deliver on your promise and follow through

6. *Appropriate boundaries:* the ability to provide information and services in a safe and productive way

in an effort to help, many make the mistake of overanalyzing clients' comments or body language or talking over them. It is important for spa therapists to be genuine and tell the truth, but they must also know when to back off.

Learn to respect clients' knowledge and to adjust your techniques to meet their needs. When engaging in conversation with clients, it is important to give them your undivided attention. Call each client by name and smile when you look at the person. You can sell products in an authoritative, exuberant, or low-key manner depending upon your style, but in business relationships, it is important to establish boundaries and follow through on any promise you make. A friendly approach is often your best approach, provided you are delivering information and services in a safe and productive way that does not invade a person's privacy or cause them to lose their dignity.

If you are trying to get clients to buy retail products, you must stay focused and talk to them. Although many spa owners are making an effort to support service providers in closing the sale by enlisting administrative personnel, this technique can actually backfire if it lacks a personal touch. An all-too-common experience I had tells the story best: After receiving several services at a day spa, I was given a "routing slip" and ushered to the front desk where the checkout person announced that several products had been recommended by the service provider who performed my treatment; however, at no point in time had the service provider actually mentioned or discussed any of the products with me.

If you use this type of approach, everyone on your staff must be enrolled in the program. Otherwise you can expect clients to feel, and rightfully so, that it is just another sales ploy.

Support Your Staff

One of the most important roles a spa owner or manager has is that of mentor. Even if your service providers understand that recommending products is a professional responsibility, it can take months for clients to buy into a program. When this happens, you must do everything possible to support your staff.

Read everything you can about selling in the spa and pass your knowledge along. Encourage continuing education. Hold discussion groups. Develop sales dialogues and role-play. Take a team approach, and ask others to share their successes to help find solutions. Bring staff together for a fun day of training and testing products and treatments out on each other. Supply lunch, dinner, or refreshments and give them all trial sizes for their own use. Invite motivational speakers and sales gurus to the spa. Attend seminars with your staff. Visit other spas and share information.

Most importantly, be aware of the specific problems your employees are having and set time aside to coach them. If they are struggling with recommending products, work with them to develop nonthreatening dialogues until they become natural. You also need to be willing to go back to the drawing board and work on your business. Is there something about your sales program or philosophy that needs adjusting? Take a critical look at your methods. Are you managing your end of the program by developing sales promotions and providing adequate training? Do you supply samples and encourage staff to introduce them in a way that is relevant to the client's needs? Remember that good sales managers are good problem-solvers.

Set Goals

Taking a thoughtful and ethical approach to sales does not mean you should limit your expectations. If your sales program is based on integrity and your compensation methods are equitable, it is perfectly reasonable to set goals that will stimulate growth. However, when dealing with employees who for the most part see themselves as healers, this can be a delicate subject. To avoid any misunderstanding, it is best to make your expectations clear at the onset of the employee relationship. We'll talk more about managing employee relations in Chapter 11; here it is enough to recognize that setting goals is a necessary part of any sales program.

To meet sales goals, some day spa owners are now enlisting administrative or additional retail sales personnel to boost or "close the sale." Team selling has its place in today's spa environment, but it also raises several issues, such as who gets the commission, if there is one, or should it be divided? If you are marketing your spa as a place of healing, how does this approach affect the therapeutic relationship?

These questions are currently under a great deal of scrutiny in the spa industry; however, similar to the way nurses support physicians, when product recommendations are based on genuine caring and concern for meeting the client's needs, qualified reinforcement by another staff member can actually encourage clients to make purchases that will benefit both them and you. It is your job to see that all staff members support your sales philosophy and are trained to work as a team.

Incentive Programs

Some people seem to be intrinsically self-motivated; but, most people require some sort of reward to get them to meet their obligations. When it comes to increasing retail revenues in the spa, giving your employees a strong incentive for meeting sales goals can mean everything in terms of achieving your financial objectives. However, any incentive program also needs to make good business sense (see Table 10-1).

Historically, retail sales compensation has been based on a commission structure, or some percentage of the actual sale, typically 10 to 15 percent on retail products in the spa industry. Today many spas are using different methods of compensation to address new sales models, such as team selling. As you figure out the best way to reward employees for their efforts, keep in mind that the amount of compensation should not jeopardize the profitability of your business.

The key to making any rewards program work is to make it a positive situation for both the employee and the spa owner. Money is a strong motivator, but it is not the only motivator. Find out exactly what inspires your staff and build it into the program. Is it time off, a trip to a destination spa, paid education, or a monetary bonus at the end of the week, month, or year?

> ### RULE #7
>
> Give your employees a strong incentive for meeting sales goals.

TABLE 10-1	DOS AND DON'TS OF A STRONG INCENTIVE PROGRAM
Do:	**Don't:**
• Explain your retail sales policy thoroughly at the onset of the relationship.	• Use manipulative or unethical practices to drive sales.
• Learn what motivates your staff.	• Use tactics that force employees to be competitive with one another.
• Keep egos in check.	• Praise one employee at the expense of another.
• Offer positive feedback and encouragement.	• Use the front desk to "close the sale."
• Hold your staff accountable for productivity.	• Threaten employees or coerce them into doing things that make them feel uncomfortable.
• Establish goals.	• Renege on your promise.
• Give employees the tools they need to be productive.	• Focus on what isn't working.
• Frame criticism constructively.	• Use straight commission compensation methods.
• Establish fair and equitable rewards.	• Withhold critical information from employees.
• Create an atmosphere where employees feel supported by one another.	• Put front desk personnel in direct competition with service providers.
• Offer positive encouragement.	• Expect employees to be intrinsically motivated.
• Ask everyone to share their positive experiences.	• Don't let disagreements among employees fester.
• Encourage staff to up-sell.	• Use a monetary reward as a quick resolution.

Innovative rewards programs, based on team selling or profit sharing, can benefit everyone. These methods encourage employees to rely on and support each other to be successful. They also require a fair method for measuring productivity. Be prepared to share sales information with employees. In the end, this information is likely to generate a more cohesive business unit.

Manage Money Anxiety

A strong incentive program and all the sales training in the world may not prepare your staff for "money anxiety." Getting clients to purchase products after they have spent a sizable amount on services can be difficult, and it is perfectly normal for staff to feel uncomfortable if a client expresses concern over the cost of products.

When faced with price objections, it is generally a good idea to make recommendations and let clients decide how much they can afford to spend. If clients seem overly concerned about pricing, it is important to listen to their concerns and help them make choices that are within their budgets, but don't defend your prices. If your prices are geared toward your target market and you are offering a fair value for the products and services you are selling, you should be comfortable with your pricing.

Up-Selling

You can use all of the techniques discussed here and in Chapters 8 and 9 to increase your clientele, but increasing the amount you sell to the same number of clients can still be a challenge. *Up-selling* is the term used to increase the size of each sale and one to which most of us can relate. Think about the last time you bought a cup of coffee. Chances are you were asked if you wanted a doughnut or muffin to go along with it. Up-selling is a common practice used by a variety of businesses. It typically includes offering the customer a number of extras, accessories, or a more expensive item that has some greater value. This is different from and should not be confused with "bait-and-switch" methods.

There are many ways to up-sell in the spa business. You can suggest an additional service that complements one in which the client is already interested, offer a higher quality product, or sell additional supplies, such as spatulas and sponges to be used with products. You can sell a series rather than a single treatment or take a lesson from retail stores and include a free gift with the purchase of a greater dollar amount.

How successful you are depends on two things: (1) your staff's ability to overcome any money anxiety issues they have and (2) your ability to provide a definite benefit to the client. From a management perspective, it is most important to assign a value that is clearly relevant and easy for employees to sell. For example, adding an enzyme to a basic facial automatically increases the effectiveness of the facial and typically costs less as an add-on. You will need to decide the best way to up-sell services in your spa, but initially it helps to write a script and demonstrate how to do it.

MERCHANDISING

Take a trip to the nearest mall. What do you see? Hundreds and hundreds of retail merchandise displays designed to entice and cajole the consumer into buying. You can learn a lot at the mall. The next time you go, take a notepad and study boutique and department stores that sell personal care products. As you browse the aisles, take note of their merchandising techniques. Are some more effective than others; if so, why?

Establish a Selling Environment

Merchandising, or how retail products are arranged and displayed on your spa shelves, sets the stage for a positive selling environment. Once again, presentation is everything.

Merchandising should be fun and visually appealing. If you have the luxury of a fantastic window space, begin there and pull clients in with interesting displays that showcase the retail products you have for sale in your spa, tying in any monthly or seasonal promotions that are currently available. Dramatic posters, dynamic words and phrases, and artistically arranged props will help you to accomplish this goal.

Once clients are inside your spa, encourage them to buy with attractive showcases, powerful before-and-after photos, and testers that give them

MALL MERCHANDISING TECHNIQUES

A trip to the mall offers a valuable lesson in merchandising. List five techniques used by retail stores in the personal care industry to attract customers. On a scale of 1 to 10 how would you rate their effectiveness? How could you use or adjust these techniques to your spa?

1. *For example, free samples, video demonstrations, etc.*   1 2 3 4 5 6 7 8 9 10

2. _____   1 2 3 4 5 6 7 8 9 10

3. _____   1 2 3 4 5 6 7 8 9 10

4. _____   1 2 3 4 5 6 7 8 9 10

5. _____   1 2 3 4 5 6 7 8 9 10

a chance to "play" with products. Selling spa retail products is a sensory experience. Clients must be able to see, touch, feel, and smell the products before they buy.

A carefully planned retail boutique that allows clients to browse and sample is the epicenter of your spa's merchandising plan. Create an enticing shopping environment by incorporating fresh flowers, scented candles, testers, and attractive product displays. Provide comfortable seating, refreshments, and reading material that invite clients to linger. Success lies in the details. But don't stop merchandising in the boutique; posters, samples, and literature strategically placed in treatment rooms, hallways, sitting areas, and restrooms extend the retail experience and are great conversation starters.

For selling to occur, you must also proactively merchandise. Introduce clients to your products by incorporating them in treatments, offering samples, and inviting them to have a mini treatment. A dedicated customer service ambassador can be instrumental in increasing sales. Consider hiring a licensed service provider with excellent sales skills for this purpose.

RULE #8

Attractive user-friendly retail displays invite clients to explore and buy.

Retail Displays

Attractive retail displays with a plentiful selection of products help promote sales (Figure 10-2). Displays should be neat, clean, and organized. Each item on your retail shelf must be justified. Does it enhance the value of your treatments and services or extend the spa experience? Retail products should be coordinated with treatments and complement the services you provide; however, there is always room for creativity. Be open to expanding your retail center with additional items your clientele might appreciate, such as handcrafted jewelry, paintings, or sculptures from local artists.

Organization

Carefully arranged retail shelves make it easier for clients to identify the products they are seeking. Use systems that make sense, such as grouping products according to skin type or condition, gender, or body parts—for example, *Dry Skin, Men's, Face,* and *Body*—and identify these with signs.

Shelf-talkers, or placards that explain the product and its use, are great sales tools and are ideal for clients who would rather browse than interact with a salesperson. When it comes to silent selling it is important to mark the price of products clearly, either on the bottom of the item or on the display. This works well for those who might be shy about asking

to promote business during that time frame. Start by examining those particular services or treatments that could use a boost and then work your daily menu of services. For example, you might add a specialty eye or advanced skin care treatment to a popular facial. On the other hand you might consider offering a service with a high-profit margin that is in great demand on weekends at a special rate during that time or other slow periods. To a certain extent this is a form of yield management, a technique that is commonly used in the airline and hotel industries to maximize revenues.

Next, consider what you can do to promote sales on a monthly basis. Are there any holiday or vendor promotions that you can plug into? Sit down and plan your calendar for the entire year beginning in January, and don't wait until the last minute to implement it. Planning and organization are critical to successful sales promotions. Creating an offer, ordering products, designing materials, purchasing paper, distributing e-mail messages, meeting ad deadlines, and mailing postcards does not happen overnight. It is critical for all promotions to be in customers' hands within a reasonable time for them to act on the offer.

Seasonal or quarterly promotions are excellent supplements to the monthly sales program and are easily coordinated with other strategies. Think in terms of winter, spring, summer, and fall treatments that add value to your monthly and weekly promotions. For example, during the summer months, you could offer a special incentive on healthy alternatives to tanning, such as spray-on tanning treatments or wax hair removal. At the same time, your monthly promotions could focus on products that help to maintain the effects of these treatments, such as body moisturizing lotions and sun protection products. A quarterly newsletter is ideal for promoting seasonal specials and can be extremely cost-effective when delivered electronically or posted on your Web site.

Don't forget to schedule a time to implement automatic sales generators, such as thank-you, reminder, referral, and birthday cards and series savings "credit cards" or membership programs. Designating a certain day of the week or month and a person responsible for accomplishing this task generally works best. In addition, teaching your staff to up-sell series and combination packages will help to encourage repeat business and generate interest in standard spa fare.

When developing any sales promotion, remember that customers need to have a real incentive to act on the offer, which means that your offer has to be a good one! The trick to profitable sales promotions is to understand what it is that your customers want—added value or a cash discount? Sometimes it can be a combination of the two. Table 10-2 will help you to get started.

Plan for Success

Yield management is a revenue management strategy specifically designed to optimize profits. This is accomplished by making highly desired services available at times that may not be in demand in a way that makes them more attractive; and alternately increasing prices on services that are in high demand at peak times. This technique is commonly used in the airline and hotel industries where the practice of yield management has become an effective revenue management tool.

The practice of yield management in the spa industry is just beginning to be explored, however, spa owners should not confuse it with discounting where you are lowering the price to make the sale more appealing. The primary purpose of a yield management program is to maximize revenue. Some of the ways in which spas are using this strategy include engaging third party providers to sell services online; limiting access to online appointments; adding value to popular services at an off peak time, such as a weekday morning, targeting a specific segment of spa-goers that are in a position to take advantage of

(continued)

Plan for Success (continued)

the offer; and alternately increasing prices on services that are in high demand at peak times, for example during peak weekend hours. Those interested in pursuing this practice are cautioned to study this technique carefully, which in some ways is viewed as price discrimination, a practice that can have adverse reactions if your clients and service providers do not recognize its value.

Sales promotions can be enhanced by tying them into your public relations program or a charitable drive, such as donating a certain percentage of profits to a worthy cause. Look at those causes you feel passionate about at the beginning of each calendar year and decide how you can make them relevant to your promotions. Two months that are easy for spas to tie into are October, which is breast cancer awareness month, a cause relevant to every female spa-goer, and May, which is skin health awareness month. Focusing on these issues can be a great way to generate free publicity as well.

SEEK SUPPORT FROM VENDORS AND OTHER MERCHANTS

If you are not getting the attention you deserve from your suppliers, ask for it. In fact, you should insist on it. The relationship with your vendor should be a reciprocal one that benefits both parties.

TABLE 10-2	IDEAS FOR WEEKLY, MONTHLY, AND QUARTERLY SALES PROMOTIONS

Weekly

1. Bring a friend in for a combination manicure/pedicure treatment on Tuesday mornings and receive a special rate or a free product, such as a polish, foot soak, or scrub. Throw in an extra value, such as a complimentary continental breakfast to make the offer more appealing.

2. Book a month's worth of weekly manicures and save a certain percentage off the regular price. Give clients incentive to book these services during slower periods by adding value to specific times and days of the week when you are not as busy.

3. Add a complimentary steam, hydrotherapy, or some other added-value service to all couples massage therapies on Monday night only. Include a gift package with a massage oil, loofah, and bath oil to extend the spa experience at home.

4. Select a slow day for a special bonus, such as a complimentary eyebrow shaping with each facial on Wednesdays. Such offers can be limited to day or evening appointments only if you would like to increase business during certain time slots.

TABLE 10-2	IDEAS FOR WEEKLY, MONTHLY, AND QUARTERLY SALES PROMOTIONS (CONTINUED)

Monthly

1. Take advantage of holidays such as Christmas, Valentine's Day, and Mother's Day to develop special spa gift packages. Be sure to include a broad enough selection to accommodate every budget.

2. Give something away to the first 10 or 100 customers who book an appointment in January of each year. There are lots of things you can give away. The trick is to choose a product or service you wish to promote or one closely tied to your USP, such as a free jar of your signature scrub. The value of the item or discount should be something you can afford to give away.

3. Give each client a free lipstick with the purchase of any makeup lesson during the month of October when make-up is on everyone's mind due to the Halloween holiday, or during any month when clients would be looking to change their seasonal makeup palette.

4. Make March men's month and promote facials and massages geared toward your male clients. Use August to focus on teens, addressing issues such as acne or skin blemishes that will affect them when going back to school.

5. Use vendor-driven promotions to add value. When vendors offer special pricing, encourage clients to buy more. For example, if they buy one of any ABC brand product, they'll receive the second one at half price.

Quarterly

The seasons are ideal for promoting higher-priced spa items or packages. Use them to target certain skin conditions that are relevant to the season and promote treatment series or bundle services rather than individual treatments.

1. *Winter:* Promote a series of exfoliating face or body treatments that are best performed when it is easier for clients to stay out of the sun. Spa packages that combine hydrating facial and body services are an ideal remedy for winter dry skin conditions. They are also a nice complement to exfoliating treatments.

2. *Spring*: Offer a series of renewal treatments or a long term hair removal program in preparation for the skin-baring summer months. As an added bonus, consider extending a series package through summer.

3. *Summer:* Promote summer skin protection products throughout the summer months or a series of sunless tanning treatments. Manicure and pedicures will be popular at this time; so don't discount them. Instead, promote products that will enhance the benefit, such as polishes, foot lotions, and scrubs between services, or include them in larger spa packages.

4. *Fall:* During this time of new regimens, such as going back to school or starting a new job, promote a new image by cross-merchandising with an image consultant and targeting makeup products. Fall is also a great time to promote treatments and products to remedy the effects of sun damage or to target school age clients battling acne skin conditions.

RULE #10

Enlist others to support you in your efforts.

In addition to product training and education, vendors should do everything possible to help you market and promote the products and equipment they distribute to you. When it comes to sales and service, that includes cooperative advertising, scheduled promotions, and supportive marketing materials, such as direct mail postcards, newsletters, sales letters, informational pamphlets, and product displays. They should also be available to offer technical support, merchandising expertise, and sales training.

If vendors are doing their job, they will make it a point to position their products in a way that appeals to your target market and helps you to reach clients. Vendors should also do the best they can to develop a solid public relations program and generate additional publicity. Take advantage of any public recognition your vendors receive by showcasing articles, celebrity endorsements, and positive media attention. Fortunately, in today's competitive sales environment, we are witnessing an increase in this type of vendor support.

Cross-Merchandise

Cross-merchandising with other businesses, such as health and fitness clubs, chiropractors, physicians, hair salons, bridal shops, photographers, restaurants, hotels, and inns, is another great way to encourage new business. Look for businesses that offer complementary services, but don't rule out a business just because it does not fit a certain criteria. If you cannot come up with a mutually gratifying "product" that appeals to the clientele of both businesses, consider sharing databases, trading services, setting up a rewards program, or offering your spa services as a perk.

RULE #11

Give clients what they want.

SATISFY CLIENT DESIRES

You've heard it over and over again, but one point cannot be emphasized enough: You must give your clients what they want.

Traditionally, spas have targeted women; however, that is changing. Today, spa owners are looking for ways to increase their profits. One of the ways spas are doing that is to fulfill the unmet needs of certain segments of the population, such as men and teens who are becoming more interested in spa services. Let's take a look at how spas can build an effective sales and customer service program that satisfies the needs and wants of these three spa market segments: women, men, and teens.

Selling to Women

It's no secret that women constitute the majority of all spa-goers. But are we really tuned in to their needs? As a spa owner, it is important to avoid complacency when it comes to women.

We spent a good deal of time reviewing the demographics of women in today's marketplace in Chapter 2. Some of the more important things we learned are that women are better educated and account for a greater number in the workforce than any other generation of women in history. They also have greater spending power and are juggling far more responsibilities than ever before. Giving them what they want before they ask for it will help you to win their loyalty.

If you already have a clientele, take a good look at the demographics of the women who come to your spa. Are there any correlations between the statistics highlighted in Chapter 2 and your spa clients? What age group do they represent? Are they mostly single or married? Working moms? If so, do you know how many children they have, and what percentage of those children are preschool age? Do they own their homes or rent? What is their average income?

All of this information will help you to target your sales and service plan to meet the specific needs of the women who come to your spa. For example, if you find that the majority of your clients are women between the ages of 30 and 40 with young children who are juggling the demands of a career with motherhood, you might want to offer an express facial or a mini massage or bundle certain packages and promotions at times when they are more apt to be able to arrange child care. If your clientele includes a number of stay-at-home moms, then you might want to implement value added packages or promotions when their children are in school.

If you are just opening a spa, study the demographics of the area and take time to understand the culture. Is there a certain segment of the female population that you wish to target? Whatever the specific demographics of your target female spa population, you will want to know what they value and adjust your marketing techniques accordingly. The following are some general tips that will help you to sell to women:

- Women value relationships, especially long-term relationships.
- Women want to be listened to and know that they have really been heard.
- Women want answers to their questions.
- Women like detailed information about the product, service, or company with which they are doing business.
- Women want to have their concerns taken seriously.

- Women enjoy camaraderie and like being part of a team.
- Women like to process things.
- Women believe in education.
- Women want their time to be respected.
- Trust is a big factor in developing relationships with women.
- Women value a personal referral from a trusted source.

TARGETING THE FEMALE SPA-GOER

Name five ways you can adjust your sales and customer service program to better meet the needs of women.

1. _____
2. _____
3. _____
4. _____
5. _____

Selling to Men

The number of spas catering to men only is increasing, as is the number of spas looking to attract men to enhance their profits. But before you attempt to jump on this marketing bandwagon, be sure you have a thorough understanding of what men want in a spa. For men to feel confident in your spa services, you will need to be well versed on male skin conditions and the best products for treating them. You will also need to know exactly what type of services appeal to them and the best way to introduce them. If this information was not addressed thoroughly in your training, read as much as you can on the topic and seek continuing education from other sources, such as advanced or secondary education programs and vendors to increase your knowledge.

Those day spas devoted exclusively to a male clientele will want to create an environment that makes men feel comfortable. Your décor will set the tone. Keep it clean, simple, and uncluttered. Use masculine colors and incorporate artifacts that appeal to men. Take a masculine approach in your brochure as well, describing the benefits and features of services succinctly and in masculine terms. But don't go overboard; stereotypical terminology could be misconstrued as offensive. Do avoid flowery language and overly technical descriptions. Men have hand-and-foot treatments, not manicures and pedicures.

If your spa is female-oriented but you are looking to attract a male clientele, designate a separate area for men only that will appeal to them. Follow the decorating guidelines stated in Chapter 5 and be sure to incorporate visuals that reinforce the efficacy of spa treatments for men, such as posters of men having facials and massage treatments, and provide literature that addresses male concerns. Stock personal care items that men require, such as razors and shaving cream, and be sure your robes and slippers will fit them. Designate a section of your menu or brochure exclusively to men. Simply renaming treatments that were originally designed for your female clientele won't do. Address skin care issues that are of specific concern to men. Making men feel welcome is all in the details.

You will also want to follow through with the same ideology that was applied to understanding the female market. If you intend to target a specific population, such as male executives between the ages of 40 to 60, you should investigate the needs and lifestyle of that particular market segment. What are their primary reasons for seeking spa services? Are they concerned with appearances or looking for ways to combat the signs of aging? Do they want to manage certain skin conditions, relax, or de-stress? What is the average income level? How much leisure time do they have? When is the optimal time for them to enjoy spa treatments? The following are some general tips that will help you to sell to men:

- Men appreciate straightforward, concise information.

- Men respect authoritative advice.

- Men like simplicity and efficiency.

- Men want to have products and services that are easily accessible.

- Men are loyal to product brands.

- Men prefer a friendly sales approach.

- Men value discretion and like to have their privacy respected.

- Men prefer a masculine approach to their personal care needs.

- Men are not necessarily concerned about the cost of products and services.

TARGETING THE MALE SPA-GOER

Name five ways you can adjust your sales and customer service program to better meet the needs of men.

1. _____

2. _____

3. _____

4. _____

5. _____

Selling to Teens

Teens are quickly becoming one of the fastest growing segments of the spa population, but not every spa is equipped or designed to handle teens. If you decide to target teenagers, it pays to have a good understanding of their habits and psychosocial needs.

Media-driven and brand-savvy, today's teens are sophisticated. They are also self-conscious and heavily influenced by their peers. This makes them interested in products and services that will enhance their appearance (Figure 10-3). All of us were teens at some point and can relate to many of the issues they have; however, times do change; so it is important to study this complex population.

Look at the magazines teens are reading, the television programs they watch, and talk to them, but don't expect them to be completely forthcoming. It takes time for teenagers to build trust. Study the fashion trends, makeup, hair styling, and skin care products that are showcased in teen magazines. Can you pinpoint what is popular with them in terms of spa services? Look to those that cater specifically to teens for more input. What's on their menu: spa parties; makeup, manicures and pedicures, waxing services; hair styling; tattooing? Some spas now target the preteen set with spa "teas" and birthday parties that include dress-up, manicures and makeup fantasies. Other popular services include makeup lessons, skin care classes, and mini-facials. There are many creative ways to pull in teens. Host a spa day for mothers and daughters, best friends, teammates, or sisters or sponsor a complete day of beauty education.

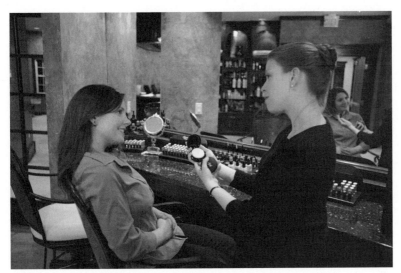

FIGURE 10-3 Teens like to keep up with the latest makeup trends.

Knowing what teens value is important, but before you put out the welcome mat, it is wise to understand how they behave in social situations. Teens can express themselves rather loudly, especially when they travel in groups. This can be disruptive to other spa guests. If you have the space and are intent on marketing to them, you might consider segregating a special area for teens. If this is not possible, consider setting one night of the month or certain days and times aside.

There is a tremendous opportunity for cross-referrals from allied health professionals in the teen market; however, a word of caution is in order here: Teens can be vulnerable, and issues may come up that you are not qualified to address. Getting into self-esteem or weight control matters can be dangerous territory. If you find yourself confronted with something you are not qualified to handle, always defer to expert advice. Team up with high school guidance counselors for more input, and invite guest speakers, such as nutrition counselors and exercise or yoga instructors, to promote self-care.

If you decide to host teen seminars or workshops in your spa, discuss liability issues with your attorney first. Providing services such as massage therapy or tattooing can be tricky. In fact, many spas have age restrictions when it comes to certain services, such as massage therapy, for teens; some age restrictions may be mandated by state and local laws. Keep the focus on making your spa a safe place for teens to bring their health and beauty concerns and safeguard your business interests by developing a policy that includes parental consent for any service you feel may be considered controversial for those underage.

The following are some general tips that will help you to sell to teens:

- Teens enjoy multitasking. Watching a video while talking on the phone or "texting" and "instant messaging" their friends is just their thing.

- Teens have special skin care concerns.

- Teens are vulnerable and complex.

- Teens want to be cared for and listened to.

- Teens look for guidance but like to maintain a sense of independence.

- Teens are heavily influenced by their peer group.

- Teens are comfortable using the Internet.

- Teens like to keep up with the latest trends and fads.

- Teens are self-conscious about their appearance.

- Teens tend to have a limited but disposable income.

- Teens lead busy lives.

- Teens may not always get enough sleep.

- Teens may not always adhere to home care programs.

TARGETING THE TEENAGE SPA-GOER

Name five ways you can adjust your sales and customer service program to better meet the needs of teens.

1. _____

2. _____

3. _____

4. _____

5. _____

BUILDING POSITIVE CLIENT RELATIONS

Giving clients what they want is an important part of establishing an economically viable business. But in the spa industry, you must do more than that—you must build positive trusting relationships with your clients.

Trust is the basis of all positive relationships and a critical factor in the spa business where service providers are intimately involved with clients. How do you get clients to trust you? In the spa business, you earn it with credibility, commitment, connection, caring, confidence, communication, and courtesy (Figure 10-4).

The elements of trust are scattered throughout this chapter and depend on your ability to: (1) establish *credibility* or sell with integrity; (2) demonstrate an ongoing *commitment* to helping clients resolve their problems; (3) establish a *connection* or bond with the client; (4) show genuine *caring*,

RULE #12

Earning the client's trust is critical in the spa business.

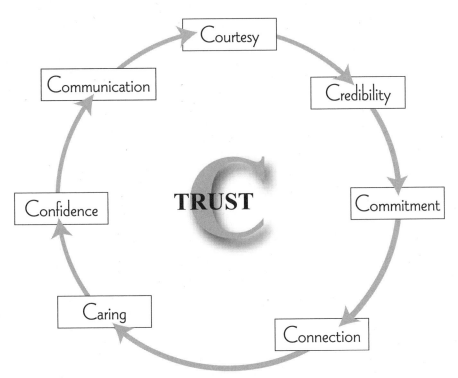

FIGURE 10-4 Trust begins with a capital C in the spa business.

empathy, and compassion for the client's goals and objectives; (5) convey *confidence* in your skills and the product and equipment that you use to conduct business; (6) develop good *communication* skills; and (7) treat each and every client with *courtesy,* dignity, and respect.

A client's trust is not earned overnight. Trust is built by doing many little things over the course of time, and it is your job as a spa owner to develop professional standards that encourage them. One of the most important factors in establishing trust occurs the moment the client steps into your spa. How clients are greeted sets the tone for the entire relationship. A warm welcome or a simple gesture, such as a smile or nod, if the front desk person is checking another client in, lets clients know you appreciate and value their business at the onset of the relationship.

Another extremely important consideration in developing trust involves your ability to handle sensitive issues, such as modesty and confidentiality. Many spa services require the client to be unclothed. This places the client in a vulnerable position. Training your staff to properly drape clients and respect their right to privacy allows clients to feel safe and maintain their dignity. Clients also need the reassurance that comes from knowing that all the personal information you collect about them will be kept confidential.

Uncovering the Client's Concerns

The initial consultation or intake interview lays the groundwork for building a mutually satisfying and trusting relationship with your client. Learn to take full advantage of it. Many service providers make the mistake of simply asking the client to fill in the blanks and never even bother to look at it. Others review the information and spend most of the consultation time offering advice. The goal of any intake form is to gather information and present the client with treatment options. However, at the beginning of any therapeutic relationship, it is more important to listen than talk.

The intake interview is the perfect opportunity to practice attentive listening and hone your interpersonal skills (Figure 10-5). Tune into the client's concerns. Why did they come, what would they like to change about their appearance or lifestyle, what services are they interested in, what expectations do they have, and are those expectations realistic? The initial intake should give you some indication of the client's lifestyle, overall health, products they use, skin care regime, and personality. Learning the best way to communicate with them will help you in your approach. Do they work best with a prescription format, reading material, or graphic presentation?

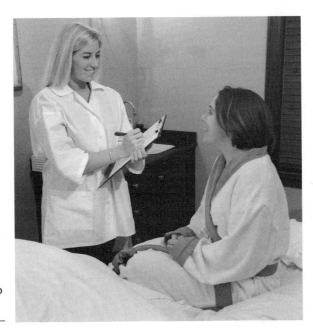

FIGURE 10-5 Tune into the client's concerns.

Listen to what clients want and take time to answer any questions they may have. Summarize their goals to make sure you have interpreted them correctly, and every time clients come in refer to your notes. Establishing and addressing the client's concerns requires an ongoing dialogue and the ability to make changes when necessary. Don't be afraid to ask them what they like and don't like and what is working and what is not. When you are truly present and clients feel they have been heard, they feel special and cared for—and they come back!

RULE #13

Listen, listen, listen!

Educating Clients

Information is a powerful sales tool that is often overlooked. Don't forget that clients come to you for professional guidance and expect you to educate them about the best products and treatments for their needs.

Before recommending any product or treatment to clients make sure you can answer any questions they may have about it. Too often, well-intentioned service providers endorse products but are unable to identify the active ingredients or explain the theory behind the technology. It is important that you demonstrate a solid understanding of the products and treatments you recommend and can explain these in simple terms the client can understand.

Clients are more knowledgeable today than ever, but they are not spa professionals. Guide them in a way that respects their intelligence and include them in the process. Education is at the core of every successful client relationship, but it must be a working partnership. Tune into the client's concerns and develop a plan together. Use the intake questionnaire as a guide and let clients know what their options are based on your spa offerings and their goals. Referrals to outside service providers are appropriate only if your spa does not offer the service.

Timing is everything, so it is important to educate clients at a time when you have their full attention. This is usually during the consultation when you are discussing treatments and after a service when you are recommending retail products for home care. Neither should take too much time. Streamline information so clients do not become overwhelmed. A written treatment plan is ideal and helpful in summarizing everything you have discussed (Figure 10-6). It should include a schedule for follow-up visits and recommended products for home care along with written instructions on when and how to use the products. The goal is to give them something tangible to refer to at home. A bookmark that takes on a prescriptive format is a great way to present a treatment plan and also serves as a constant reminder of your spa business. Be sure to include your telephone number and let clients know when you are available to answer any questions.

Clients need motivation and reassurance, but they should not be coerced into purchasing anything they do not want or need. Aggressive, pushy tactics will only alienate the client; so put the quota aside and train staff to offer samples if the client is not ready to buy everything suggested to them. Perhaps you will sell a cleanser or corrective treatment first and gradually introduce the entire product line. Learn to gauge the client's interest, and don't dictate a completely new program unless you are convinced the client is ready for it. Some clients are completely dedicated to a particular product line and may never be interested in purchasing retail products from you; so don't jeopardize valuable service dollars over a jar of cleanser.

You can do many other things to let clients know you are invested in education. Conduct workshops, classes, or seminars; and invite guest speakers. Write a newsletter, provide literature from manufacturers, or develop your own fact sheets and charts to explain procedures if none are available. When you demonstrate educational leadership, clients know you have their best interests at heart, and you have a much better chance at earning their trust.

RULE #14

Education is at the core of every successful client relationship and sales program.

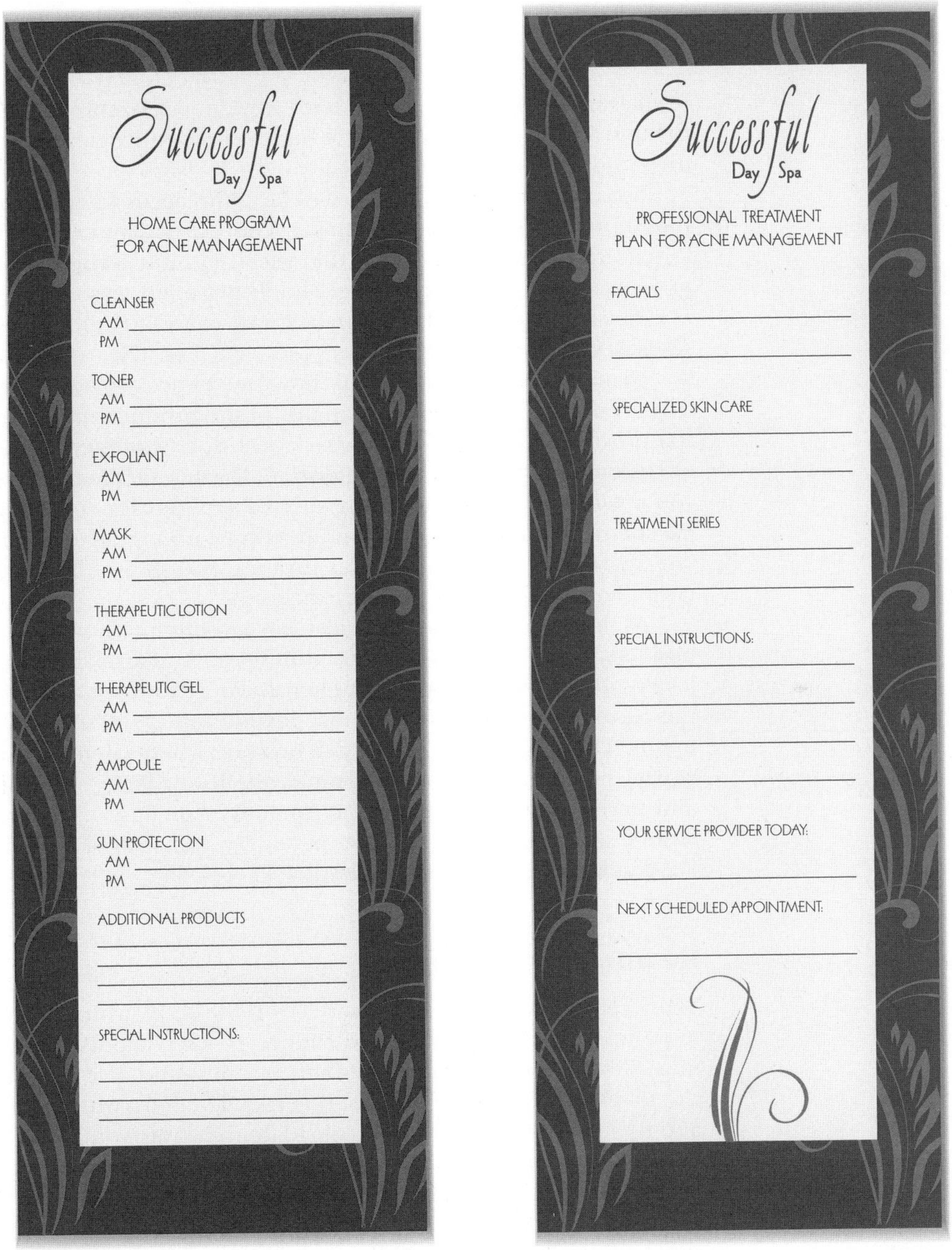

Successful
Day Spa

HOME CARE PROGRAM
FOR ACNE MANAGEMENT

CLEANSER
AM _____
PM _____

TONER
AM _____
PM _____

EXFOLIANT
AM _____
PM _____

MASK
AM _____
PM _____

THERAPEUTIC LOTION
AM _____
PM _____

THERAPEUTIC GEL
AM _____
PM _____

AMPOULE
AM _____
PM _____

SUN PROTECTION
AM _____
PM _____

ADDITIONAL PRODUCTS
_____
_____
_____
_____

SPECIAL INSTRUCTIONS:
_____
_____
_____
_____

Successful
Day Spa

PROFESSIONAL TREATMENT
PLAN FOR ACNE MANAGEMENT

FACIALS
_____
_____

SPECIALIZED SKIN CARE
_____
_____

TREATMENT SERIES
_____

SPECIAL INSTRUCTIONS:
_____
_____
_____

YOUR SERVICE PROVIDER TODAY:
_____

NEXT SCHEDULED APPOINTMENT:
_____

FIGURE 10-6 A written treatment plan.

RULE #15

If you want clients to remain loyal, you must be dedicated to giving them a superior level of quality care and excellent customer service time after time.

CLIENT RETENTION

It takes months, even years, of hard work and a sizable amount of capital to build a solid clientele. In these highly competitive times, protecting that investment should be a top priority.

Spa owners can hardly afford to be complacent when it comes to client retention. Nor should they be naïve. There are many reasons for a client's initial visit to your spa. Perhaps they received a gift certificate or responded to a special offer. But there are generally two main reasons they come back: (1) they respect your professional expertise; and (2) they benefit from the services you provide.

In many respects, clients still "buy" the service provider, and it is trust in their expertise, along with the quality of the products and treatments your spa provides, that brings them back. But don't underestimate the impact of customer service on client retention. If you want clients to remain loyal, you must be dedicated to giving them a superior level of quality care *and* excellent customer service time after time. Your staff is the most important ingredient in delivering this promise and should be trained to make customer satisfaction the top priority.

As the spa owner, you must also pay attention to how you operate your business. Good business policies, honesty, and integrity help to build client loyalty these days. Beyond this, clients will be looking at everything from the cleanliness of your spa, to how flexible you are in scheduling appointments. The spa business is a service business where clients should naturally expect prompt, courteous, personal attention. Make your policies clear and never let a client leave your spa angry or upset. Train your staff to handle any problems that arise promptly and with skill and diplomacy. We'll talk more about this in Chapter 11.

Reward Good Clients

Many spas provide top-notch services these days, which makes it all the more important to reward good clients. To keep clients coming back, you must show them that you value their business and give them some incentive to return. Train your staff to treat regular clients with extra special care and use every opportunity available to demonstrate your generosity. Events such as client appreciation days, exclusive bonuses, and gifts help to make clients feel special. It is also important to supply them with samples; honor them on birthdays, anniversaries, and other special occasions with a personal gift; point out series savings packages, and give them advance notice of any sales promotions or discounts you offer. A personal thank-you and reward for referring new business is another way to show your appreciation and should be used every time a client recommends a new customer to your spa. Treating clients well lets them know you do not take their business for granted.

Follow-Up

Other simple measures can be taken to let clients know you care. A simple note or phone call often does the trick; however, if you are like most busy spa owners, you are probably thinking, "When will I find the time to do that?" Don't be afraid to delegate this task to qualified personnel but do provide a structured protocol.

Following up with clients is a great way to maintain the connection and is easily accomplished by establishing a designated call-in and call-out hour (Figure 10-7). Given the increasing complexity of spa services, it is important for clients to be able to get in touch with you should they have a reaction to a treatment or product, or a question about their home care regimen. As spas take on more of a therapeutic role, it is also important for you to let clients know that you are concerned about their well-being. When clients have a new or more aggressive treatment, a quick follow-up to see how they are doing can mean all the difference in building trust in your services. Think about how good you feel when a doctor or nurse calls to check in after a delicate medical procedure.

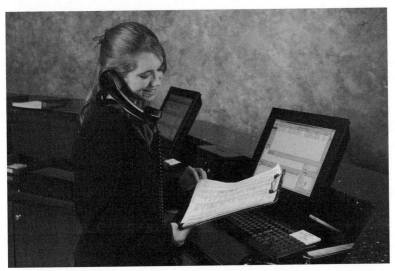

FIGURE 10-7 A quick phone call goes a long way in building client relations.

Solicit Feedback

Asking clients for their input is another great way to improve client retention. You can use several methods to solicit client feedback. Some of the more common ones include suggestion boxes, client surveys, and focus groups; however, it can be difficult to get clients to participate in these activities. Giving the client some incentive, such as a free service for participating in a focus group or a discount coupon for answering a survey, can increase the response rate.

It is also important to develop surveys and customer service checklists. Many times, clients would like to offer their input but are too rushed at the end of a service to fill out a lengthy questionnaire. If they did not have the best experience, they may also be concerned with retaining anonymity. A simple postcard that can be returned at their leisure, the opportunity to respond to a direct e-mail, or a survey posted on your Web site can make it easier for clients to provide honest feedback.

When creating surveys or customer service evaluation forms, keep them simple. It should not take longer than 10 to 15 minutes for the customer to complete such forms. In fact, the shorter they are, the better. Questions that require yes and no answers or provide multiple-choice options are the easiest to analyze and the least confusing for the respondent, provided the questions are straightforward. If you lack experience in developing surveys, consider hiring a professional or use specialized software and prepackaged formats.

At times, you will want to give clients free rein to report on their experience. A strategically placed suggestion box or guest journal that invites clients to offer their comments can help to accomplish this goal. You can also add an area for this purpose on surveys and checklists.

The main objective is to find out what you are doing right and what needs improvement. Ask clients how they feel about the quality of services, variety of treatments, frequency of treatments, friendliness and competence of your staff, cleanliness of your spa, their favorite treatments, views on pricing, and their perceptions on how easy it is to make appointments and check in and out of your spa. Also, ask what they would like to see added to your spa menu. Anything that relates to operating your spa business is subject to scrutiny.

Providing clients with an opportunity to tell you what they like and don't like makes them feel they have a say in how you operate your business and goes a long way in keeping them satisfied.

THINK IT OVER

A strong sales program is at the core of every profitable spa business and should be nurtured with creativity, passion, and a long-term commitment to providing clients with excellent customer service. Your ability to gain the client's trust is an integral part of developing good client relations and increasing sales. As in all healthy long-term interpersonal relationships, this requires a great deal of tender loving care.

Continued efforts to understand, improve, and create new methods for satisfying the customer's needs are an integral part of a healthy sales and customer service program. Be honest and deliver services in a professional manner, invite client feedback, and make yourself available. This type of reciprocal behavior builds strong, caring, and mutually gratifying relationships, especially in the spa business.

RULE #16

Long-term relationships require tender loving care.

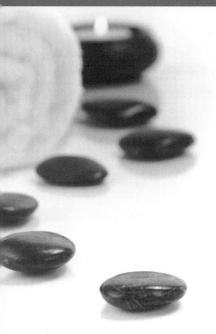

MAINTAINING YOUR BUSINESS

Why do some businesses seem to flow effortlessly? The answer to that question is a simple one—organization. Successful business owners and managers plan carefully. They have systems and policies for dealing with virtually every aspect of management and operations. By determining methods for handling situations before they arise, they are in a better position to manage them well.

As you establish policies and procedures for maintaining your spa, it is important to remember that the spa business is no longer a level playing field. The smaller day spa owner is now in the position of competing with seasoned corporate and medical professionals who can afford to hire highly qualified business administrators and consultants to put policies and procedures in place. To remain competitive, spa owners must adopt professional standards for handling all business matters.

YOUR MISSION

The first step in establishing policies and procedures is a mission statement. Your mission speaks directly to the vision or plan you have for developing a profitable spa business. This is different from the mission statement developed for a consumer brochure discussed in Chapter 9, which is more closely tied to your spa concept and treatment philosophy. While the statement made in a consumer brochure may contain an explanation of your policy on customer service and the qualifications of your staff, it is largely focused on marketing your spa business to the public.

In contrast, the vision you have for developing your spa business sets the tone for the type of operation you will run and lets those in your employment understand the direction in which you are headed and the basic principles or foundation on which your business goals are based. This message should be incorporated into your employee manual or handbook and in your business plan, with an emphasis on how you intend to grow your company into a profitable business. It should make a clear statement about how two of the most important ingredients in your success, namely your customers and employees, fit into the scheme of things.

Today, more so than ever, businesses are being asked to maintain higher standards of integrity when it comes to employee and client relations. Running a business with integrity is hard work. Developing a mission statement that expresses your personal business values, embraces the contribution of your employees, and addresses the standard of care you demand in meeting client needs is an important part of establishing a successful business and maintaining integrity (Figure 11-1).

Successful
Day / Spa

Mission Statement

Successful Day Spa is dedicated to providing clients with quality personal care products and innovative spa services that address their individual health, beauty and wellness concerns.

Education is at the core of our business model and is the measure of our success. *Clients* who understand the value of our products and services, *employees* who feel supported in their quest for knowledge, empowered to manage tasks independently, and who seek to attain new levels of responsibility; along with *partners* who honor our mission to maintain a safe, ecologically conscious and prosperous spa environment are the mainstay of our business.

As the founders of Successful Day Spa we believe that when we act in a socially responsible manner, respect individual differences, sell with integrity, educate from the heart, value the contribution of each individual, maintain the highest standards of quality control and customer service, and foster good will in the community, we are in an excellent position to promote the true essence of health, beauty and wellness—one that allows each and every person who enters our spa to grow healthier in mind, body and spirit. It is this plan to expand the company with skill and diplomacy that will ultimately establish Successful Day Spa as a leader in the global spa community.

Successful Spa Founders

FIGURE 11-1   Example of a Company Mission Statement.

SPA POLICIES

A mission statement is a good place to begin defining your business goals, but many systems must be put in place to help you each those goals. Tackling business policies and procedures is a time-consuming and often strenuous undertaking that requires day spa owners to be well versed on a variety of human resource and business administration topics. Breaking these down into smaller tasks can help you turn what often seems like a monumental project into one that is more manageable.

The best approach is often a simple one. Start with the basics, such as the days and hours your spa will be open, and how to book an appointment and move on to policies that will help day-to-day operations go smoothly, for example, how cancellations, late arrivals, and no-shows will be handled; your policy on refunds and exchanges; what recourse clients have if they are dissatisfied with a product or service; your policy on tipping; and which methods of payment will be accepted (Figure 11-2). Many spas institute additional measures to guard against financial loss, such as requesting a credit card or partial payment to reserve an appointment. If you adopt this policy be sure this information is made available to clients booking appointments by phone, via the internet and/or in the spa. It should also appear in any printed material that describes your policies such as your brochure.

Spa etiquette is a major factor in providing guests with a pleasant experience, so it is important to let spa guests know how to behave when they come to your spa. Will you allow children in the spa? Ban the use of cell phones and other electronics? Do you require special attire to be worn for certain services? Are guests expected to arrive early to fill out any necessary questionnaires or forms? Client comfort, safety and privacy should always be a top priority when establishing these policies.

Once you have identified your basic policies, take a long look at them. Are all of the policies you have created ones which you can stand behind? How strict are you willing to be in enforcing them? If you are unable to enforce your policies or plan to bend the rules for some, you will have a tough time maintaining credibility. This does not mean that you cannot establish a hierarchal system whereby the first time clients unwittingly commit a violation they receive a polite warning, and the second time the rule is enforced; however, it does mean that whatever precedent you set should be made clear to all of your employees, and you will need to stick to it. All policies should be prominently featured in a strategic location of the spa, for example, in a framed photo display at the front desk.

Successful
Day Spa **Spa Policies**

Scheduling Appointments

All appointments must be made in advance and may be scheduled online, over the phone at 987.654.3210, or in person with our Spa Concierge. We recommend scheduling your appointment well in advance of the desired date. A credit card is required to reserve your appointment.

Cancellations

All of our spa services are carefully coordinated to deliver the best possible experience for each guest. If for any reason you must cancel your appointment we ask that you kindly provide us with a 24 hour notice. Cancellation of individual services made less than 48 hours in advance are subject to a 25% cancellation fee. Cancellation of spa packages made less than 48 hours in advance are subject to a 50% cancellation fee. Failure to provide us with any notice of cancellation will result in a 100% charge for the scheduled service.

Cancellation of private parties and special events are subject to additional fees as specified in the terms of the agreement.

Payment & Fees

We accept cash, checks, and all major credit cards.

There is a $25 charge for any returned check that requires additional banking fees.

SPA ETIQUETTE
Check-In

Please arrive 15 minutes prior to your scheduled appointment to gently unwind and prepare for your service. First time spa guests are asked to arrive 30 minutes prior to their scheduled appointment to familiarize themselves with the spa and fill out a confidential client questionnaire.

Personal Storage & Valuables

Individual women's and men's lockers are available for our guests. However, Successful Day Spa cannot assume responsibility for any lost or stolen items. For security purposes we request that guests refrain from bringing anything of value into the spa.

Code of Conduct

Our goal is to provide a safe and comfortable environment for each guest. All of our practitioners are licensed and trained to conduct all services in a dignified and respectful manner. We respect your right to privacy and will not disclose any information beyond that which is required within the scope of the therapeutic relationship. Please let us know if you have a preference for a male or female service provider when scheduling your appointment.

FIGURE 11-2 Example of Spa Policies.

Maintaining our Serenity

To ensure that each guest has a relaxing experience we request that you turn off your cell phone and refrain from using any electronics in the spa. For your convenience wireless internet service is available in our café where a private area is also designated for cell phone use.

Safety

To ensure a restful experience for all of our guests we kindly ask that you leave pets and children under 12 at home. For safety reasons, all children 16 years or younger must be accompanied by an adult.

Gratuities

A gratuity is not included in the price of our services. Gratuity is left to the discretion of our guests and should be based on personal satisfaction. For your convenience, envelopes are available at the front desk for this purpose. A gratuity may also be included in your service check or charge.

Late Arrivals

All of our appointments are coordinated to provide the maximum benefit to each guest. Should you arrive late for your appointment please note that you may opt to shorten your treatment if time allows or you may choose to reschedule your appointment. All late arrivals are subject to full charge.

Refunds or Exchanges

Merchandise accompanied by a sales receipt may be returned for spa credit only within 30 days of purchase. Please note that personal care products must be unopened and in their original packaging to receive credit.

GENERAL INFORMATION

Hours of Operation

Sunday 12:00 noon to 6:00 pm
Monday 8:00 am to 8:00 pm
Tuesday 8:00 am to 8:00 pm
Wednesday 8:00 am to 8:00 pm
Thursday 8:00 am to 8:00 pm
Friday 8:00 am to 8:00 pm
Saturday 8:00 am to 6:00 pm
Please note our last appointment is taken one hour before closing.
To make reservations for a Private Party or Event please contact our Spa Event Coordinator at extension 22.
www.successfuldayspa.com
987.654.3210

Series Packages & Special Promotions

All of our facials, advanced skin care massage therapies, manicures and pedicures are available in series saving packages. Please ask the appointment coordinator for details when you make your reservation. We also offer a number of seasonal promotions which may be viewed on our website or delivered directly to you via our newsletter subscription.

FIGURE 11-2 Example of Spa Policies. (*continued*)

Products

We carry an exclusive line of Successful Skin Care™ products along with the Top Age Management Name Brand, Acne Management Name Brand and Top Organic Name Brand.

Gift Certificates

Successful Day Spa gift cards & gift certificates are available in any denomination and may be purchased online, by phone at 987.456.3210, or in person. Instant gift certificates are available for any occasion and may be purchased 24 hours a day, 7 days a week via our internet shopping cart. All of our gift cards and certificates may be redeemed for a period of up to five years from the initial date of purchase.

Private Parties

Successful Day Spa invites you to plan your next event or social gathering in the comfort and serenity of our private Spa Party Suite. The spa may be reserved for private parties, business or group outings, and other special events by appointment only and is subject to a deposit to reserve the date. Our Spa Event Coordinator is available to help you with all of your party needs, including catering, flowers, a chocolate fountain, party banners, guest favors, etc. For more information please visit our website or call us at 987.654.3210.

Location

123 Chic Main Street, Urban Oasis, SPA 45678 www.SuccessDaySpa.com 987.654.3210

Directions

From points *North* take the express highway to Route Nirvana, Exit 8. Turn left off of the ramp and follow the road until you come to Blissful Meadow Drive. Successful Day Spa will be the second building on your right.

From points *South* take the express highway to Route Nirvana, Exit 8. Turn right off of the ramp and follow the road until you come to Blissful Meadow Drive. Successful Day Spa will be the second building on your left.

From points *East* take the highway to Route Paradise, Exit 6. Turn left off of the ramp and follow the Path to Wellness. At the next left turn right onto Blissful Meadow Drive. Successful Day Spa will be the second building on your right.

From points *West* take the highway to Route Paradise Exit 6. Turn right off the ramp and follow the Path to Wellness. At the next right turn left onto Blissful Meadow Drive. Successful Day Spa will be the second building on your left.

Please note: these policies are meant as an example only, spa policies will vary according to individual business needs.

FIGURE 11-2 Example of Spa Policies. (*continued*)

Establish User-friendly Business Systems

As you create systems and policies for running your business, it is extremely important to remember that you are in business to do business and that business must be profitable to survive. Never lose sight of the fact that you need to make it easy for clients to do business with you. This can be a challenge, especially for spa owners with high ideals who view their spa as a sanctuary from which to escape the real world. As much as spa owners may wish to preserve a stress-free and relaxing environment, in our hurried society, convenience is the name of the game.

There are several things you can do to make sure your spa is convenient. Provide several payment options, such as cash, check, debit, and charge cards, and allow clients to include gratuities (if you accept them) when paying by check or charge card. Let clients know you respect their time by giving them options to purchase gift certificates and book appointments online. If economically feasible, set up a system that allows clients to purchase retail products via an Internet shopping cart on your Web site. This will make it easier for them to replenish the professional products you sell.

It is also important to establish hours of operation that are convenient for your clients, not for you. If you find that your staff and clients are pressed for time and space, look for ways to offer services simultaneously by having service providers team up to offer multiple services during the same time slot. This is often easier than you think: Imagine a simple manicure being given during a facial treatment or a simultaneously performed manicure and pedicure treatment. Several treatment combinations can work successfully. There are many other ways to accommodate those on the go, such as self check-in and checkout options. Although such strategies may feel uncomfortable at first, if these options are something your clients want, it is important to provide them.

Convenience does not mean a lack of personalized attention. This is especially important when it comes to the telephone. Whenever possible, spa owners should provide direct access to a "real person." A personal service business that rarely has a person answer the phone could be construed as lacking quality customer service. Nevertheless, you will most likely have the need to incorporate a voice mail system. Voice mail is considered an ordinary part of doing business today, but the quality of experience in using these systems varies widely. Make your voice mail system as user-friendly as possible for the caller. Let the caller know exactly why you are unavailable, when you will return the call, or when they can speak with you directly.

If your business relies on clients who are coming from a distance, consider the use of an 800 number; toll-free phone service has come down in price over the years. This option has given many day spas in targeted market areas, such as coastal or resort communities, looking to promote a destination-type spa atmosphere or attract a transient clientele a great deal of marketing leverage as they take advantage of national print and Web-based publications to promote their services.

Gratuities

Establishing a policy on tipping is critical in the spa business. Many spa guests are confused about what, if any, gratuity is appropriate. While some spas are doing away with gratuities to accommodate newer models of compensation and the higher cost of treatments, others who are reluctant to give up what is typically a burning issue for those who receive them (primarily service providers) are building a gratuity charge into the cost of treatments. If your spa does not allow tipping, this should be stated in a highly visible location in the spa, typically at the front desk or wherever services are paid and on your price list or brochure. If your spa allows tipping, you will need to develop a more detailed policy.

It is extremely important for spa owners to understand that tips are considered part of an employee's taxable income, and as such, they are obligated to report them to the IRS. If you handle your own payroll, the IRS can supply you with all of the information needed to perform this task, including payroll tax report forms 4070 and 4070A used expressly for this purpose. Many spa owners opt to have their payroll service provider handle this responsibility. Whatever method you choose, you will need some mechanism for tallying and tracking tips.

Generally, cash tips are disbursed daily. Some spas actually supply small envelopes that clients may use for this purpose and have the front desk person distribute them to service providers at the end of the day or shift. It is then the service provider's responsibility to report this income back to the spa owner on IRS form 4070. In turn, the spa owner is responsible for reporting the tip income to the IRS and collecting the appropriate taxes from the employee's wages. The IRS offers employers several options for performing this task which can be researched online at *www.irs.gov*.

If you allow clients to include tips in checks or charge card payments, you will need to use a different method to track and distribute them. Many spa owners elect to include the tip amount in the service provider's payroll check on whichever schedule they are paid.

Gift Certificates

Many spas derive a sizable amount of revenue from the sale of gift certificates, particularly around holidays. What is difficult for most spa owners is tracking and fulfilling the value of those gift certificates, some of which are never redeemed. A good financial software program is imperative for tracking all gift certificate sales, but it will not prevent you from losing money.

A huge volume of gift certificate sales can place the spa owner in the precarious position of collecting large sums of money for products and services to be delivered in the future. There is an additional risk for those who issue gift certificates for specific services instead of a set dollar amount

Plan for Success

Gratuities or tips are considered part of an employee's taxable income, and as such must be reported to the IRS. Establishing a method for reporting taxes is critical for any spa that allows tipping. All spa owners are encouraged to review *IRS Publication 3144 Tips on Tips, A Guide to Tip Income Reporting for Employers* for this purpose. The IRS also publishes a guide for employees, *IRS Publication 3148 Tips on Tips: A Guide to Tip Income Reporting for Employees Who Receive Tip Income.*

if the cost of providing those services rises before they are delivered. For example, if you sell a gift certificate for a specific type of facial at a set value, when that facial goes up in price, you actually lose money.

Inevitably all gift certificates are equivalent to cash; however, that cash is really not available to the spa owner until the client uses it for service and all expenses associated with it have been paid. Creating a policy for handling that cash until its value is redeemed is important for spa owners who may otherwise be tempted to spend it unwisely and pay for it later. Some spa owners set up special accounts to handle gift certificate revenues, such as money market or interest-bearing checking accounts to avoid loss.

Spa owners should also be aware of laws that apply to the redemption of gift certificates. The Uniform Disposition of Unclaimed Property Act set forth legislation or *escheatment* laws for dealing with unclaimed property, including gift certificates. Under this act, individual states are allowed to set specific time limits on a business's obligation to honor gift certificates before reporting the income to the government as "unclaimed property."

Today, these laws are changing, with many states adopting new policies on the sale of gift certificates. For example, new laws in Massachusetts allow the merchant to keep the value of the gift certificate after a period of seven years rather than reporting it as unclaimed property, provided the date of issue and an expiration date appear on the gift certificate. Gift certificates written without these dates are redeemable in perpetuity. Previous law in Massachusetts required businesses to set a limit of two years before turning gift certificate money over to the state as unclaimed property.

Individual states may have varying requirements, such as insisting that a set expiration date appear on the gift certificate or, alternatively, requiring that no expiration date be applied and the gift certificate be honored ad infinitum. If your state is not one of them, and there is no other law preventing it you may want to adopt the latter policy anyway to promote good public relations. Another issue to be resolved is how much of the gift certificate amount value must be spent before the client can demand "cash back." In some instances you may also need to define what constitutes a gift certificate, such as a plastic gift card or a paper gift certificate. When in doubt, check the individual laws that apply in your state.

CLIENT MANAGEME NT

Managing client relations is a crucial facet of running a spa business. It should be guided by an in-depth policy covering such issues as how the telephone is answered, how clients are greeted when they enter the spa, how long they are kept waiting for services, how confidential information is handled, and how clients are indoctrinated, draped, and ported from room to room.

A standard protocol for communication and service delivery that includes all of these items will help you to build a better business. For example, a prime concern for clients on the go is often the time spent waiting to receive services or check out. As a spa owner, you will need to determine how long it is appropriate to keep clients waiting and what actions might help to alleviate such a problem. If your staff constantly runs past scheduled appointments or your front desk is understaffed, can you really expect clients to respect a statement like "we know your time is important"? If you know it, show it by implementing systems that will help to eliminate the problem. For example, use pagers that alert service providers when their next client has arrived and train everyone to perform the same treatment in exactly the same amount of time.

Client Record Keeping

Careful record keeping is essential to maintain good client relations. Service providers see many people in varying frequency, making it impossible to remember all of the details about every single client. A good software program managed by a qualified administrator will help your staff to retain important client information and stay on top of business goals. Make sure you invest in one that provides detailed summary reports and take time to evaluate them on a regular basis. Do records indicate that your staff has a good client retention rate, receives frequent referrals, and demonstrates client satisfaction? Is this supported by sales records that indicate clients are showing progress, listening to staff recommendations, and purchasing products? Such data is vital to maintaining a successful spa business and should be shared with your staff.

Although it is perfectly understandable for spa owners to be concerned with maintaining security, allowing service providers to have access to client files and computerized reports will help your staff do their job better. If you are uneasy about how best to balance security and service, speak to your IT service provider or software vendor about establishing systems that give your technicians the information they need to do their job yet provide adequate security measures. Spas cannot let concerns about service providers stealing client information keep them from maintaining professional standards; however, if you are still uneasy and feel this could be an issue in your spa, consult with your business attorney about establishing policies and legal agreements that protect your interests as well as the confidentiality of client information. Include these policies in your employee manual or handbook. You should also take additional precautions to back up important data. In addition, password protection is advised when dealing with confidential information.

Client Profiles and Consent Forms

Client profiles and consent forms are two of the most important documents spa owners possess. The initial intake form or questionnaire is used to gather pertinent client information and develop a client profile or history that will help service providers to do their job better and increase client satisfaction. It is also used to alert the service provider to anything that might put the client at risk, such as an allergy to a particular product or substance or a medical condition that could prevent the client from engaging in certain spa treatments.

Similar to patient history forms used by medical personnel, the client profile contains personal information that should be kept confidential. Should clients misrepresent their status—for example, by failing to inform you they are taking a medication that could put them at risk when undergoing certain spa treatments,—this form could become a critical part of your defense against any legal claims should the client suffer damages related to services performed in your spa.

An effective intake form, questionnaire, and client profile, as we learned in Chapter 10, lay the groundwork for building a mutually satisfying and trusting relationship with the client. They should supply the service provider with important client information: clients' reasons for visiting the spa; their goals and expectations; services they are seeking; products they use; any pertinent medical conditions or medications they are using; a general idea of their overall health, lifestyle, and stress level; and nutritional habits that could affect treatment or pose a contraindication to treatment. These forms can also help the spa owner assess marketing effectiveness by asking how new clients heard about the spa. Some spas incorporate particular policies that could impact the responsibilities of either party, such as clients' financial responsibility if they cancel or miss an appointment or that the spa makes no claim as to the results of treatment and assumes limited liability.

Additional treatment notes should be maintained to document how the client responds to a particular treatment, indicate any allergic reactions, record the client's likes or dislikes, and list what products were used or purchased. In some cases, a benign comment or personal anecdote may be helpful to the service provider for the purpose of bonding with the client; however, it is best not to make references to privileged remarks that could have serious consequences, such as a note that contains intimate details about a client's personal life.

Consent forms are used to protect the spa business owner against liability for treatments that pose some risk and are generally used for more aggressive or complicated treatments, such as chemical peels. Research the use of such forms carefully and make sure that the responsible staff member

Plan for Success

Spa owners are advised to have all consent and intake forms reviewed by qualified legal counsel before implementing them and are reminded to check with the appropriate licensing boards in their state as to whether or not treatments requiring consent can be performed in the spa under the scope of their license.

introduces the consent form to clients in a nonthreatening way that clearly defines the purpose, breadth, and scope of the treatment and any possible repercussions or home care that may be required. Because this document is instrumental in protecting the spa business owner against liability, those responsible for implementing its use should be well trained.

Confidentiality

With the number of sophisticated treatments and equipment used in spas growing, the need to obtain detailed personal and medical client information has increased. It is critical that this information and all client records be kept confidential.

Maintaining a client's right to privacy is a matter of professionalism that should be standard practice in all spas. The treatments clients have, frequency of their visits, and other personal data that is shared with you and your staff is privileged information. This is particularly important for day spas affiliated with medical professionals. In this case, maintaining patient privacy and compliance with federal regulations such as the Health Insurance Portability and Accountability Act (HIPAA) should be stressed to all spa personnel working directly with the physician and handling confidential patient files. If you do not understand HIPAA rules and regulations as they apply to your spa practice, seek competent legal advice.

As a spa owner, it is ultimately your responsibility to protect client confidentiality by maintaining strict security policies. All paper files should be kept in a locked file, and computerized files should have restricted access that is only available to key personnel.

Coping with Challenging Customers

We talked at length about the ingredients that go into delivering quality service in Chapter 10, but even with the best customer service policies in place, dealing with the public can be challenging. Over the course of your career, you are bound to run into a variety of situations that require a great deal of patience, skill, tact, and diplomacy.

Clients come in all personalities and psyches—those who like to let you know how much they know, those who will test the limits of every policy you have, those who need more attention than you can seemingly provide, and those who are just plain problematic or complain about everything. It is your job to develop policies that prevent problems before they arise and, when unavoidable, to train staff to handle difficult situations in the most diplomatic way possible. At times, this may require the use of outside professional help.

Plan for Success

The Health Insurance Portability Act (HIPAA) was developed by the Department of Health and Human Services (HHA) to protect the rights of individuals with regard to obtaining information about their health in a medical setting. This law states that any communication that takes place in a medical setting must be kept confidential.

Because spas and medical spas collect important privileged medical information about clients and patients, all spa owners are warned that any breach of confidentiality can have serious legal and liability consequences.

Educating staff on HIPAA regulations should be included as part of a responsible risk management program. For more about HIPAA rules and regulations go to *www.hhs.gov/ ocr/hipaa*, the official Web site of the Department of Health and Human Services.

Many of the problems that arise with clients can be prevented by maintaining appropriate boundaries. Let your employees know that you expect them to maintain a friendly demeanor toward clients in the spa, but in most circumstances, it is best not to develop friendships with clients. This may not help you to win a personality contest, but it will let your staff know where you stand on these critical issues.

You should be clear about where the role of your spa staff begins and ends. Giving advice that they are not qualified to dispense or hired to give is inappropriate. Remind your spa service providers that they are not psychologists, marriage counselors, or physicians, and make it clear that they should not advise on issues that are beyond the scope of their spa license. It is also important to teach your staff to maintain appropriate physical and emotional boundaries. Go back to Chapter 10 and review the section on sensitivity training. Anything that could be construed as inappropriate or sexual misconduct has the potential for liability.

Spa personnel also need to maintain appropriate boundaries when engaging in casual conversation and should be careful not to ask clients personal questions. While clients will often volunteer information, it is important for all spa staff to be tactful and discreet. If a client shares personal information in passing that does not mean that it is okay to share it with the rest of the staff. Train staff to listen politely and avoid gossiping and/or expressing opinions that could make clients uncomfortable.

Some clients will, of course, "push buttons," and no staff member should be humiliated or embarrassed in the name of customer service. As a spa owner, it is your job to set the right example. While service providers perform services, they are not servants. Teach your staff to recognize abusive behavior and provide positive assertiveness training to help them cope with difficult situations.

HIRING EMPLOYEES

Hiring employees is often a nerve-wracking process for those who do not have a background in human resource management. How will you attract competent workers to your day spa? Finding employees who are a good fit requires a thoughtful marketing strategy that clearly identifies the qualities you are looking for, and that positions your spa as one that offers career-minded employees a great job opportunity.

Most spa businesses begin the hiring process by placing an ad. Classified ads can be found in newspapers, trade journals, employment agencies, trade organizations, training schools, and various other job banks on the Internet.

Before you place an ad, it is extremely important that you have a good understanding of employment laws. The federal government's Equal Employment Opportunity Commission (EEOC) and your state employment office are good places to start. Many books are available to guide you in creating unbiased employment ads, interview questions, and job application forms. In addition to these references, you may want to seek the help of a qualified human resources, or HR, consultant. As a final precaution, you should have all related job application forms, interview questionnaires, and employee documents reviewed by a competent business attorney who is well versed in employment law.

Once you are apprised of the law, make a list of the qualifications the ideal candidate will possess. Are you looking for someone with experience or a novice you can train? Is your spa an extremely busy place that requires someone with lots of energy? A help-wanted ad should let prospective candidates know exactly what you are seeking. This may include a variety of technical and personal qualifications. For example, if you are looking for a front desk manager who has strong interpersonal, communication, administrative, and computer skills, say so. You might specify that your spa needs an esthetician who can perform basic and advanced skin care treatments, take direction, handle the demands of a varied clientele, and work as part of a team. Add to this any benefits that are available to employees, such as health insurance or a 401k plan. A carefully written ad will help you to attract the right people to your spa business.

Interviewing Candidates

Interviewing job candidates is a time-consuming process. If you are bombarded with hundreds of qualified candidates, narrow the list down to a select few whose cover letters and resumes address the qualifications you are looking for and who have additional traits you consider beneficial to the position. Presentation is an important factor in this initial phase; so pay special attention to the details. Has the candidate taken the time to ensure the cover letter and resume are grammatically correct, neat, legible, and error-free? If the candidate is not inquiring about a position as a result of a direct ad, do they ask what the correct procedure is for applying for a job and follow through as requested? These things can tell you a lot about a person before you even speak to him or her. Once you have found several candidates who meet your criteria, pre-qualify them with a quick telephone screening. This will save you from wasting everyone's valuable time if the match is clearly not one that will work for one reason or another.

When meeting face-to-face with a candidate, be prepared with a list of questions, but remember that it is illegal to ask a person questions about

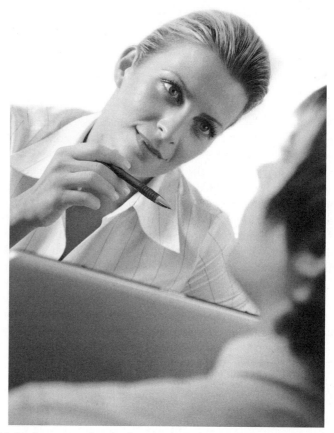

FIGURE 11-3 Be prepared with a list of qualified questions when interviewing potential employees.

marital status, number of children, medical conditions or health problems, disabilities, sexual preference or gender, religion, race, color, ethnic heritage, age, or date of birth (Figure 11-3). To be fair, all candidates should be asked the same questions in the same order.

Generally, employers are interested in three key areas: experience, skills, and attitude. You can often learn more about these by asking open-ended questions such as: "What are your strengths and weaknesses?" or "What did or didn't you like about your previous position?" Some interviewers like to present specific situations and ask candidates how they would handle them. This gives candidates an opportunity to provide information in their own words.

QUALIFYING JOB CANDIDATES

When qualifying candidates, use the following general categories to guide you:

- Career goals—where does the candidate want to be in five years?

- Work style—does the candidate enjoy working as part of a team or alone?

- Organization—how does the candidate organize his or her day?

- Honesty—can the candidate speak to the information furnished on his or her resume?

- Licenses—can service providers supply a current license for the position for which they are applying?

- Personal presentation—does the candidate conduct him or herself in a professional manner?

- Philosophy—does the candidate uphold the same values in terms of customer service and work ethic?

- Product preferences—does the candidate like the products you are currently using?

- Employment history—has the person held jobs for a considerable length of time, or does he or she seem to go from one spa to the next in quick succession?

- Compensation—does the candidate have specific salary requirements?

- References—can the candidate supply at least three references?

Take your time when interviewing prospective employees. Hiring someone out of desperation rarely works. If you are impressed with a candidate, bring him or her back for a second interview. Test the skills of service providers by having them give you or another member of the staff a treatment. Front desk personnel hold an extremely important position in the spa; so you will want to make sure they are up to speed. Consider hiring people for this position on a "temporary to permanent" basis that allows you to test their skills during a trial period. It is also a good idea to introduce qualified candidates to other key members of your staff. And it is only fair to give the candidate an opportunity to ask you questions as well. This can actually be a telling experience and may bring about answers to questions that you would not ask yourself.

If you have specific policies and procedures for employees on which you are not willing to be flexible—sales quotas, housekeeping chores, attendance at early morning staff meetings, or a team approach, for example—be up-front about them. In most cases, it is helpful to supply the candidate with a complete job description. After a second interview, it is also wise to give candidates an opportunity to review your employee manual or handbook before making a formal offer. This will help you to uncover any objections they may have.

As a spa owner, remember that you have the right to be selective about the people to whom you entrust your clients and your business. Spas handle personal information and provide clients with intimate services; therefore, it is also important to conduct a background check on employees before hiring. Use a reputable and licensed professional or service that adheres to the letter of the law for this purpose, and always request written permission to check references or conduct an investigation first. More and more employers are concerned with drug use when completing a background check; laws vary from state to state when it comes to drug testing. Check the regulations in your state before going down this path.

Although all of this may seem like a lot of work, in the end you will be glad that you took the time to conduct a thorough interview. In the spa business employees not only need to have good technical skills, they must enjoy working with people on an intimate basis, be trustworthy, and communicate effectively.

Job Descriptions

The importance of job descriptions cannot be overstated. Clear directives help to prevent misunderstandings and allow employees to meet obligations successfully. Start with an outline of each position in your spa (Figures 11-4 and 11-5). This should include a detailed list of all the duties and responsibilities that each employee, including service providers, support staff, and administrative personnel, are required to perform. It is equally important to develop a salary range for each position—that is, what you are prepared to pay each person on your staff performing that specific job. Next to each job description, list the qualities a qualified candidate will possess to perform this job successfully in your spa, and review these requirements periodically. Have the job requirements remained the same or changed? Does anything need to be added or

Successful Day Spa — **Job Description for Front Desk Manager**

The Front Desk Manager will have at the minimum an associate's degree in Business Management and/or three-to-five-years management experience in a day spa or salon environment. The person in this position reports directly to the spa manager. He or she is responsible for performing the following duties and is subject to additional requirements as specified in the employee manual for Successful Day Spa.

- Schedule appointments.
- Check in and check out spa guests.
- Handle customer service issues.
- Maintain a log of all customer service complaints.
- Report customer complaints to the owner or spa manager on a weekly basis or promptly when necessary.
- Manage cash register.
- Provide the spa owner with daily, weekly, and monthly sales reports.
- Maintain retail inventory.
- Interface with vendors and generate purchases orders.
- Supervise and train other administrative personnel.
- Resolve technology problems.
- Maintain a log of all technology problems associated with administrative equipment, such as computers, telephone, fax, copier, printer, and Internet connectivity.
- Coordinate marketing collateral and track related inventory.
- Act as liaison to marketing manager or consultant.
- Track promotional efforts.
- Maintain the security of client information and files.
- Attend monthly staff meetings.

*Note that these job descriptions are fictitious and are not meant to be inclusive. Job descriptions and requirements will vary based on the individual business needs, size, and type of the spa facility you operate.

FIGURE 11-4   Example of a job description for Front Desk Manager.

Successful Day Spa   **Job Description for Level I Esthetician**

Level I estheticians are required to hold a current esthetician license in the state of the spa. Estheticians report directly to the spa manager. They are responsible for performing the following duties and are subject to additional requirements as specified in the employee manual for Successful Day Spa.

- Conduct initial intake interview with client.
- Review applicable consent forms with client.
- Analyze skin types and conditions before treating any client.
- Update client records every time a client visits the spa.
- Record results of treatment on specified treatment form after each spa visit.
- Perform basic facials.
- Perform wax hair removal.
- Perform make-up application.
- Perform hand and foot treatments.
- Sanitize treatment room after each treatment.
- Replenish linens in treatment rooms at the beginning of each day or shift.
- Restock back bar at the end of each day or shift.
- Recommend skin care products to clients for home care.
- Fill out a home care form for each client and review this with the client at the end of each treatment.
- Report any problems immediately to management staff.
- Sell a minimum of $2,000 in retail products monthly.
- Maintain an 80 percent client retention rate.
- Refer clients to other service providers.
- Confirm their schedule monthly with the front desk manager.
- Attend monthly staff meetings.
- Attend a minimum of three continuing education classes per calendar year.

Note that these job descriptions are fictitious and are not meant to be inclusive. Job descriptions and requirements will vary based on the individual business needs, size, and type of spa facility you operate.

FIGURE 11-5   Example of a job description for a Level I Esthetician.

deleted? Always double-check this information before presenting it to a job candidate.

Once you have hired an employee, the first order of business should be to review the job description with them and have them sign it. If problems arise later, you will have acknowledgement that they were informed of the duties and responsibilities of the position. Job descriptions can also provide a useful basis for evaluating an employee's performance.

EMPLOYEE RELATIONS

If customers are the most important asset in any business, then where do your employees stand? Employees are your closest business alliance and a crucial element in successful business operations. Choose them wisely and treat them well.

A lot goes into employee relations. In fact, managing employee relations is likely to take up most of your time. As in any strong interpersonal relationship, consider this a wise investment. Employee relationships, like clients, must be nurtured with tender loving care.

Managing Employees

Managing employees is a full-time job that requires strong leadership, communication and business skills. Many theories, books, and management tools can help you to develop effective management strategies and leadership qualities, but first you must decide if you want to assume the role of manager in your spa.

Spa owners who are new to the industry may prefer to maintain an executive position and hire others, such as a spa director, to perform direct management duties. But for those coming from the position of a service provider, making the decision to switch to a full-time management role or trying to juggle management duties and perform treatments simultaneously can be a significant source of conflict. If you are undecided about what your role should be, go back to Chapter 1, take a second look at the character traits of a successful entrepreneur, and then conduct the business skill analysis.

Focusing your attention on one role may well be the deciding factor in the success of your business; however, even if you opt to work strictly in a management capacity, you may still have a need to outsource several of your responsibilities. This is perfectly normal. A good spa manager may be adept at handling a number of day-to-day operations, but it is foolish to expect a single person to act as accountant, financial advisor, technology guru, human resources manager, marketing manager, and public relations director. Delegating some of these responsibilities and implementing strategies that make the manager or director's job easier is usually the best way to keep business running smoothly.

Employee Manual

Small day spa owners may feel an employee manual is unnecessary. This could not be further from the truth. A small intimate staff may feel like friends or family, but they are not. Close relationships with your employees won't protect you from litigation should conflicts arise. While you should always seek to maintain positive relations with your employees, remember that business is business. At the risk of sounding cynical, it is important to note that more than one spa business owner can attest to being "burned" by a trusted employee who they also considered a friend.

All businesses need guidelines or standards of acceptable behavior that are practiced consistently and without prejudice. The employee manual is a general policy guide for managing employee relations (Figure 11-6). It should address important issues, such as the procedure for calling in sick or late; time allotted for vacation, sick leave, family leave, or bereavement; severance pay; expectations for assisting other staff; benefits such as health insurance or discounted services; promotions; salary increases; and employee performance evaluations.

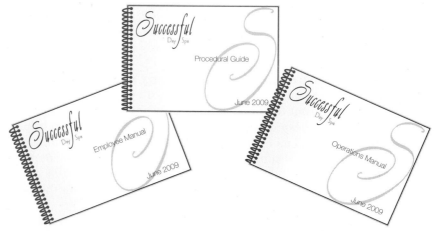

FIGURE 11-6 An employee manual, an operations manual, and procedural guide are critical to running a successful day spa.

Ideally, an employee manual or handbook will contain input from your employees. Beware that under certain circumstances an employee handbook may be treated as a contract; so it is important to include a clause that states otherwise and includes a reference to the "at-will" relationship between employer and employee. This is the understanding that an employer/employee relationship can be severed *at will* with or without due cause, although it should be noted that the at-will rule can be challenged by an employee. Other agreements, such as a non-compete agreement, should be handled separately. These should outline the specific arrangement you have with an employee.

As a business owner, it is your responsibility to provide an employee manual or handbook that details your policies and informs employees of their rights and responsibilities at the start of the employment relationship. When writing an employee manual, it is best to consult with a human resources professional who is well versed on creating appropriate and unambiguous language. Hire a qualified business attorney familiar with employment law to review your employee manual to ensure compliance with federal regulations and the specific labor laws in your state. This should be reviewed periodically as laws change.

By law, an employee manual should be accessible to employees at all times. However, it is also wise to have employees sign a statement that they have seen and read your employee manual or handbook. Keep these documents in a secure place, preferably off-site. Should you have to fire someone for insubordination or uphold your policies on a legal matter, this document is likely to come in handy.

Your employee manual may not cover every single situation that could possibly arise, but a well-written employee manual can help you to establish clear boundaries and ultimately avoid many foreseeable problems.

Procedural Guide or Manual

The procedural guide or manual provides specific guidelines for how spa services are conducted (Figure 11-7). Guidelines are extremely important in achieving consistent results and maintaining quality control. Additionally, when used as part of a complete training program, procedural manuals can help to prevent accidents and decrease the cost of providing services. For example, by specifying strict adherence to intake questionnaires and consent forms, stressing the correct sterilization procedures and universal precautions, and dictating the exact amount of product to be used for each treatment.

When developing procedural manuals, it is best to include your staff in the process. Empowering employees generally leads to a sense

TOPICS COMMONLY ADDRESSED IN THE EMPLOYEE MANUAL

A mission statement

Absences and late arrivals

An "at-will" clause

Benefits (retirement plans, employee discounts on services and products, continuing education, etc.)

Client records

Confidentiality

Definition of full- and part-time employees

Disciplinary action

Dress code

Emergency procedures

Employee grievances

Employee notices/communications

Family leave

Gratuity reports

Harassment policy

Health insurance

Hiring and selection process

Incentive programs

Incremental or tiered pay scales

Leave of absence

Lunch and break times

Observed, paid, and unpaid holidays

Opportunity for advancement or promotions

Organizational hierarchy

Overtime

Pay periods and pay dates

Performance evaluations

Professional conduct

Request for timeoff

Safety standards

Sick leave

Substance abuse

Tardiness

The company's commitment to equal opportunity laws

The training process

Trial evaluation periods

Vacation time

Work schedules

Workers' compensation

of ownership and compliance with policy. If you have strong beliefs about a particular method, introduce your beliefs with supporting documentation and invite employee feedback. Keep an open mind and conduct trials for all procedures. Once you have agreed on a protocol, spell it out clearly using a step-by-step outline and simple language, complete with diagrams. Certain circumstances, such as compliance with OSHA standards, will require you to enforce your rules strictly. In the end, informing employees exactly how to perform a procedure benefits everyone, including the client, who can rely on the consistent high quality of your services time after time.

Operational Guide

The operational guide is another useful tool that is helpful in training employees and answering many of the ordinary questions that arise

Successful Day Spa

Step-by-Step Procedure for Successful Day Spa Signature Facial

Products:	Skin Specific Successful Private Label Line
Room Setup:	Prepare facial bed with warm blankets. Tranquility aromatherapy infusion
Supplies:	Cleanser, toner, Successful organic exfoliating enzyme, treatment mask, massage oil, moisturizing cream and sunblock, cotton pads, facial sponges
Step 1.	Cleanse skin with skin-specific cleanser and toner.
Step 2.	Analyze skin.
Step 3.	Steam skin while performing relaxing shoulder and décolleté massage.
Step 4.	Perform facial exfoliation.
Step 5.	Apply treatment serum.
Step 6.	Use appropriate massage cream or hydrophilic oil to perform lymphatic drainage massage described in the Massage section of the procedures manual.
Step 7.	Remove residual massage cream.
Step 8.	Apply treatment mask with fan brush.
Step 9.	Perform relaxing hand and foot massage.
Step 10.	Remove mask.
Step 11.	Apply toner and moisturizer.
Step 12.	Apply eye cream.
Step 13.	Apply sun protection.

FIGURE 11-7 Procedural guides are essential to maintaining quality control and should include step-by-step instructions for each treatment performed in your spa.

in managing day-to-day operations, such as how to use spa or business equipment including steamers, microdermabrasion, hydrotherapy, telephone, computers, printers, and credit card and fax machines. Many equipment vendors automatically supply basic operating instructions, but it is important to embellish these with specific directions, such as the proper greeting when answering the telephone or the correct method for cleaning spa equipment and restocking supplies after each use.

In addition, step-by-step procedures for day-to-day operations, such as ordering products, opening and closing the spa, conducting emergency evacuation procedures, and calling for assistance with plumbing, electrical, or technology problems will help your business to run smoothly and ensure that it is "business as usual" should the responsible person be out sick. A list of every piece of equipment along with the date of purchase, vendor, serial number, customer service telephone number, contact person, terms of the service contract, and other relevant information and a log of any problems that have occurred is another strategy that will help you to stay on top of mechanical problems.

These policies and procedures are particularly useful in day spas that operate in shifts or have more than one front desk person. Successful businesses typically house all of these important documents in a binder that is strategically located at the front desk to provide easy access to all who need them.

Training

A spa's reputation is built on providing clients with consistent and reliable quality service; so I am always a little apprehensive when a spa makes a statement that a service will vary in some way based on the "technician's style." While each service provider may have a "unique style," all spa services should deliver the same results using a consistent format and method of delivery.

Training all of your employees to use the same methods within the same time frame keeps clients from feeling they have been shortchanged. It also allows clients to feel confident that any technician on your staff can perform the same service. As a spa business owner, this provides the added security of knowing that you are not at the mercy of any one service provider.

There is another reason to promote proper training. Procedures are complicated today, which increases the risk involved. An additional concern is that not all spa personnel have the same basic training or depth of experience required to perform more sophisticated treatments. Some spa owners resent this: Shouldn't employees come equipped with the knowledge needed to perform spa services? Yes and no. Spa owners should expect employees to have basic skills, but beyond this, it is perfectly normal for individuals to have different levels of skill, experience, and backgrounds. In any profession, there is a learning curve. This holds true whether your employees are new to the spa profession or new to your spa.

It is always in your best interest to make sure service providers are aware of the benefits, features, and contraindications to any treatment conducted in your spa, since the ultimate liability falls on your shoulders. Be open to providing instruction in your methods and allow for adequate supervision time. Many employers automatically specify a three-month trial period where employees are monitored by a senior staff member with whom they meet at a regularly scheduled time each week. This is a great way to discourage bad habits and encourage those you want to promote. It can also be a great way to bond with new personnel.

At the minimum, training should involve an initial indoctrination period that includes a review of your policy, procedure, and operations manuals with the spa director or front desk manager, followed by a demonstration of each procedure the employee is expected to perform. A test of the employee's skills before he or she is allowed to work on clients is advised and can easily be performed by giving treatments to other staff members. Ideally, this should be followed by direct supervision at regularly scheduled intervals with a senior staff member and an open-door policy to address any problems that arise.

Training staff takes time, energy, and money, but it is well worth it. Welcome the opportunity to train staff in your methods since this can have a positive effect on client satisfaction. Invest in procedural manuals, continuing education, and vendor-driven classes to increase your staff's knowledge. Make it fun, interesting, and rewarding, and include employees in the decision-making process by offering a selection of classes and workshops. Establish teams to create and test-run new treatments and meet to solicit feedback from the rest of the staff.

Team teaching, peer-centered learning, and mentoring programs can increase the retention rate and help to make learning fun. Do not lose sight of the fact that the spa business is experiential in nature; so it is important for employees to "experience" any new treatment before trying it out on clients. Have a practice night where staff members work on each other and follow up with a special reward, such as a gift certificate to a nice restaurant or theater tickets when the team reaches a set sales goal. Don't forget the importance of cross-training. Everyone on your staff should have at least a general idea of what their colleagues are doing to refer clients for other services. These benefits will let employees know their efforts to learn new techniques are appreciated. Well-educated and empowered employees, shaped and molded to fulfill the needs of your unique business, are the key to your spa's success.

Team Building

We hear a lot about "team building" and "coaching" today. When it comes to creating a profitable spa business, the importance of developing a cohesive team cannot be stressed enough, but building a team takes time and patience (Figure 11-8). Don't expect a fragmented group to become

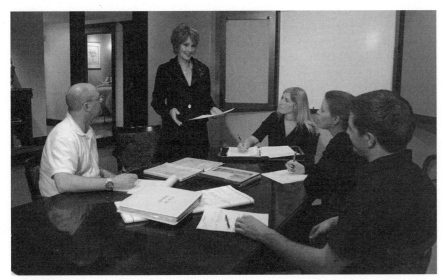

FIGURE 11-8 Time spent training and building a cohesive team is well worth the effort.

unified overnight. In an industry that has long rewarded individuals for "entrepreneurial" traits, the concept of a team does not come naturally. If you are in transition from a commission-based pay structure or have purchased or currently own a spa business that has previously relied on "independent contractors" and "booth renters" to build business, creating a team will be especially challenging. Anticipate objections and be prepared to try a variety of approaches. You may have to ease in new staff members or build an entirely new team but in the end, you will have a unified team that can rely and depend on each other to deliver positive client-centered outcomes.

Team building may sound like a game, but it is hard work and depends on a number of factors, such as trust, cooperation, and camaraderie. Successful team building comes from a dedication to common goals, developing respect for individual differences, showing compassion in difficult situations, and sharing responsibility.

Motivating Employees

As the team leader in your spa, it is ultimately your job to lead and motivate your staff. Because spa owners and managers generally have one-to-one interaction with employees on a daily basis, they are in an excellent position to develop positive nurturing relations with their staff and to motivate them to perform their jobs to the best of their ability.

QUALITIES OF A COHESIVE TEAM-CENTERED STAFF

- Respect for individual differences
- Dedication to common goals
- A willingness to share the responsibility and workload
- Cooperation among staff
- Compassion in difficult situations
- Trust that team members can rely and depend on each other

A lot of employers tell me they perform acts of kindness regularly, such as buying lunch or bringing flowers, to motivate their staff. Such advice is doled out frequently by well-meaning consultants, and of course, these are kind and generous things to do; however, lunch and flowers won't mean much to your employees if they do not feel valued, honored, respected, and listened to, or if they are left coping with faulty equipment, poor work conditions, and a sparse clientele.

If you are truly invested in motivating your employees to perform to the best of their ability, find out what it is they want from you and make an honest attempt to deliver it. You may be surprised by what you learn. Beyond decent wages, benefits, and safe working conditions, employees generally want:

- Clear policies and procedural guidelines that give them a voice in how things are done
- Job descriptions that list exactly what is expected of them
- Positive communication between management and staff
- A method for resolving conflicts fairly
- Systems that make their work easier
- Equipment that functions properly
- A well-stocked dispensary
- Adequate lunch and break time
- Reasonable spa policies

- Management that is accessible
- Follow-through on expressed concerns
- Marketing and sales promotions that bring in clients
- Incentive programs that give them an opportunity to make more money
- An opportunity to advance in the company
- Recognition for a job well done
- Continued education

In short, employees want many of the things reserved for building trusting relationships with clients; they want to be valued, respected, cared for, listened to, and treated with kindness, compassion, and courtesy. How will you accomplish all that?

Learning to motivate your staff may require continuing education on your part. Perhaps you will take a class or seek a coach or mentor to guide you. Many leadership programs, books, and resource guides offer good advice. You will need to find out what works best for you.

A number of team-building exercises and programs that can be used in the spa have already been mentioned, such as peer-centered learning, mentoring, and team-based incentives. When trying different techniques, remember to make adjustments that make sense for your business and employees, and don't be afraid to bring in outside professionals for help when needed, such as business coaches and consultants and human resource, communication, and counseling experts to work with your team.

The use of personality indicators is a popular team-building strategy that works well in some businesses. When used to bring attention to individual differences and communication styles or to acknowledge the unique contribution of each member of the team, this technique can bring about positive changes; however, it is wise to tread cautiously and enlist a qualified professional to administer such programs. The goal is to promote diversity and learn to work with others, not to provide excuses.

Coaching is another popular technique used to generate positive behaviors. If this technique appeals to you, set time aside for individual supervision but don't wait until an employee is in crisis or receives a poor evaluation to implement the program. Chances are your staff will have difficulty sharing a problem with you if you have not taken time to build a solid relationship with them. Those who are less accessible may choose to assign this duty to other competent personnel, such as a spa director or senior staff member.

This leads to what is, all too often, a common management problem—delegating authority. If you have ever held a position in middle management where you have been caught between employees and the owner or CEO, you can appreciate the frustration and havoc that can ensue. It is human nature to go to the person who is in authority; so if you undermine the person you have charged with the power to do your bidding, such as a spa director, you send a strong message to the entire staff and to the person caught in the middle. If you give staff members the authority to handle certain situations, stand behind them and show them that you value their good judgment. If you have created policies and procedures that are fair and reasonable and training that supports these efforts, this should not be hard to do.

Good leaders, like good managers, are good problem-solvers. They are not afraid to empower their employees or support those they have placed in authority. They are also willing to look at themselves critically and admit when they need help. You cannot go wrong if you strive to be fair, keep your word, show respect for your employees, encourage excellence, practice positive communication skills, maintain appropriate boundaries, set a good example, speak kindly, and praise often.

Evaluating Employee Performance

Many small business owners dread evaluating employees, but there are benefits to the evaluation process. Regular performance evaluations give managers an opportunity to check in with employees, build rapport, and offer support. In return, management often receives valuable insight from employees regarding their own style, organization and performance. This creates a win-win situation that ultimately builds trust and increases client satisfaction.

Everyone wants the exchange to result in a favorable report. To encourage the best possible outcome, all evaluations should be fair and equitable. For example, each employee should be held to the same standards as a colleague holding the same position. How and when employee performance will be reviewed should be defined clearly at the onset of employment. The employee manual is a good place to include this information and to let employees know exactly what criteria will be used to judge their performance.

The key to a productive evaluation is having a set agenda. It is generally a good idea to provide the employee with a written report beforehand. This allows both parties the opportunity to come to the meeting prepared to discuss issues openly. Most companies use a standard evaluation form for this purpose, which can be adjusted to suit the individual needs of your spa. Industry trade associations are often a good resource for evaluation forms and may also be able to direct you to human resource consultants with experience in the spa industry.

Plan for Success

When evaluating service providers, note that while teamwork is highly regarded in most spas, a good deal of the work performed by service providers is done in isolation. This is where you will need to rely on more objective computerized data such as client retention and referral rates.

EVALUATING EMPLOYEE PERFORMANCE

Consider the following general criteria for evaluating a spa service provider's performance.

- Individual performance (skills and technical knowledge)

- Productivity level (ability to perform specified number of treatments within the time allotted)

- Product knowledge (understanding of ingredients and purpose of products)

- Staff relations or teamwork (ability to get along well with others)

- Customer relations (client retention and referral rate)

- Client administration (compliance with initial intake, record-keeping, and consent forms)

- Retail sales (ability to meet set goals)

- Work habits (punctuality, cleanliness, and ability to follow instructions and take direction)

- Professionalism (appearance, skill level, attitude, and personal development)

Job descriptions, computerized sales reports, and company policies can also help you to establish objective performance standards. For example, incorporating an employee's responsibility to be on time, report problems with equipment, show courtesy to clients and other staff, and demonstrate a willingness to work as a team are easily incorporated into evaluation forms. You will need to develop individual evaluation forms for all of your workers, including managers, administrators, support staff, and service providers.

As you assess your employees' performance, remember that we all have different ways of doing things and frame your remarks in a kind way that allows employees to maintain their dignity. Speaking in terms of strengths and weaknesses is a good way to show employees that you recognize their positive attributes. If you see that someone with potential is struggling to do a good job, use that willingness to learn and take the time to coach them. Remember that it typically takes at least six months for an employee to adjust to a new position. Direct supervision by a skilled superior can make all the difference in generating success and is generally worth the time that would otherwise be spent recruiting a new employee.

All evaluation forms should be in writing, and completed reports should be filed for each staff member, regardless of the size of your spa operation. In the event of a dispute or the inevitable moment when you have to fire someone, this information will be important.

TEST YOUR CRISIS MANAGEMENT SKILLS

Develop a plan for managing a crisis before it happens. To test your skill, how would you handle the following situations? The government resources that follow these scenarios may be helpful.

1. Employees have reported that a steam machine has been malfunctioning. That same machine burns a client during a treatment. The client reports to you that the employee has informed her you were aware of the problem but have procrastinated on fixing it, and now she intends to sue.

2. Your spa director reports that the front desk manager has smelled alcohol on the breath of several employees upon their return from lunch.

3. A front desk person is caught stealing money from the "tip envelopes" designated for service providers.

4. An employee blatantly disregards treatment protocols and insists on doing it her way, proudly waving the banner of "I know better" to the rest of your staff.

5. An unexpected visit from the state board finds that you are not in compliance with state sanitation codes. This report is public information and is published online.

6. You find out that one of your employees, with whom you have a noncompete agreement, intends to open a spa two miles down the road and has invited several colleagues currently in your employment to join her.

7. One of your clients claims to be the subject of inappropriate touching during a spa treatment.

8. One of your employees charges your spa director with racial discrimination after being given several menial tasks to perform not listed on her job description.

9. A discharged employee, terminated for repeated unexcused absences and tardiness, makes a case for age discrimination when she learns that several coworkers have missed an equal number of workdays and have also been late on more than a few occasions.

10. After receiving a positive review, an employee requests a raise that is more than the standard incremental increase and threatens to quit if you do not comply.

Handling Difficult Situations

Lots of problems can be avoided by understanding and adhering to fair labor laws and safety standards and by supplying your employees with specific job descriptions and clearly defined policies. But even the best run businesses are bound to encounter a difficult situation occasionally. When that time comes, will you be prepared? Know your rights when it comes to firing an employee, dealing with inappropriate behavior or employee misconduct, and defending yourself against false claims.

Government Regulations and Legal Resources Offices

- Equal Employment Opportunity Commission
- Federal Fair Labor Standards Act
- The Equal Pay Act
- The Age Discrimination in Employment Act
- The Pregnancy Discrimination Act
- The Immigration and Control Act of 1986
- Occupational Safety and Health Act (OSHA)
- The Civil Rights Act
- Americans with Disabilities Act

COMPENSATION

Spas are labor intensive with salaries typically representing their biggest expense. As the spa industry continues to undergo enormous change, it seems that virtually every spa owner is struggling with the issue of best practices in compensation. Amid concerns over narrow profit margins and a preoccupation with what everyone else is paying, there is also the worry that as a small business, they cannot compete with larger chains and medical spas that offer more inclusive compensation and benefit packages.

From the job seeker's perspective, compensation is an equally emotionally charged subject. Because spa service providers and managers often have a wide range of skills and come from varied backgrounds, it can be difficult to establish an equitable system that makes everyone happy.

How do you determine a fair level of compensation? Should spa salaries be based on a candidate's actual experience with regard to the position for which they are applying; related experience that may prove helpful in their work as a spa technician or manager; or a predetermined pay scale based on your ability to pay? Is compensation negotiable in any way? When put to the test, spa owners tend to have varied opinions.

Let's say you have two candidates applying for the position of esthetician on your staff. Esthetician Candidate #1 is a high school graduate with little work experience. She has graduated from a basic esthetics course that required her to obtain a 600-hour certificate necessary to be eligible to take the state board exam and acquire a license. She has a part-time job in a day spa scheduling appointments on the weekend. Esthetician Candidate #2 has graduated from the same 600-hour esthetics course but went on to obtain a certificate from an advanced medical aesthetics training program where she acquired additional skills. Candidate #2 also has a bachelor's degree in business management. Prior to pursuing a career in esthetics, she held a sales position with a Fortune 500 company. Should both candidates receive the same starting salary? Herein lays the problem that so many day spa owners are faced with today. It is perplexing, but there is no reason to let emotions get in the way of creating a fair and equitable pay system based on the actual job requirements.

Tiered salary levels or incremental-based pay scales provide a solution for many. These systems employ a classification system, such as Level I, II, or III, each with its own set of criteria and requirements for advancing to the next level. Using this model, an entry-level practitioner might start out performing basic services at an hourly rate of between $12 and $15, with the opportunity to increase income by selling retail products or receiving a bonus based on meeting team sales goals. Advancing to a Level II might occur when the person becomes eligible to perform more advanced treatments, perhaps after a certain period of time spent working for the company and participating in a peer mentoring or continued education program, with an automatic option to start at this level for those graduating from advanced training programs. Wages at this level might jump to between $15 and $18 per hour, again with the opportunity to increase take-home pay by selling retail products. Level III might be achieved after an employee has been with the company for a certain number of years and has contributed to a peer mentoring or continuing education program. Wages at this level might increase to between $20 and $25 per hour, with the opportunity to receive additional retail sales commissions.

These examples are not meant to be absolute standards; they are hypothetical and should be adjusted according to the price of your services, what you can afford to pay, and the cost of living in your area. I have addressed the issue of estheticians here, but you will need to establish similar parameters for each service provider, manager, administrative employee, and support staff. There are many ways to be creative with such a system. For example, you might consider adjusting wages according to the number of continuing education credits a service provider accrues per year or generate a system that incorporates profit sharing.

New Models of Compensation

Developing a method of compensating employees that allows your spa to be profitable yet attracts career-minded and competent personnel is one of the biggest challenges you will face. From inception, most day spas adopted the salon model of compensation, in which service providers have typically been paid 40 to 60 percent commission of the total intake of services performed. What has become increasingly more apparent is that this model no longer supports the goals of today's team-oriented spa operation, which has very different financial obligations.

The problem with commission-based pay structures is that they leave little opportunity for increased profits, growth, or expansion. If service providers receive a high percentage of the service fees with no obligation to contribute to the costs associated with providing that service, they have little impetus to change or to become invested in team-based models where profits are shared. This model generally attracts those service providers willing to build their own clientele, provided they can schedule their own hours and assume limited responsibilities. Traditionally, these employees have had other means for obtaining benefits, such as health insurance. In the beginning, this method of compensation may have seemed like a good deal to spa owners burdened with the high cost of a start-up operation and who may not have been able to afford much in the way of benefits; however, as business increases and service providers earn higher salaries, the majority of spa owners realize they have severely curtailed their ability to maintain a profitable business and have attracted employees over whom they have little control. In many respects, commission-based pay is tantamount to supporting others in running their own business while you incur all of the risk and do most of the work. This outdated method of compensation leaves the spa owner with limited means to develop benefit packages that would allow them to compete for and attract qualified professionals with a different work ethic.

Faced with hard choices, many are adopting new standards and models. Some are attempting to fix the commission structure by lowering commission rates and using tiered commission schedules that require employees to increase sales volume to receive higher percentage rates. Others are developing pay scales that offer service providers a flat or fixed rate percentage of each service performed. In addition, many are incorporating product surcharges and applying team or tiered commission rates to retail sales. These systems may provide some relief for those struggling to find more equitable pay systems, but in the long run, they are not likely to promote the type of team-based environment and profitability needed to bring day spas to the next level of professionalism.

Those unhappy with variations of the same theme are charting new territory, replacing commission-based compensation with newer methods such as hourly-based pay that includes benefit packages. These methods are being complemented with additional commissions based on retail sales, profit sharing, and bonuses that give employees an opportunity to increase their individual profitability. Many of these are based on the productivity of the entire staff, a practice that promotes team efforts. In addition, some day spas are incorporating incremental salary and benefit increases that inspire a long-term employee commitment. Such practices are giving new hope to those who are struggling to make a profit and encourage a more professional status in what has become an increasingly competitive market.

Independent Contractors and Booth Renters

A word of caution is in order for those who might be tempted to adopt two of the more popular methods that are used to engage workers in the beauty industry: booth renters and independent contractors.

The term *booth renter* refers to an independent practitioner, such as an esthetician or massage therapist, who rents a designated space or room within another business entity, such as a salon, skin care clinic, or day spa for a set monthly fee. Booth renters are responsible for performing all of the duties and have all of the responsibilities associated with self-employment, such as paying their own taxes, purchasing insurance and ordering their own products; however, it should be noted that arrangements between spa owners and booth renters vary. For some spa owners, the idea of additional guaranteed income has made this an appealing option, but it is fraught with legal, insurance, licensing, and business concerns, which in many cases can be more trouble for the spa owner than they are worth. Before engaging in this type of business relationship, it is important to determine if it is lawful in your state. Check all state regulatory agencies for spa owners that apply, including the boards that supervise and license the service providers who will be renting space from you. It is also important to seek the advice of a qualified business attorney to determine if leasing space in this manner makes sense for your business and to assess all legal contractual, insurance and tax requirements.

Independent contractors are individuals who perform specific services at a rate of compensation they set and control. Compensation and other terms are generally specified in a mutually agreed-upon contract. Independent contractors have their own telephone number and their own business cards. They can perform the services they provide in whichever way they see fit and are free to work for a number of different businesses. Spas hire a variety of independent contractors such as accountants, attorneys, and information technology, marketing, and spa consultants. Under the terms of independent contractor status, these people receive a 1099 tax form for the fees they earn and are responsible for paying their own income taxes.

Problems arise when spas compensate people, who are in reality employees, as independent contractors to avoid paying mandatory employment taxes, such as Social Security, federal and state taxes, and workers' compensation insurance. Should those spa employees, such as service providers, underreport their income or fail to file or pay taxes altogether, the government loses money. This is actually illegal and a situation that may attract the unwelcome attention of the IRS. If a spa is found guilty of intentionally misusing the independent contractor status, the IRS can demand back payment of payroll taxes plus interest and penalties. This has led to an increased policing of the industry and has contributed to spas adopting policies that provide service providers with benefits commonly associated with professional employment status. If you ultimately decide to engage service providers as independent contractors you will want to have your attorney review the terms of your contract carefully. The issue of professional liability insurance for both independent contractors and booth renters is a prime concern. But such liaisons can have other repercussions that are not immediately obvious to the new spa owner; for example, they can

Plan for Success

Spa business owners who engage independent contractors must abide by the legal definition of the term as outlined by the IRS. The IRS uses three general categories to determine independent contractor status: behavioral control, financial control and the relationship between the two parties. An explanation of these criteria, along with a complete description of what constitutes an employee, can be found in several IRS documents for employers, including IRS Publication 15, *Circular E, Employer's Tax Guide* and IRS Publication 15A, the Employer's Supplemental Tax Guide. A quick overview of these criteria can also be found in IRS Publication 1779, a simple easy to read brochure that can be downloaded from the IRS Web site *www.irs.gov*. If you need help determining the status of a worker, IRS Form SS-8, "The Determination of Worker Status for Purposes of Federal Employment Taxes & Income Tax Withholding" is available for this purpose.

affect the resale value of your spa. Study all angles of this type of business arrangement carefully before moving forward.

Employee Benefits

Benefits are an important factor in retaining good employees. While a small business may not be able to afford all of the perks associated with a larger corporate facility, they are often in a position to find out exactly what their employees want and to be more flexible when it comes to meeting those requests.

Most employees prefer to work for a well-run organization that gives them a say in how things are done. At the same time, they expect to earn enough money to maintain a decent standard of living. The two need not be in opposition. Take time to understand what employees want from you. Keeping employees happy results in less turnover and satisfied customers and in the long run lowers the cost of doing business.

A good benefits package is often at the top of the list of what employees want and at times may be more important than a higher rate of pay. The high cost of health care has made health insurance a priority in terms of benefits. Paid time off, such as vacation days, holidays, sick leave and family leave, are also important. Retirement plans such as a 401k, life and disability insurance, and continuing education are other benefits that tend to attract more career-minded employees. These benefits are typically offered only to full-time employees, but the truth is employers can choose to offer benefits to part-time employees as well. In the spa business, where part-time employees are often a large percentage of the staff, this can make a huge difference in staff retention.

Right now you are probably thinking, "Sure, easy enough for her to say, but how can I afford to offer these types of benefits to everyone starting out?" You may need to shop around for an insurance agent who specializes in working with small businesses, but it is possible for small day spas to offer group health insurance and other insurance benefits, such as life insurance and disability insurance. The Small Business Service Bureau (*www.sbsb.com*) is just one example of an organization designed to help business members realize some of these goals. Trade organizations, bank representatives, other small businesses, and day spa owners are other good resources for referrals. Accountants and attorneys that work with small business owners are usually aware of new laws that can help small business owners and typically have access to a wide network of insurance and business consultants.

The important thing to remember is that if you hire a lot of part-time people just to save money, you are sending the wrong message. I frequently hear from disgruntled spa employees who are working several part-time jobs to make ends meet. Health care costs are often a major expense for them, and they are frustrated when health insurance and other benefits are not offered to them because of their part-time status. Those who are looking to make a career in the spa business are generally willing to buy into plans that would give them job security. If this is not an option, they tend to become disenchanted and move on. In the end, spa owners lose quality workers who could help them to build a better business.

If you want good employees, you must demonstrate that you value them. Perhaps the best advice you can receive is to work on your business and develop a compensation system that allows you to be more profitable. This will give you the leverage you need to offer a creative benefits package and attract quality career-minded people to your spa. The bottom line is that if you choose to be in business for yourself, don't expect your employees to bear the burden of that risk.

EMPLOYEE BENEFITS

A good employee benefits package generally includes:
- Decent wages
- Health insurance
- Paid vacation time
- Paid holidays
- Paid sick leave
- Family leave
- Continuing education
- A retirement plan
- Personal days
- Profit sharing

TAXES

Taxes are one of the more complex business matters facing spa owners. To gain an overall understanding of your tax obligations, it is recommended that you begin with a review of *IRS Publication 334, Tax Guide for Small Businesses.* If you are a more visual learner, the IRS also provides several video tutorials which can be viewed online. Other educational programs may be available through locally sponsored IRS affiliates. For more information go to www.irs.gov, the official Web site of the U.S. Internal Revenue Service.

While it is important for small business owners to be aware of tax laws, there is no question that tax issues are complicated. The following information is offered as a general overview to guide you in researching some of the more frequently asked questions business owners have; however, it is not meant to be a replacement for expert professional advice. Tax laws are subject to change and individual business circumstances vary. It is generally in your best interest to retain the professional services of a qualified business attorney and tax accountant, preferably a Certified Public Accountant, who has a good understanding of the spa business and stays on top of changing tax laws and requirements to help you understand and manage your individual tax obligations. Additional help such as a skilled bookkeeper is recommended to keep your spa business operating smoothly on a daily basis.

Tax Identification

Your first obligation as a spa business owner is to obtain a tax identification number. The IRS uses two important numbers to identify taxpayers: the Social Security (SS) number and the Employer Identification Number (EIN).

Your Social Security number is your individual taxpayer number. If you are a sole proprietor with no employees this number may be sufficient for tax purposes, however this scenario is not typical. Most spas have employees which will require them to obtain an EIN, also called a federal tax identification number. But even if you operate your business as a sole proprietor with no employees, you may need an EIN for other reasons, for example, to open a bank account for your business.

The IRS supplies two forms for tax identification purposes, the *SS-5 Form*, which is used to obtain an individual Social Security number and *Form SS-4* which is used to obtain an Employer Identification Number. Both forms are available directly from the IRS by phone or fax, and can also be downloaded from the IRS Web site.

Business Taxes

As a business owner you will be required to pay several taxes including federal and state taxes on the income that your business generates. Your tax obligations are based on the type of business structure that you select, for example whether you operate your business as a sole proprietor, partnership, corporation or limited liability company. The forms required and tax responsibilities for each entity vary and should be reviewed as part of the overall process when electing a business structure. Your business attorney and tax accountant are the best resources for making these very important tax related decisions and can alert you to other tax requirements that may apply to your individual business circumstance, such as local real estate or excise taxes. Additional tax obligations such as self-employment, payroll taxes, sales tax, etc. as outlined here are usually required. Be sure to calculate all of these payments into your budget to avoid a negative cash flow.

Self-employment tax

Anyone operating their own business is required to pay a *self-employment tax*. This tax allows self-employed individuals such as independent contractors, and the owners of business entities which are structured as a sole proprietor, partnership or limited liability companies to become eligible to receive the same Social Security retirement, disability, survivor benefits and hospital insurance or Medicare, that is available to employees.

The self employment tax rate is based on net earnings and is calculated as a percentage of Social Security and Medicare taxes. For example in January 2008 that figure was 15.3 percent (12.4 percent Social Security tax plus 2.9 percent Medicare tax).

Self-employment tax information is submitted using IRS Schedule 1040. When supplying this information to your accountant it is important to report all income. Failure to do so or to under-report your income can result in serious consequences, such as tax penalties and lower Social Security benefits upon retirement.

Filing Tax Returns

All businesses must file tax returns. Your tax return provides the IRS with a detailed account of your income and expenses for a certain time period which is defined as either a *calendar* or *fiscal tax year*. The IRS uses several criteria for determining a business' tax year. This is largely based on the type of business structure and accounting method you elect. For example, spa businesses, operating as sole proprietors, partnerships, limited liability companies and S-corporations, usually file income tax returns according to a *calendar year*, which consists of 12 consecutive months, beginning on January 1 and ending on December 31 of any given year. If your business operates on a *fiscal year*, you may end your tax year on the last day of the month of your choice with the exception of December. Businesses operating on a calendar year are required to file all tax returns by April 15 of every year, unless that date falls on a Saturday, Sunday or legal holiday, in which case taxes are due on the next consecutive business day. Businesses that operate on a fiscal year are required to file all tax returns on or before the 15th day of the fourth month after the close of their fiscal year and are allowed the same grace periods for weekend days and holidays. These items should be reviewed carefully with your accountant to avoid any late fees or penalties.

If you are a new business owner you should be aware that technology has made it easy to file tax returns via the Internet but it is has not eliminated the need to maintain detailed records, nor has it replaced the need for professional accounting and bookkeeping services. Knowledge of the type of records and receipts you must keep, and the selection of an accounting method and tax year are important business decisions that should be reviewed in detail with your accountant prior to commencing business. Precise data entry by a bookkeeper skilled in the *generally accepted principles of accounting* discussed in chapter 3 is another important part of tax record-keeping that should not be overlooked.

Estimated Tax Payments

If you are a self-employed individual and expect to owe the government taxes you are required to make *estimated tax payments*. These taxes are based on previously reported income and are due quarterly on April 15, June 15, September 15 and January 15 of each tax year.

There are two separate forms for submitting estimated tax payments: *Form 1040-ES,* which is used to report federal taxes and *Form 1-ES,* which is used to report state tax. Estimated tax payments can have a significant impact on the cash flow of a small business however failure to make estimated payments can result in penalties. There are several payment options available through the IRS to help you stay ahead of these important tax obligations. Your tax accountant can help you to select the right payment method for your business needs.

Employee Tax Forms

Business owners who hire employees are responsible for correctly classifying and reporting the tax status of those individuals. There are several important IRS forms used for this purpose: *Form W-4, Form W-2* and *Form I-9.*

Form W-4, the Employee's Withholding Allowance Certificate, must be filled out by each employee. The information supplied on this form determines the amount of taxes that are to be withheld from the employee's paycheck and is determined by the employee's filing status, for example, whether they are single, married, or married withholding at a single rate. Employees may also specify a certain number of dependents on this form, for example children or elderly parents, for whom they are financially responsible, and for which they are allowed certain deductions.

Form W-2, the Wage and Tax Statement form, summarizes the employee's total earnings (including wages, tips and other compensation) and the amount of taxes that were withheld during a specified calendar year. The employer is required to deliver a copy of form W-2 to each employee by January 31st of the following year, for example, if the calendar tax year ends on December 31, 2008, the employer must issue a W-2 for that period by January 31, 2009. The information provided on this form is intended to aid the employee in filing their own tax returns and should correspond to the information reported on regularly scheduled payroll checks received by the employee. A copy of this form must also be furnished to the IRS. A third copy should be maintained for the employer's records.

Form I-9 is used to verify the employment and identity of every person working in the United States. Employers are mandated by law to keep a copy of this form on file for each employee for a period of three years from the date of hire or one year from the date employment ends, or whichever comes later. I-9 forms are available through the U.S. Citizen and Immigration Service (USCIS). For more information visit the USCIS Web site (www.uscis.gov).

Nonresident and Resident Alien Workers

Employers should be aware that nonresident or resident aliens working in the U.S. are also obliged to pay income taxes to the IRS. An *ITIN,* or *Individual Tax Identification Number* is available for this purpose and may be accessed through the IRS. Additional information regarding resident and nonresident alien workers can be obtained from the IRS and the U.S. Immigration and Naturalization Service (INS).

Independent Contractors

Spa business owners that make use of independent contractors are not responsible for calculating their tax obligations. As we learned earlier, this is the responsibility of the individual service provider; however any business owner who pays gross receipts of more than $600 annually to any independent contractor is responsible for filing *IRS Form 1099*, which reports the gross amount paid to that person for the tax year. A copy of this form must also be delivered to the contractor for their records by the end of January for the previous year.

Employee Tax Deductions

There are several deductions which must be taken from an employee's paycheck for tax purposes. These include Federal Income Tax, Federal Insurance Contributions Act or FICA taxes (Social Security and Medicare tax) and State Income Tax. These deductions are based on the withholding allowance specified by the employee on form W-4 and are calculated according to information supplied by the IRS and the Department of Revenue (DOR) in each state. Although this task can be accomplished manually, most business owners use software, a payroll service provider, and/or accountant to process payroll deductions for them.

If you are a new business owner, it is important to note that employers must match the FICA tax deducted from an employee's salary and are also required to submit a report of these and federal income tax payments to the IRS on a quarterly basis. *Form 941* is used for this purpose. Individual state income tax requirements vary. To learn about your state tax obligations contact the Department of Revenue in your state. Direct links to each state office are available from the IRS Web site and may also be accessed through the Federation of State Tax Administrators.

Miscellaneous Employee Deductions

Employers may deduct other expenses from an employee's paycheck such as health insurance and individual retirement plan benefits. These items are not considered employee tax deductions however they do offer the employer certain tax advantages which should be reviewed with your tax accountant.

Federal Unemployment Tax

The Federal Unemployment Tax Act (FUTA) requires employers to pay an additional Federal Unemployment Tax. This tax is a joint tax program between the state and federal government that is used to compensate employees who lose their jobs. There are a number of qualifying criteria associated with this tax which should be reviewed with your accountant; however, unlike FICA taxes, it is important for employers to understand that the employee is not required to contribute to payment of this tax. All FUTA taxes are paid solely by the employer who must file an Employer's Annual Federal Unemployment Tax Return (Form 940) by January 31 of the following year for this purpose.

Sales Taxes

If your spa sells retail products you will probably need to collect a state and perhaps local tax on those items. This usually requires a resale certificate or sales permit; however local and state sales tax laws vary, as do rates, and there are a few states that do not require any sales tax. Certain items, such as food and clothing, may also be exempt.

To determine the laws that apply to your spa you will need to contact local and state revenue offices in your locale. If you have more than one spa and these are located in different states it will be important for you to research all applicable laws. The Federation of Tax Administrators is an organization of state tax officials that provides research and information on state tax laws. The FTA can be a valuable resource when it comes to comparing, contrasting and reviewing state laws.

If you decide to engage in e-commerce you will be faced with a different situation. Although the Supreme Court has determined that unless a business has a physical presence in the state in which they are retailing they do not have to collect taxes, these rules are being challenged. Before setting up shop online, it is important to review your sales tax obligations with a competent tax attorney especially if you ship products out of state. You may also want to shop around for a software program that will automatically calculate retail tax for you.

Deferred Income Tax

In the spa business deferred income tax generally applies to the sale of gift certificates. As we learned earlier, gift certificates pose a unique problem for spa owners who are often faced with huge revenues from the sale of holiday gift certificates. This can have serious tax consequences for the spa business owner who fails to develop a method for tracking and handling the cash associated with these sales. If you do not understand your tax obligation as it applies to the sale of gift certificates, it is imperative that you seek the professional advice of an accountant who is familiar with the spa business and tax laws in your state; someone who can also help you to set up a system of accountability. Otherwise, you may find yourself in the unfortunate position of owing a huge amount of tax dollars, a situation that could put your business in serious jeopardy.

Tax Deductions

The IRS allows business owners to take a number of tax deductions. These are outlined in *IRS Publication 535, Business Expenses* which includes an account of the various deductions allowed, such as employee benefits, transportation, education, travel, meals and entertainment, supplies, advertising, utilities, etc. It is worth the time for every business to review this publication; however, it is important to know that deductions are subject to certain limitations and laws on this subject do change. A good tax accountant can help you to stay on top of these laws, but you must also do your part. Business owners looking to maximize their deductions must keep careful records and should be prepared to substantiate all of their claims in the event of an audit.

Plan for Success

Ignorance is no defense against the law when it comes to taxes. Failure to comply with any of your tax obligations, for example, file a tax return(s), make tax payments on time; or any attempt to intentionally defraud the government by supplying false or erroneous information can have serious legal consequences that may result in penalties, fines and/or imprisonment.

INVENTORY CONTROL

Managing inventory is one of the most important operations involved in maintaining an efficient spa business. The goal is to have enough stock on your shelf to conduct business, but not so much that it paralyzes your cash flow. Until products and supplies are sold or used to perform a service, they are actually inhibiting your cash flow and should be considered a liability. Again, go back to the top 20 reasons businesses fail (see Chapter 3) and learn to look at those products sitting on your retail display shelves and in your dispensary as cash that is waiting to turn into income.

At the onset of business, you will need to rely on sales projections to manage inventory, but as your business develops, understanding how much to stock requires a careful analysis of your turnover rate. The turnover rate refers to the amount of time it takes to replace your original inventory. This means you need to have a good idea of what's selling and what's not.

Generally, the "80/20 rule" applies: 80 percent of your profit is likely to come from 20 percent of the products on your shelf. Learn which products these are and keep them on hand. Stock the bare minimum of those that are not good sellers. Get rid of products that aren't selling, but before you do, make sure you understand the reason they are not selling. It may have more to do with where the product is positioned on your display or the fact that your staff is not promoting a particular treatment than it does with effectiveness. If you discover that an item simply is not a winner, reduce the price for quick sale since it is actually costing you more to store it than it is worth in terms of depreciation and overhead. On the other hand, if you find that a product is jumping off your shelves, investigate why. Retail products can generate significant revenue, especially if they are the subject of major advertising efforts. It is just as important to track the consumption of service supplies. If you find that back bar products are dissipating without an increase in service revenue, it could mean that employees are wasting product. Cross-referencing the ratio of product to treatments will help you to get to the bottom of the situation quickly.

Make the Most of Technology

A good software program is critical to controlling inventory (Figure 11-9). Too often spa owners have fantastic software programs that they are not using to the full extent of their capabilities. Inventory is one area where a good software program can save both time and money. Computerized systems can alert you to maximum or minimum levels and prompt automatic purchase orders. To avoid miscalculation, assign one or two people, such

Code #	Number of Items on Hand	Inventory Description	Number of Items Sold September 2005	Number of Items Sold to Date
		Inventory Control Report: September 2009		
		Date of Report: October 1, 2009 10:00:00 AM		
1001	7	Successful Purifying Cleanser	45	402
1002	9	Successful Cleansing Milk	40	374
1003	15	Successful Cleansing Gel	44	363
1004	19	Successful Purifying Astringent	26	269
1005	16	Successful Skin Freshener	19	249
1006	20	Successful Hydrating Mist	25	175
1007	15	Successful Super Exfoliating Enzyme	55	450
1008	9	Successful Gentle Skin Polishing Grains	50	478
1009	5	Successful Invigorating Gommage	40	392
1010	20	Successful Daily Moisturizer	33	376
1011	7	Successful Night Repair Cream	47	411
1012	11	Successful Oil-Free Hydrating Lotion	52	427
1013	19	Successful Collagen Complex	68	508
1014	23	Successful Blemish Lotion	75	465
1015	10	Successful Sun Protection SPF 15	28	425
1016	6	Successful Sun Protection SPF 30	34	449
1017	7	Successful AHA Lotion	33	408
1018	14	Successful Vitamin C Serum	81	560
1019	25	Successful Vitamin A Moisturizing Gel	77	554
1020	13	Successful Vitamin E Oil	65	488
1021	12	Successful Lemon Grass Body Scrub	70	575
1022	16	Successful Shea Butter Body Lotion	39	412
1023	21	Successful Purifying Clay Mask	38	365
1024	17	Successful Hydrating Mask	30	442
1025	16	Successful Sensitive Skin Mask	55	493

FIGURE 11-9 A computerized system will help you to maintain your inventory efficiently.

as a spa manager and front desk assistant, to control the system and charge one person with the responsibility for approving all purchase orders. In addition to these safeguards, you will need to follow up with a physical count. Generally, this is performed on a quarterly basis for those selling retail products. A PDA, or handheld computer, can be useful for this purpose and eliminates the need for duplicate entries (Figure 11-10).

Once you have your inventory system under control, it is important to be conscious of expiration dates. If a product expires before you can

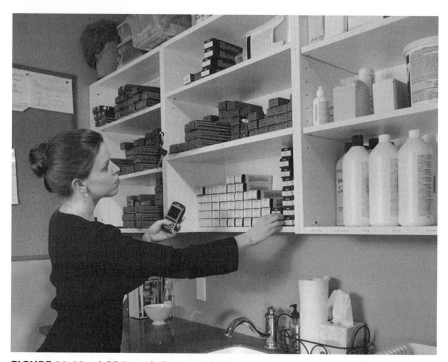

FIGURE 11-10   A PDA can help to conduct inventory more efficiently.

sell or use it, you have thrown money out the window. This applies to both back bar and retail products. An orderly dispensary and organized retail shelves will help you to track stock. Again, limit the number of staff members in charge and hold them accountable on a monthly basis. Busy spas with less space may need to conduct this task more frequently. Larger spas that operate seven days a week for extended hours may need to make other adjustments or use more employees, such as day and evening managers, to perform these tasks.

Establish Security Measures

Although you want to think that you can trust all of your spa guests and staff members, theft can be an issue. To avoid losses, develop a security system for inventory early on. Keep your dispensary and expensive retail products locked and develop a protocol for opening shipments and restocking shelves. Unfortunately, spa owners have uncovered a variety of creative thieves, including those who steal from unattended shipping boxes, powder rooms, and display shelves with limited visibility. Keep only an adequate supply of products in treatment rooms, locker and change areas, and restock regularly. If you use remote displays, place only empty boxes in those areas and devise ways to attach testers directly to displays so they are not easily removed.

Maintain Good Vendor Relations

Maintaining productive relationships with suppliers is imperative to inventory control. We discussed vendors at length in Chapter 6, but the basics are worth repeating. To keep inventory flowing smoothly, you should have a clear understanding of the lead time needed to process an order and subsequently receive shipments. Establish a realistic safety margin for keeping your spa well stocked. Not having the right product on your shelf at the right time will cause you to lose money. Make sure your suppliers are reliable. Are there minimum order requirements? Do they waive freight charges or reduce them if your order is over a certain weight or amount? What is the policy and process for returning damaged goods? Are additional shipping costs involved?

Suppliers typically run sales promotions or specials. It is a good idea to take advantage of these sale prices if it makes sense, but never stock more than you can realistically sell or need. You could wind up losing money if you are unable to sell products at the full price.

QUALITY CONTROL

Providing clients with quality treatments and excellent customer service over an extended period of time can be difficult. How will you motivate your staff to continually provide superior quality?

We have already discussed many of the checks and balances that go into quality control, such as adequate training, policy and procedural manuals, and continuing education. If you are running logs on customer complaints and equipment breakdowns, review them regularly. This will give you a good idea of where you need to make improvements. Don't forget to talk to your employees. There is no replacement for the feedback you get from staff.

It is also important to ask clients directly what they think about your products and services. Surveys and focus groups, as discussed in Chapter 10, are ideal for soliciting client input (Figure 11-11). Secret shoppers can also help to uncover strengths and weaknesses in your operation and may even help to motivate employees to do their best, especially when you let them know you intend to use these techniques.

More objective measures of quality control can be obtained from analyzing the many computer reports your software program generates,

Successful
Day Spa

Successful DAY SPA
123 Chic Main Street
Urban Oasis, SPA 45678

Successful
Day Spa
sophisticated beauty therapies

Dear Guest:

Thank you for visiting Successful Day Spa. We hope your experience was positive, and look forward to seeing you again soon.

It is very important to us that all of our clients are satisfied with the treatment they received. Please take a few minutes to let us know how we did by completing this survey and returning it to us by mail or drop it off at the front desk on your next visit.

Thank you,

Sally Spalady

Sally Spalady
Successful Day Spa

HOW DID WE DO?

We value your input. Please take a few moments to rate your interaction with our staff and the quality of your spa visit.

	Excellent	Good	Fair	Poor
Customer Service Staff				
• Appointment Scheduling	☐	☐	☐	☐
• Courtesy	☐	☐	☐	☐
• Helpfulness	☐	☐	☐	☐
Service Providers				
• Professionalism	☐	☐	☐	☐
• Knowledge	☐	☐	☐	☐
• Attitude	☐	☐	☐	☐
Quality of Treatment				
• Promptness of Service	☐	☐	☐	☐
• Facial	☐	☐	☐	☐
• Massage	☐	☐	☐	☐
• Body Treatment	☐	☐	☐	☐
• Hair Styling	☐	☐	☐	☐
• Manicure	☐	☐	☐	☐
• Pedicure	☐	☐	☐	☐
• Hair Removal	☐	☐	☐	☐
• Make-Up	☐	☐	☐	☐
Spa Facility				
• Atmosphere	☐	☐	☐	☐
• Cleanliness	☐	☐	☐	☐
• Comfort Level	☐	☐	☐	☐

Would you recommend us to others? ☐ Yes ☐ No

What did you like about your treatment? _____

Did you feel your needs were met? _____

Did you feel your expectations were met? _____

If you could change anything about your experience, what would it be? _____

What could we do to improve your next visit to our spa? _____

Name: _____
Address: _____
Telephone: _____
Date of Service: _____
E-mail: _____

Please return completed questionnaire to the front desk. If you are in a hurry please mail this postage-paid mailer back at your earliest convenience.

Thank you for your time. All spa guests who respond to this customer satisfaction survey are eligible for a monthly spa give-away to be awarded on the first day of each month.

FIGURE 11-11 Customer satisfaction survey.

such as client retention and referral rates or by implementing an independent evaluation program.

RAISING PRICES

A careful review of your financial statements will quickly determine when you need to raise prices. This should include a thorough review of quarterly profit and loss statements and a break-even analysis that calculates the cost of each service the spa provides. Fixed costs, such as your rent, will not fluctuate on a quarterly basis. So unless the variable costs—for example, the cost of purchasing a particular retail or back bar product used to perform a treatment—suddenly increases dramatically, price adjustments are generally best implemented on a yearly basis.

When analyzing the cost of each service, look at all figures carefully. This should include a complete assessment of each individual treatment in terms of the cost of direct and indirect labor (wages, taxes, insurance, and benefits for service providers, administrative employees, and support staff), materials (products and equipment), and overhead expenses such as rent and utilities, repair and maintenance, insurance, marketing and advertising, linens, laundry, and housekeeping. If you have not calculated these figures, go back to Chapter 3 and review this information using the worksheets provided. The information relating to profit margins and ROI discussed in Chapter 6 will also be useful. After carefully looking at all of these figures, the question to ask is: Are you making enough money on each product and service you sell? If the answer is no, is that because your expenses have increased or because you are not managing finances well? Be fair. The time to raise prices is when your costs increase—that is, the cost of the product, the cost of performing the service, and/or the cost of doing business; however, it is also important to measure your prices against those of your competitors and compare them to industry standards to be sure that you are not selling yourself short.

Raising prices does not mean you have to raise all your prices. You may only need to raise prices for services where cost has increased or on those more popular treatments. Again, consider the 80/20 rule. Raising prices for those treatments and products that are in greater demand will keep profit margins at a reasonable rate. Solicit input from staff and weigh this against sales figures. Does this coincide with information provided by client surveys that indicate your prices are too high or too low?

If you ultimately decide to raise prices, it is always best to give clients fair warning. Many spa owners use this as an opportunity to encourage clients to have treatments at lower rates before the price goes up. It is also wise to ensure clients that they will continue to receive the same high level of quality care they have come to expect. Do not be surprised if you lose some customers, but do not let the thought of losing a few customers deter you from increasing your prices when necessary. Like everything else, the cost of doing business increases.

EVALUATING YOUR SUCCESS

Most business owners are likely to equate success to profit, however success can mean different things to different people. For some, it is the satisfaction of fulfilling a real need in the community. For others, it is about doing what they love to do. You will need to set your own standard. When evaluating your success, use your vision as a guide. What were your original goals? Have you accomplished these goals? What would you like to accomplish next? Use the SWOT analysis presented in Chapter 3 to take stock of your business from year to year and reinvest profits to realize those goals that are still unmet.

As your business develops, it is important to enjoy the fruits of your labor, but it is also important to spend profits wisely. Will you use your profits to provide employees with more benefits, establish a profit sharing or continuing education fund, increase marketing and advertising efforts, or purchase another piece of equipment? Think in terms of those things that, in addition to improving your business, will benefit everyone on your team. The bottom line is that you must continue to realize a profit to sustain your vision.

Revising Your Vision

If you have not been as profitable as you would like to be, don't give up—make changes! Starting a business is hard work and in most cases does not result in instant wealth. A great deal of responsibility will rest on your shoulders, and you are bound to make a few mistakes. Don't be too hard on yourself. Those who are unwilling to admit something is not working will not last long. Successful business owners are those who are willing to look at their methods critically and make adjustments as needed. You *can* turn your business around if you are willing to grow and revise your vision!

THINK IT OVER

As you continue on your spa journey, take time to nourish your entrepreneurial spirit regularly. Use the exercises at the beginning of this book and take an hour out of each day to care for yourself: walk, run, swim, dance, meditate, enjoy a massage, or simply do nothing. As a small business owner, it is vital to practice stress management every day.

It is equally important to learn new things. Attend spa trade shows and join industry associations. Take an active role in the small business organizations available in your community and participate in business conferences outside of the industry. Develop a support network among other business owners on whom you can rely. Show up every day with a good attitude and a willingness to work hard. Be honest and pay attention, but most of all enjoy your work! A career in the spa business is full of exciting possibilities that are equally rewarding and invigorating to all who aspire to a life of health, beauty and wellness.

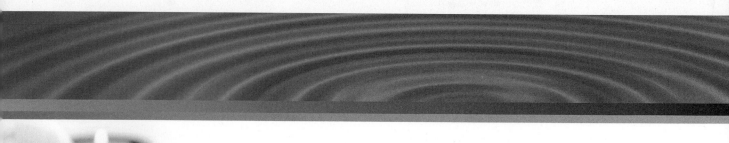

BIBLIOGRAPHY AND RECOMMENDED READINGS

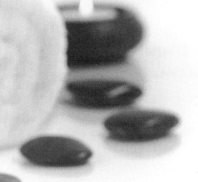

Barletta, Martha. *Marketing to Women.* Chicago: Dearborn Trade Publishing, 2003.

Belch, George E., and Michael A. Belch. *Advertising and Promotion: An Integrated Marketing Communications Perspective.* New York: McGraw-Hill, 1998.

Bennett, Peter D., ed. *Dictionary of Marketing Terms,* 2nd ed. Chicago: NTC Business Books, 1995. Published in conjunction with the American Marketing Association.

Berke, Conrad. *Entrepreneur Magazine: Successful Advertising for Small Businesses.* New York: John Wiley & Sons, 1996.

Berkowitz, Erin N., Roger A. Kerin, Steven W. Hartley, William Rudelius, George E. Belch, and Michael A. Belch. *Marketing,* 5th ed. New York: McGraw-Hill, 1997.

Bly, Robert W. *Power-Packed Direct Mail:* How to get more leads & sales by mail. New York, NY: Henry Holt and Company, Inc. 1995.

Cohen, Paula, and Susanne S. Warfield. *Legal & Liability Issues of a Medical Spa.* Ridgewood, NJ: Paramedical Consultants, 2004.

Covey, Stephen R. *The Seven Habits of Highly Effective People: Restoring the Character Ethic.* New York: Simon & Schuster, 1989.

Culp, Judith et al. *Milady's Standard Esthetics Advanced, First Edition.* New York: Milady, a part of Cengage Learning, 2010.

D'Angelo, Janet, et al. *Milady's Standard Comprehensive Training for Estheticians.* New York: Thomson Delmar Learning, 2003.

Delaney, Patrick R., Barry J. Epstein, Ralph Nach, and Susan Weiss Budak. *Wiley GAAP 2004: Interpretation and Application of Generally Accepted Accounting Principles.* New York: John Wiley & Sons, 2003.

Dodd, Annabel Z. **The Essential Guide to Telecommunications,** 3rd ed. Upper Saddle River, NJ: Prentice Hall, 2002.

Donlan, Vicki with Graves, Helen French. *Her Turn: Why It's Time For Women To Lead In America.* Westport, CT: Praeger Publishers, 2007.

Dyer, Wayne. *The Power of Intention.* Carlsbad, CA: Hay House, 2004.

Gambino, Henry. *Marketing & Advertising for the Salon.* New York: Thomson Delmar Learning, 1996.

Gerber, Michael E. *The E Myth Revisited: Why Most Small Businesses Don't Work and What to Do About It.* New York: HarperCollins Publishers, 1995.

Gerson, Joel, et al. *Milady's Standard Fundamentals for Estheticians.* New York: Thomson Delmar Learning, 2004.

Gerson, Joel, D'Angelo, Janet, Deitz, Sallie, Lotz, Shelley, Frangie, Catherine M. and Halal, John. *Milady's Standard Esthetics Fundamentals 10th Edition.* New York: Delmar, Cengage Learning, 2009

Gray, John. *Men Are From Mars, Women Are From Venus.* New York: HarperCollins Publishers, Inc. 1992.

Hill, Pamela. *Milady's Aesthetician Series: Ensuring An Optimal Outcome in Skin Care.* New York: Thomson Delmar Learning, 2006.

Hill, Pamela. *Milady's Aesthetician Series: Microdermabrasion.* New York: Thomson Delmar Learning, 2006.

Hill, Pamela and Bickmore, Helen R. *Milady's Aesthetician Series: Advanced Hair Removal.* New York, 2008.

Hill, Pamela and Culp, Judith. *Milady's Aesthetician Series: Permanent Makeup: Tips and Techniques.* New York: Thomson Delmar Learning, 2007.

Hill, Pamela and Sterling, Christian. *Milady's Aesthetician Series: Medical Terminology, A Handbook for the Skin Care Specialist.* New York: Thomson Delmar Learning, 2006.

Hill, Pamela and Todd, Laura. *Milady's Aesthetician Series: Advanced Face and Body Treatments for the Spa.* New York: Thomson Delmar Learning, 2008.

Kentie, Peter. *Web Design Tools and Techniques,* 2nd ed. Berkeley, CA: Peachpit Press, 2002.

Leavy, Hannelore R., and Reinhard R. Bergel. *The Spa Encyclopedia.* New York: Thomson Delmar Learning, 2003.

Lees, Mark. *Skin Care: Beyond the Basics, Third Edition.* New York, Thomson Delmar Learning, 2007.

Lesonsky, Rieva. *Start Your Own Business.* Irvine, CA: Entrepreneur Media, 2001.

Medcroft, Stephen. *Telecom Manager's Survival Guide: The Essential Reference for Telecommunications Systems, Solutions, and Cost Control.* New York: American Management Association, 2003.

Miller, Erica. *Day Spa Operations.* New York: Thomson Delmar Learning, 1996.

Miller, Erica. *Day Spa Techniques.* New York: Thomson Delmar Learning, 1996.

Pettigrew, Judy Hoyt. *Women Mean Business: The Secret of Selling to Women.* New York: Creative Consortium Books, 2000.

Peale, Norman Vincent. *The Power of Positive Thinking.* New York: Prentice-Hall, Inc., 1952.

Phillips, Carole. *Milady SalonOvations in the Bag: Selling in the Salon.* New York: Thomson Delmar Learning, 1995.

Popcorn, Faith, and Lys Marigold. *EVEolution—The Eight Truths of Marketing to Women.* New York: Hyperion, 2000.

Quinlan, Marylou. *Just Ask a Woman: Cracking the Code of What Women Want and How They Buy.* New York: John Wiley & Sons, 2003.

Steingold, Fred S., and Ilona M. Bray. *Legal Guide for Starting & Running a Small Business.* Berkeley, CA: Nolo, 1999.

Tolle, Eckhardt. *The Power of Now.* Novato, CA: New World Library, 1999.

Tolle, Eckhardt. *A New Earth: Awakening to Your Life's Purpose.* New York, NY Penguin Group, A Plume Book, 2006.

Underhill, Paco. *Why We Buy: The Science of Shopping.* New York: Simon & Schuster, 1999.

Yudkin, Marcia. *Internet Marketing for Less than $500/year: How to Attract Customers and Clients Online without Spending a Fortune,* 2nd ed. Gulf Breeze, FL: Maximum Press, 2000.

U.S. GOVERNMENT AGENCIES

Bureau of Economic Census

Bureau of Labor Statistics

Census Bureau

Center for Disease Control (CDC)

Consumer Product Safety Commission (CPSC)

Department of Commerce (DOC)

Department of Education (DOE)

Department of Health and Human Services (HHS)

Department of Justice

Department of Labor (DOL)

Department of Labor, Women's Bureau

Department of Revenue (DOR)

Department of Treasury, Internal Revenue Service (IRS)

Equal Opportunity Employment Commission (EEOC)

Environmental Protection Agency (EPA)

Food and Drug Administration (FDA)

Federal Trade Commission (FTC)

Health and Human Services

Immigration and Naturalization Service (INS)

Internal Revenue Service (IRS)

National Center for Complementary and Alternative Medicine (NCAM)

National Center for Education Statistics

National Trademark Office (U.S. Patent and Trademark Office)

Occupational Safety and Health Administration (OSHA)

Small Business Administration (SBA)

ORGANIZATIONS AND STUDIES

American Institute of Architects (AIA)

American Advertising Federation

American Association of Advertising Agencies

American Business Brokers Association

American Institute of Certified Public Accountants

American Marketing Association

Association for Asian Research

American National Standard Institute (ANSI)

American Society of Appraisers

American Society for Aesthetic Plastic Surgery

Better Business Bureau

Center for Women's Business Research

The Day Spa Association (DSA)

The Day Spa Association, *First Compensation & Benefits Survey,* April 2005

The Day Spa Association, *Day Spa Benchmarks: A Blueprint for Success,* April 2003

The Day Spa Association, *The Evolution and Future of the Day Spa Industry*

The Day Spa Association, *The Marketing Demographics of A Day Spa Goer,* Winter 2004–2005

Federation of Tax Administrators

Green Spa Network

Insurance Information Institute (I.I.I.)

International SPA Association (ISPA)

The International SPA Association's (ISPA), *2003 Spa-goer Study*

The International SPA Association's (ISPA), *2004 Spa Industry Study*

The International Spa Association's (ISPA), *2006 Consumer Trends Report*

The International Spa Association's (ISPA) *2008 Spa Industry Update*

National Association of Certified Valuation Analysts

National Coalition of Estheticians, Manufacturers/Distributors & Associations (NCEA)

National Association of Women Business Owners (NAWBO)

Natural Marketing Institute (NMI) 2007 LOHAS Consumer Trends Database

Service Corporation of Retired Business Executives (SCORE)

Small Business Service Bureau

The Society of Dermatology Skin Care Specialists

The Society of Plastic Surgical Skin Care Specialists

The Society of Permanent Cosmetic Professionals

JOURNALS

Adweek

American Demographics

American Spa

Cosmetic Surgery Times

DAYSPA

Dermascope

Entrepreneur

Global Cosmetic Industry

Les Nouvelles Esthetiques

Luxury Spa Finder

LOHAS

Marketing News (AMA)

Massage & Body Work

Medical Spa Report

Pulse (ISPA)

Skin, Inc.

Spa Finder

Spa Healthy Living Travel & Renewal

Spa Management

Women's Business

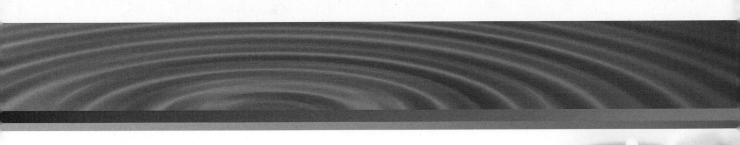

INDEX

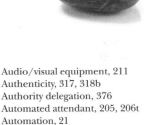

'b' indicates boxed material; 'f' indicates a figure; 't' indicates a table